VACCINES

FRONTIERS IN DESIGN AND DEVELOPMENT

Copyright © 2005
Horizon Bioscience
32 Hewitts Lane
Wymondham
Norfolk NR18 0JA
U.K.

www.horizonbioscience.com

British Library Cataloguing-in-Publication Data

A catalogue record for this book is available from the British Library

ISBN: 1–904933–09–2

Printed and bound in Great Britain by The Cromwell Press

Contents

Contents

Contributors

Jean-Pierre Abastado
IDM
LUTI, University Pierre et Marie Curie
Paris
France

Mohammad Al-Khalili
IOMAI Corporation
Gaithersburg, MD
USA

Jeffrey Almond
Research and Development Department
Aventis Pasteur
Marcy l'étoile
France

Claude André
Scientific and Medical Department
Stallergènes SA
Antony Cedex
France
candre@stallergenes.fr

Jean-Christophe Audonnet
Vaccinomics and Virology
MERIAL
Lyon
France
jean-christophe.audonnet@merial.com

Russell Basser
CSL Ltd
Parkville
Victoria
Australia
russell.basser@csl.com.au

Pamela L. Beatty
Department of Immunology
University of Pittsburgh School of
Medicine
Pittsburgh, PA
USA

Joseph Bresee
Viral Gastroenteritis Section
Respiratory and Enteric Virus Branch
National Centre for Infectious Diseases
Centers for Disease Control and
Prevention
Atlanta, GA
USA

Nicolas Burdin
Immunology Research
Aventis Pasteur
Marcy l'Etoile
France
nicolas.burdin@aventis.com

Cecil Czerkinsky
INSERM EMI
Faculté de Médicine-Pasteur
Avenue de Vallombrose
Nice
France
czerkins@unice.fr

Anne S. De Groot
EpiVax, Inc.
Providence, RI
USA
AnnieD@EpiVax.com

Stirling Edwards
CSL Ltd
Parkville
Victoria
Australia

Larry R. Ellingsworth
IOMAI Corporation
Gaithersburg, MD
USA

Contributors

Olivera J. Finn
Department of Immunology
University of Pittsburgh School of
Medicine
Pittsburgh, PA
USA

ojfinn@pitt.edu

David C. Flyer
IOMAI Corporation
Gaithersburg, MD
USA

Ian H. Frazer
Centre for Immunology and Cancer
Research
Princess Alexandra Hospital
Woolloongabba
Queensland
Australia

Roger Glass
Viral Gastroenteritis Section
Respiratory and Enteric Virus Branch
National Centre for Infectious Diseases
Centres for Disease Control and
Prevention
Atlanta, GA
USA

Gregory M. Glenn
IOMAI Corporation
Gaithersburg, MD
USA

gglenn@iomai.com

Michel Goldman
Department of Immunology
Hôpital Erasme
Brussels
Belgium

Ali M. Harandi
Gothenburg University Vaccine Research
Institute (GUVAX)
Gothenburg
Sweden

Jan Holmgren
Gothenburg University Vaccine Research
Institute (GUVAX)
Gothenburg
Sweden

Paul-Henri Lambert
Centre of Vaccinology
Department of Pathology
University of Geneva
Switzerland

paul.lambert@medecine.unige.ch

Claude Leclerc
Unité de Biologie des Régulations
Immunitaires
INSERM
Institut Pasteur
Paris
France

cleclerc@pasteur.fr

Julie A. McMurry
EpiVax, Inc.
Providence, RI
USA

Laleh Majlessi
Unité de Biologie des Régulations
Immunitaires
INSERM
Institut Pasteur
Paris
France

Jules Minke
MERIAL SAS
Lyon Gerland Laboratory
Lyon
France

Philippe Moingeon
Research and Development
Stallergènes
Antony
France

pmoingeon@stallergenes.fr

Alessandra Nardin
IDM
LUTI, University Pierre et Marie Curie
Paris
France
anardin@idm-biotech.com

Hervé Poulet
MERIAL SAS
Lyon Gerland Laboratory
Lyon
France

Duncan Steele
Initiative for Vaccine Research
Department of Immunization, Vaccines
and Biologicals
World Health Organization
Geneva
Switzerland
steeled@who.int

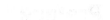

Preface

Vaccines based on live attenuated pathogens, inactivated whole pathogens or purified capsular polysaccharides have been, over the last decades, extremely successful in preventing a large number of common infectious diseases. More recently, both prophylactic and therapeutic vaccines have begun to be developed to control chronic infectious diseases associated with viruses, intracellular bacteria or parasites. Vaccination approaches are also being used or considered for numerous targets beyond infectious diseases, including cancers, autoimmune diseases, allergies and neurodegenerative or metabolic diseases. In most circumstances, these innovative vaccines are molecularly defined, and aim at stimulating immune effector or regulatory mechanisms in an antigen-specific manner.

This book reviews the challenges and opportunities linked with the development of some of these new vaccines. In this regard, four frontiers can be schematically identified:

- *The knowledge frontier*: the rational design of adjuvants and vaccines can benefit from our better understanding of the nature of proinflammatory or regulatory signals controlling both innate and adaptive immune mechanisms.
- *The technology frontier*: on the basis of this emerging scientific knowledge, new delivery systems, adjuvants, antigen identification tools and vector systems can be proposed.
- *The target frontier*: prophylactic and therapeutic applications of vaccination can be considered for essentially any disease in which the immune system is involved.
- *The development frontier*: in the context of a growing regulatory pressure, the cost and complexity of innovation, defined as a capacity to design, develop, manufacture and distribute new vaccines, can be tackled only by complex collaborative networks.

As illustrated by the various contributors to this book acting on these various frontiers, the field of vaccine development faces significant hurdles. It also carries major hopes that safe and efficient molecular vaccines will be made available to both developed and developing countries in the near future. Now is a time when a 'frontier spirit' is needed.

Philippe Moingeon
January 2005

Chapter 1

Driving Forces in the Development of Innovative Vaccines

Philippe Moingeon

Abstract

Schematically, four frontiers to the development of innovative vaccine can be identified, including:

1 *The knowledge frontier*: our current understanding of innate immune mechanisms, antigen processing and presentation, immune memory, and pathogen–host interface provides the ground for rational approaches to vaccine and adjuvant design.
2 *The technology frontier*: vaccine development is facilitated by genome mining as a mean to identify target antigens, new protein expression systems, rationally designed adjuvants and vector systems, needleless administration devices, as well as new tools to monitor immune responses.
3 *The target frontier:* the (re)emergence of old and new infectious pathogens creates a need for new prophylactic vaccines. Therapeutic vaccines are being developed against a variety of targets, including chronic infectious diseases, allergies, cancers, as well as metabolic and neurodegenerative diseases.
4 *The development frontier:* vaccine development faces a more stringent regulatory environment. Societal acceptance, as well as production and distribution issues (e.g. large-scale manufacturing of biologicals, cost containment, availability to developing countries) have also to be taken into account.

In order to cope with these challenges, all actors involved in vaccine development (i.e. research institutions, industries, government agencies, funding entities) have to align in support of global public health strategies. Collectively, such combined and coordinated efforts should lead in the forthcoming decade to an increased vaccine coverage against a growing number of infectious and non-infectious diseases, in both industrialized and developing countries.

RESIDUAL NEEDS IN VACCINOLOGY

Conventional vaccines have been extremely successful in preventing a large number of infectious diseases. Generic vaccines based on live or inactivated whole pathogens, or surface polysaccharides have allowed, in the last 50 years, to prevent a number of infectious diseases, including smallpox, measles, polio, or meningitis associated with *Hemophilus influenzae* and *Neisseria meningitidis*, to name a few. Such vaccines were designed to elicit neutralizing or bactericidal antibodies against surface-expressed molecules on viruses or bacteria. Largely due to a growing regulatory pressure, new vaccines in development are rather based on well-defined molecular immunogens, as opposed to whole attenuated or inactivated pathogens. These 'molecular vaccines' encompass, for example, recombinant proteins, peptides, lipopeptides, plasmid DNA, or recombinant viruses based on viral vectors known to be safe in humans. Such vaccines, however are in general poorly immunogenic, and should be associated with an adjuvant. In this regard, adjuvants such as aluminum salts have been successfully used for many years to elicit strong antibody responses, but adjuvants are still lacking to elicit strong cellular (Th1) responses in humans.

Using existing technologies, significant progress has been made in the last few years towards the development of vaccines against oncogenic human papillomaviruses, herpes simplex virus 1 or *Staphylococcus aureus*. Vaccines against a number of chronic infectious diseases, for which both humoral and cellular immune mechanisms should be stimulated, are yet to be developed. Such chronic infections can involve viruses (e.g. HIV1 or hepatitis C virus), bacteria (e.g. *Mycobacterium tuberculosis, Chlamydia pneumoniae*), or parasites (e.g. *Plasmodium falciparum*). An additional challenge is that some of these vaccines should ideally control the infection at mucosal surfaces. Thus, new routes of administration, and new antigen presentation platforms should be developed to stimulate mucosal immunity. Interestingly, in the last few years, additional targets beyond infectious diseases are being considered for antigen-specific immunodulation (e.g. cancer, autoimmunity, allergies, neurodegenerative or metabolic diseases). In most of these approaches, the vaccine is rather used therapeutically, instead of aiming at preventing the disease.

On this basis, a field force analysis of the environment in which new or improved vaccines are currently being developed is shown in Figure 1.1. This schematic representation helps to identify four distinct frontiers, namely:

- The 'knowledge' frontier: recent scientific advances helping to understand in molecular terms the physiology of the immune system, and its interface with pathogens or cancers, will facilitate the rational design of new vaccines, immunotherapeutics, adjuvants and vector systems.
- The 'technology' frontier: new technologies provide innovative approaches for both the identification of target antigens, and a better presentation to the immune system (new antigen presentation platforms, formulations, vectors/adjuvants/delivery systems), possibly via non-invasive routes.
- The 'target' frontier: new targets for vaccination are being explored, including emerging infectious pathogens, cancers, diabetes, rheumatoid arthritis, multiple sclerosis, atherosclerosis, Alzheimer disease, allergies to either tree, grass pollen, or house dust mites, etc. The development of combination vaccines, associating immunologically pertinent molecules originating from multiple pathogens is also critical in order to protect against multiple diseases with a limited number of injections.
- The development frontier: new vaccines have obviously to be efficacious, but there is also a growing demand for documenting safety in very large human cohorts. Little tolerance for even rare adverse events is making societal acceptance of prophylactic vaccination more difficult. Overall, the regulatory framework for vaccine development is becoming more demanding, and the cost and duration of vaccine development are increasing dramatically. Manufacturability of the vaccine, cost containment, and inclusion into existing or future worldwide immunization programs represent additional challenges for the various stakeholders involved in vaccine development. In this regard, public–private partnerships are necessary to assemble the skills, expertise and resources to develop, manufacture and distribute vaccines of the future.

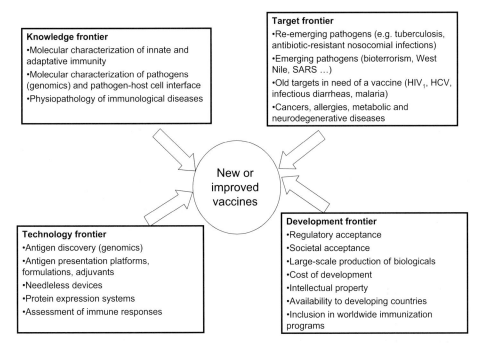

Knowledge frontier
•Molecular characterization of innate and adaptative immunity
•Molecular characterization of pathogens (genomics) and pathogen-host cell interface
•Physiopathology of immunological diseases

Target frontier
•Re-emerging pathogens (e.g. tuberculosis, antibiotic-resistant nosocomial infections)
•Emerging pathogens (bioterrorism, West Nile, SARS ...)
•Old targets in need of a vaccine (HIV$_1$, HCV, infectious diarrheas, malaria)
•Cancers, allergies, metabolic and neurodegenerative diseases

New or improved vaccines

Technology frontier
•Antigen discovery (genomics)
•Antigen presentation platforms, formulations, adjuvants
•Needleless devices
•Protein expression systems
•Assessment of immune responses

Development frontier
•Regulatory acceptance
•Societal acceptance
•Large-scale production of biologicals
•Cost of development
•Intellectual property
•Availability to developing countries
•Inclusion in worldwide immunization programs

Figure 1.1 Current frontiers in vaccine development. Current opportunities and challenges for the development of new or improved vaccines encompass four distinct categories, listed here as the knowledge, technology, target and development frontiers, respectively.

The importance of these various forces and the manner in which they shape innovation in vaccine development will be discussed in the present review.

THE KNOWLEDGE FRONTIER

Early proinflammatory events and innate immunity

It is now established that immune responses mediated by polymorphic B and T cells following pathogen insults (adaptive immunity) largely depend on the quality and accuracy of the initial 'danger' signals perceived by innate immune cells in contact with the pathogen (Janeway *et al.*, 2002; Takeda *et al.*, 2003). Thus, a number of new vaccines should ideally mimic or induce early proinflammatory events leading to innate immunity. Importantly, innate immune mechanisms involved in pathogen recognition have now been deciphered in molecular terms: APCs are known to express on their cell membrane a variety of receptors for so-called pathogen-associated molecular patterns (PAMPs) molecules, such as lipopolysaccharides (LPS), bacterial DNA, viral RNA, flagellin, etc. Such receptors include for example Toll-like receptors (TLRs) capable of conveying proinflammatory signals following engagement with cognate ligands expressed by infectious pathogens. Biological ligands (e.g. CpGs oligonucleotides, MPL) and synthetic analogs of TLR agonists are being evaluated for their adjuvant properties (see below).

In parallel, it is now recognized that non-conventional T lymphocytes exhibiting a limited polymorphism in their capacity to recognize antigens can participate to the development of protective adaptive immunity: NKT cells express an invariant TCR (α24/Vβ11 in humans) and share common features with both NK cells and conventional

T cells (Kronenberg *et al.*, 2002). Gamma/delta T lymphocytes (γ/δ T cells) represent 5% or less of circulating lymphocytes, but are locally concentrated in the skin, gut and reproductive tract mucosae. As such, these cells potentially play an effector role in controlling cancers (Ferrarini *et al.*, 2002) and intracellular infectious pathogens (Carding *et al.*, 2002). Collectively, synthetic activators of non-conventional T cells can represent powerful adjuvants due to their capacity to reveal interesting immune effector functions (e.g. cytotoxicity, cytokine production) associated with such cells. NKT cells have a capacity to produce high levels of regulatory cytokines (i.e. IL-4, IFNγ) when stimulated by α glycosyl ceramide or synthetic analogs (Giaccone *et al.*, 2002). Gamma delta T cells can be specifically activated by either organic phosphoesters, alkylamines or nucleotide-conjugates (Sireci *et al.*, 2001).

T cell responses

Vaccines were designed in the past with the aim to elicit antibodies against infectious pathogens. For vaccines directed against intracellular pathogens, or for most therapeutic vaccines, it is now recognized that both regulatory and effector properties mediated by $CD4^+$ and $CD8^+$ T lymphocytes should be harnessed. Thus, vaccines designed specifically to elicit strong cellular immune responses should both facilitate antigen entry in the cytosol, or in the lysosomal compartment of professional antigen-presenting cells (APCs) such as dendritic cells or macrophages, and induce maturation of APCs so that they express the costimulatory molecules needed to optimally prime naïve T lymphocytes (Pardoll, 2002; Moingeon, 2002). To date, there are no well-established strategies to elicit antigen-specific $CD8^+$ cytotoxic cells in humans, and this in itself constitutes a major limitation in our efforts to develop efficient vaccines against HIV1 or cancer (Moingeon, 2002).

The multiplicity of differentiation pathways associated with distinct 'helper' capacities for $CD4^+$ T cells is also better understood. Following antigen stimulation, $CD4^+$ T cells can differentiate into either Th1 and Th2 helper cells, which exhibit distinct patterns of cytokine secretion, driving the immune response towards cellular immunity or antibody production respectively (Mosmann *et al.*, 1996; Carter *et al.*, 1996). Recently, different subsets of regulatory T cells have been identified, including $CD4^+$ $CD25^+$ T reg, Tr1, and Th3 cells. Such T cells regulate T and B lymphocyte activation, either directly by cell–cell contact or through the production of immunosuppressive cytokines such as TGFβ (Th3 cells) or IL-10 (Tr1 cells) (Bluestone *et al.*, 2003; François, 2003). The dose of antigen, the cytokine milieu, the presence of costimulatory molecules, the involvement of specialized subsets of dendritic cells, or the route of administration all appear to play a role in controlling the 'orientation' of $CD4^+$ T cell responses following vaccination and this information is likely to become of critical importance in the design of future vaccines.

Immune memory

One of the main objectives of vaccination is to elicit long-term immune protection so that the initial encounter with the pathogen induces a strong anamnestic response controlling efficiently subsequent infections. There is now more information available on memory T and B lymphocytes as specialized cells capable to persist throughout the body following initial antigen stimulation. Such memory cells are extremely important for vaccination in that they rapidly acquire effector functions such as killing of infected cells (for $CD8^+$ memory T cells), providing help to B and $CD8^+$ T cells (for $CD4^+$ memory T cells), and secreting neutralizing or bactericidal antibodies (for plasma cells). The establishment of

B cell memory by long-lived plasma cells (Manz *et al.*, 2002) leads to the rapid induction of elevated titers of high affinity antibodies (IgG and IgA) following secondary antigen exposure. Two major memory T cell subsets called central (CD45RA,CD62L^{high}CCR7$^+$) and effector cells (CD45RO,CD62L^{low}CCR7$^-$), have been described, which exhibit different homing properties to peripheral lymph nodes and non-lymphoid tissues, respectively (Lanzavecchia *et al.*, 2002). Resting central memory T cells likely represent a reservoir for the generation of new effector memory T cells. Conversely, following antigen clearance, some effector memory T cells appear to convert into central memory T cells. Thus, to establish T cell memory, Th1 vaccines should ideally increase the burst size of T cell primary responses to establish a pool of central memory T cells. This could be achieved by enhancing the initial antigen load and persistence (Ochsenbien *et al.*, 1999). Adjuvants eliciting the production of cytokines such as IL-7, or IL-15 (acting as survival and homeostatic signals) are also predicted to enhance T cell memory.

Mucosal immunity

Mucosa-associated lymphoid tissues (MALT) such as intestinal Peyer's patches (PP) represent specialized structures within the mucosal epithelium, where professional APCs (e.g. Langerhans-like cells, M cells) capture pathogens and/or antigens, and initiate immune responses (Walker, 1994). The induction of mucosal immunity depends critically on the route and site of vaccine administration, largely as a consequence of compartmentalization in the mucosal immune system (Csencsits *et al.*, 2002). Vaccines eliciting strong systemic immunization also induce to some extend immune responses at mucosal surfaces. In order to elicit mucosal immunity, antigens are being administered as liposomes, biodegradable microspheres, or live vectors with a strong tropism for M cells (e.g. attenuated *Shigella, Salmonella, Listeria*, BCG, *Vibrio cholerae, Lactobacillus,* adenovirus, poliovirus) (Clark *et al.*, 2001; Wu *et al.*, 2001). These vaccines can be administered by systemic or mucosal (e.g. nasal or rectal) routes (Eldridge *et al.*, 1991; Zhou *et al.*, 1995). Cholera toxin (CT, from *Vibrio cholerae*), or the related heat labile toxin from *E. coli* (LT) appear to represent potent mucosal adjuvants, resulting in a Th2 response with local production of sIgA, as well as high titers of seric antibodies (mainly IgG1 in mice) (Rappuoli *et al.*, 1999).

THE TECHNOLOGY FRONTIER

Genomics, bioinformatics and structural biology

Genomics has already affected in a dramatic manner our approach to the identification of target antigens for vaccination purposes. Systematic genome sequencing efforts have led to the identification of complete nucleotidic sequences for most infectious pathogens, including *E. coli, M. tuberculosis, P. falciparum, Staphylococcus aureus*. Bioinformatics and sequence comparison allow to identify pathogen-specific DNA sequences, as well as 'pathogenicity islands' encoding for virulence factors, or surface proteins, both of which represent potential targets for vaccines. Following *in silico* selection, genes of potential interest for vaccination purposes can be expressed as proteins using for example an *E. coli* or yeast expression system (Sodoyer, 2004) to immunize animals. Alternatively, since not all genes can be successfully expressed as proteins, another strategy is to immunize directly with plasmid DNA, prior to conducting challenge experiments with the initial pathogen. Using this approach, the whole antigen repertoire from a bacteria can be screened in animal models for the presence of protective antigens (i.e. inducing protective immune responses) within one year. Genomics based approaches were successfully used to identify new target antigens for vaccines against *Helicobacter pylori, Chlamydia pneumoniae* or *Neisseria meningitidis* group B, to name a few (Grifantini *et al.*, 2002).

Bioinformatics, coupled to structural biology can also help improving target antigens, most particularly with respect to T cell stimulation. Within the protein sequence of a given antigen, T cell epitopes can be identified based on consensus amino acid motifs representing anchor residues for the association with major MHC class I or MHC class II molecules (D'Amore *et al.*, 1995; Rammensee *et al.*, 1997). On the basis of structural information regarding the interaction between MHC class I (or class II molecules), peptides, and T cell receptor complexes (Reinherz *et al.*, 1999), two types of modifications can be undertaken to 'enhance' T cell epitopes, i.e. to make them more immunogenic. A first one consists in changing residues involved in the interaction between the peptide and the MHC groove, to increase the affinity of the interaction. Such an approach has been used successfully to enhance the immunogenicity of T cell epitopes within the tumor-associated antigen gp100 (Parkhurst *et al.*, 1996; Rosenberg *et al.*, 1998). Another approach consists in altering amino acids likely to be seen by T cell receptor complexes. For example, a point mutation within the Cap1 HLA-A2 restricted immunodominant epitope from the CEA tumor antigen was shown to increase substantially its capacity to stimulate human PBMCs *in vitro* (Zaremba *et al.*, 1997). Importantly, in both cases, T cells thus stimulated cross-react with the natural peptide. Similarly, in murine systems, a point mutation in a kb-restricted VSV8 peptide leads to a modified peptide capable to induce positive selection of new T cell precursors within the thymus (Sasada *et al.*, 2000). Together, T cell epitope 'enhancement' strategies allow potentially to create immunogens capable of expanding T cell repertoires in neonates (so-called 'thymic' vaccination), and stimulating pools of naive T cells or memory T cells more efficiently in adults (Sasada *et al.*, 2000; Fukui *et al.*, 2000; Tangri *et al.*, 2001).

Antigen presentation platforms

Considerable research activity is undertaken to identify new antigen presentation platforms (Table 1.1). Inactivated pathogens, recombinant proteins or peptides, with or without adjuvants are rather inefficient in terms of inducing Th1 responses. As stated above, vectors capable to express the antigen inside professional APCs appear to elicit potent T cell responses, at least in animal models. Vaccines based on plasmid DNA elicit strong antibody and T cell responses in animals, including non-human primates. In contrast, DNA vaccines failed to elicit antibodies in humans, even if cellular responses (CTLs) have been induced when using milligram quantities (Wang *et al.*, 1998; Calarota *et al.*, 1998). Several attempts to further enhance immune responses elicited by DNA vaccines, have been made, using new formulations with cationic lipids, electroporation, or incorporation of cytokine genes in the construction, but with limited results so far. Non-pathogenic viruses carrying inserted genes from pathogens or tumor-associated genes are usually very efficient at targeting APCs. Viral vectors used in human studies include attenuated pox viruses (vaccinia or avipox viruses) or adenovirus (Bonnet *et al.*, 2000). Lipopeptides, presenting peptidic antigens in association with a lipid moiety, have also been synthesized and tested as candidate vaccines against HBV, HPV and HIV1 infections in order to induce T cell responses (Livingston *et al.*, 1997; Klinguer *et al.*, 1999). Transgenic plants (i.e. plants genetically engineered to express antigens from various pathogens) are also considered

Table 1.1 Selected technologies and their impact on vaccine development

Technology	Comments	References
Plasmid DNA	Elicits good antibody and cellular immune responses in animals. Tested in humans (HIV1, malaria, cancer), in whom it induces mostly cellular responses (no antibody responses). Can be formulated with cationic lipids or adsorbed onto gold particles subsequently shot into the patient (gene-gun). Encouraging results with prime-boost immunization schemes associating DNA and pox viruses	Calarota *et al.* (1998)
Viral vectors	The canarypox (ALVAC) has been used in more than 1500 patients. ALVAC based viral recombinants were shown to elicit both humoral and cellular responses in humans. Fowlpox, vaccinia, NYVAC, MVA represent other pox viral vectors tested in humans. Adenovirus is immunogenic in itself and cannot be used for reiterated administration. Retroviruses bear safety issues, with a risk of random integration in the host cell genome	Bonnet *et al.* (2000), Klein (2001)
Lipopeptides	Peptidic antigen coupled to lipid moiety. Induction of T cell responses against the HBV or HPV viruses. Currently tested in humans as a candidate vaccine against HIV1	Livingston *et al.* (1997), Klinger *et al.* (1999)
Transgenic plants	Potatoes, tomatoes, bananas engineered to express antigens have successfully been used for oral immunization of animals. A concern is the risk of tolerance induction in humans following oral administration of the antigen. Plants are also used as expression systems to produce large amounts of recombinants antigens, antibodies (or fragments thereof such as ScFvs)	Arntzen *et al.* (1997), Sodoyer *et al.* (2004)
Adjuvants/formulations	Many attempts are being made to develop adjuvants capable to elicit T cell responses or to stimulate mucosal immunity. Emerging need for adjuvants eliciting regulatory T cells. Importance of rational design on the basis of our understanding of proinflammatory signals	Schijns (2000), Moingeon *et al.* (2001)
Cellular vaccines	Dendritic cell-based vaccines have been tested in cancer patients. In this approach, tumor lysates, or tumor-associated antigens, in the form or DNA, RNA, protein or peptides are loaded *in vitro* on DCs readministered to patients. Recently subcellular organelles specialized in antigen presentation (exosomes) have been used for immunization purposes	Nestle *et al.* (1998), Lodge *et al.* (2000), Schuler *et al.* (2003)
Devices	Needleless devices used to administer antigens through new routes. This includes patches, spring or helium-powered devices, aerosols for powdered vaccines or micro-needles for transdermal/epicutaneous immunization	Moingeon *et al.* (2002) Levine, (2003)

as a support for vaccination through the oral route, and have so far generated encouraging results when tested in animals (Arntzen, 1997).

In the last few years, several groups have considered using dendritic cells (DCs) directly as an antigen presentation platform (reviewed in Schuler *et al.*, 2003). In the latter approach, monocyte-derived dendritic cells are expanded *in vitro* and subsequently loaded with antigens (presented as peptides, proteins, RNA or recombinant viruses). In cancer patients, some of these DC-based 'cellular' vaccines were shown to elicit tumor-specific T cell responses, leading to tumor infiltration by immune cells, and in some cases detectable tumor regression (Nestle *et al.*, 1998; Lodge *et al.*, 2000, Schuler *et al.*, 2003).

More recently, purified organelles (termed exosomes) which contain MHC class I and II molecules, as well as costimulatory molecules for T cells have been considered as a support to vaccination (Zitvogel *et al.*, 1998). Exosomes isolated from dendritic cells loaded with tumor-associated antigens are currently being evaluated as a vaccine in cancer patients with melanoma or lung cancer.

On the basis of numerous clinical studies, it is now assumed that no single vector, if used alone, can elicit optimal cellular responses in humans. Thus, the trend today in order to elicit broad (i.e. humoral + cellular) immune responses, is to associate multiple vectors, as part of mixed immunization regimens: in such heterologous prime-boost vaccination schemes, the antigen is presented to the immune system using a 'priming' vector. A second vector is used as a boost to present the very same antigen. Collectively, such mixed immunization regimens have been shown to elicit stronger antibody, lymphoproliferative and CTL responses in humans. Associations between DNA and poxviruses, or vaccinia and canary pox appear to be particularly promising in order to induce broad immune responses (Hodge *et al.*, 1997; Marshall *et al.*, 2000; Ramshaw *et al.*, 2000). Interestingly, the order in which these vectors are used is critical: priming with a poxvirus and boosting with plasmid DNA is poorly immunogenic when compared with the reverse combination (Ramshaw *et al.*, 2000; Eo *et al.*, 2001).

New adjuvants

Adjuvants such as aluminum salts, and to a more limited extent, calcium phosphate, are successfully being used in commercialized vaccines in order to elicit humoral responses. A major residual issue is to identify an adjuvant stimulating strong T cell responses in humans, including cytotoxic T lymphocytes. Chemical adjuvants such as ISCOMS, emulsions (e.g. IFA, SBAS2, SBAS4, MF59, Montanide ISA51 or 720, Detox), bacterial products (e.g. MPL) or cytokines (e.g. IL-2, IL-12, GM-CSF) have all been tested in humans and shown to enhance antigen-specific T cell responses (mostly lymphoproliferative, with fewer reports of MHC class I-restricted T cell responses) (reviewed in Moingeon *et al.*, 2001). It is however very clear that the magnitude of Th1 responses obtained with such adjuvants is not sufficient to confer protective or curative immunity against most infectious pathogens or cancers. Fairly recently, a shift from an empirical to a more rational approach to adjuvant development was made possible by the better understanding of proinflammatory events leading to the activation of both innate and adaptive immune responses (Schijns, 2000; Moingeon *et al.*, 2001). An ideal Th1 adjuvant should attract professional antigen-presenting cells, most particularly dendritic cells, in proximity of the antigen. It should also facilitate antigen entry inside the cell, allowing processing in the cytosol and presentation in association with MHC class I molecules at the cell surface. Several receptors expressed on antigen-presenting cells can be targeted to allow such cross-priming. This includes receptors involved in the capture of apoptotic bodies or dying cells (such as CD14, $\alpha v \beta 5$, CD36), scavenger receptors, receptors for heat-shock proteins, or mannose/fucose receptors (Moingeon *et al.*, 2001). Importantly, a Th1 adjuvant should also provide signals leading to both DC maturation and T cell costimulation. DC maturation can be achieved by mimicking some of the 'danger signals' provided by pathogens, for example using synthetic CpG oligonucleotides to engage Toll-like receptors TLR9. Also, adjuvants stimulating regulatory T cells should be developed, as part of therapeutic vaccines against either allergies or autoimmune diseases, in order to inhibit both Th1 and Th2 responses. Bacterial products such as purified protein derivative

(PPD) from *M. tuberculosis*, filamentous hemagglutinin (FHA) from *Bordetella pertussis*, cholera toxin subunit B, *Lactobacillus*, and *Mycobacterium vaccae* could be considered as candidates in this regard.

New administration devices

New needle-free or modified needle-based devices are being developed to increase vaccine safety, acceptability and therefore treatment compliance (Levine, 2003). Devices include microneedles with antigen dried-coated onto it, or jet-injectors based on spring or compressed gas to propel the vaccine through the skin. With such new administration systems, the antigen can be administered either in a liquid form, or as a powder (e.g. adsorbed onto a microscopic gold particle, as in the Powderject system). Attempts are also being made to develop aerosol delivery of powder vaccine formulations, using a nebulizer (Moingeon *et al.*, 2002). Advantages of such devices include ease of use (allowing self-administration), administration of smaller doses of the vaccine and possible dry powder formulation (which reduces refrigeration requirements). Such devices can also potentially increase efficacy due to improved tissue distribution of the antigen when administered for example through either mucosal (nasal or oral), subcutaneous or intradermal routes. Using patches, transcutaneous immunization strategies are developed, which rely upon the application on intact and hydrated skin of a mixture of the antigen and an adjuvant (usually the CT or LT holotoxins) with the aim to target and activate skin Langerhans cells. When tested in humans, transcutaneous immunization was found to elicit a mixed Th1/Th2 immune response (Hammond *et al.*, 2001).

THE TARGET FRONTIER

Chronic infectious diseases

Vaccines have been extremely successful in preventing a number of infectious diseases. Additional vaccines are still needed to control emerging or re-emerging infectious diseases (Table 1.2). There is today a major interest in controlling chronic infectious diseases, using either prophylactic, or therapeutic vaccination (Seder *et al.*, 2000; Klein, 2001; Moingeon *et al.*, 2003). Chronic viral infections in need of a vaccine encompass HIV1, herpes simplex 1 and 2, oncogenic (e.g. type 16 and 18) human papillomaviruses, hepatitis C virus, respiratory syncytial virus, cytomegalovirus, Epstein–Barr virus. Similarly, bacterial infections with *Helicobacter pylori, Neisseria meningitidis* type B, *Chlamydia pneumoniae* or *Mycobacterium tuberculosis* still require that new or improved vaccines are developed. Efficient vaccines against parasites (e.g. *Plasmodium falciparum, Leishmania major*) are yet to be developed. For such chronic infectious diseases, it is broadly admitted that an ideal vaccine should elicit both a humoral and a cellular immune response, to prevent new cell infection and eliminate infected cells, respectively (Seder *et al.*, 2000; Klein, 2001). Recently, in the context of bioterrorism issues, improved vaccines targeting smallpox or *Bacillus anthracis* became the focus of renewed interest. Two additional categories of infectious diseases are also calling for new vaccines to be developed: (i) infectious diarrheas, involving pathogens such as *Shigella* species, *Salmonella paratyphi*, rotavirus, and (ii) nosocomial infections, associated, for example, with *Staphylococcus aureus*, *Pseudomonas aeruginosa*, or enterococci species, for which prophylactic vaccines and passive immunotherapies are being developed (Moingeon *et al.*, 2003).

Major efforts are still required to develop specific combinations addressing in a single shot the needs of specific populations. For example, combination vaccines designed

Table 1.2 The target frontier for new vaccines

Target	Comments/status	References
Chronic infectious diseases (mostly viral targets)	Prophylactic and therapeutic vaccines should aim at eliciting broad immune responses (both cellular and humoral responses) in order to eliminate infected cells and prevent reinfection. Candidate vaccines tested (or being tested) in humans target HCV, HIV1, HSV1, HPV, *Helicobacter pylori*, etc. There is currently good hope that an HPV vaccine based on virus-like particles, and possibly a subunit vaccine (gD + adjuvant) against HSV$_1$, could reach the market within the next 5 years	Moingeon *et al.* (2003), Stanberry *et al.*, (2003)
Emerging infectious pathogens	Vaccines against emerging targets can capitalize on well-proven approaches (e.g. whole inactivated pathogens). Emerging targets include a new coronavirus associated with SARS, as well as West Nile, and H5N1 'avian flu' viruses.	Holmes *et al.* (2003), Ferguson *et al.* (2003), Tyler *et al.* (2001)
Nococomial infections	A conjugate vaccine against *S. aureus* was shown to exhibit a partial efficacy in patients undergoing hemodialysis. Candidate vaccines against *P. aeruginosa* are being tested in patients with cystic fibrosis and appear to delay lung colonization. Passive immunotherapy is being tested against *Enterococcus faecium* and *E. faecalis*, as well as *Staphylococcus epidermidis*	Schinefield *et al.* (2002)
Bioterrorism (smallpox, anthrax)	Cell-adapted smallpox is being developed as a second-generation vaccine against smallpox and is being tested in humans for safety and immunogenicity. A dominant negative mutant of the protective antigen (PA) from *B. anthracis* is considered as a component of a subunit vaccine against anthrax. Numerous subunit vaccines are being developed against hemorrhagic fever viral infections (e.g. Ebola or Marburg viruses): a prime-boost immunization protocol associating DNA and adenovirus is being tested in a phase I study of a candidate Ebola vaccine. Antibodies against NP (nucleocapsid) and the envelope glycoprotein protect mice against infection with the Hantaan virus	Bronze *et al.* (2003)
Parasitic diseases (*Plasmodium falciparum, Leishmania major*)	Several vaccines against *Plasmodium falciparum*, tested in humans as prophylactic vaccines, could be used in endemic areas to boost natural immune responses. The RTS,S/SBAS2 vaccine was shown to protect malaria-naïve volunteers against sporozoite challenge, and elicited antibody and short-lived CD8$^+$ T cell responses against CSP1 in semi-immune adults living in an endemic area (Gambia). Multiple subunit vaccines, administered as recombinant proteins or DNA, with or without immunostimulants (CpG, IL12) induce some protection in murine models of *Leishmania* infection. Whole killed *Leishmania* + BCG was found to lack efficacy in a WHO-supported clinical study. Interest also in targeting a 15 kDa protein in sandfly saliva, to protect against *Leishmania* infection	Moorthy *et al.* (2004)

Category	Description	References
Cancers	Candidate vaccines aim at eliciting broad immune responses against multiple tumor-associated antigens in order to eradicate residual cancer cells and prevent recurrence following surgical resection of primary tumour. First-generation vaccines were based on cell lysates or autologous irradiated cancer cells. New molecular cancer vaccines against melanoma (Mage 1, Mage 3, gp100, gangliosides), and colorectal (CEA, KSA, p53), breast (STn, mammoglobin, Her2neu, ESO1), lung (gangliosides) or prostate (PSA) cancers are being tested in humans	Rosenberg (1997), Moingeon (2001)
Allergies and autoimmune diseases	Vaccines are designed to elicit regulatory (suppressive) immune responses and to reorient inappropriate existing immune responses. Studies in humans have evaluated candidate vaccines against dust mite, pollen or cat allergies. Vaccines based on proteins or peptides designed to induce oral tolerance against rheumatoid arthritis, diabetes or multiple sclerosis have been tested in humans with mixed results	Rolland et al. (1998), Tian et al. (1999), Steinman (2001), Bach (2001)
Neurodegenerative diseases	A vaccine eliciting antibodies against the β-amyloid peptide has been tested in humans with Alzheimer disease. The development of such a vaccine has been put on hold due to the induction of severe encephalitis as a consequence of the immune response	Schenk (2002)
Metabolic diseases	Exploratory vaccines are being developed against atherosclerosis, diabetes, hypertension	
Drug addition (e.g. nicotine, cocaine)	A vaccine facilitating smoking cessation is being developed to elicit specific antibodies to nicotine, thereby preventing it from crossing the blood–brain barrier. Such a vaccine, likely to be used in relapse prevention, was shown to be immunogenic in rats. A phase I safety trial of a cocaine vaccine has been successfully conducted in humans	Hall (2002), Mettens et al. (2002)
Antifertility vaccines	Several antigens from ovocytes, sperm are being considered as targets to induce neutralizing antibodies. Vaccines based on GnRH and β-HCG have been tested in humans, with some evidence of clinical efficacy	Delves et al. (2002), Mettens et al. (2002)

for infants should protect against respiratory infectious diseases, and comprise conjugate vaccines (i.e. bacterial polysaccharides coupled to carrier proteins) in order to increase the immunogenicity of capsular polysaccharides from *N. meningitis* (type A, C, Y, W_{135}), or *Streptococcus pneumoniae* (Jodar *et al.*, 2002). Combination vaccines for adolescents should prevent sexually transmitted diseases associated with HIV_1, HPV, HSV, or *Chlamydia trachomatis*. Vaccine combinations to be developed for travelers or for specific geographical zones should ideally protect against enteropathogenic bacteria, viruses associated with hemorrhagic fevers, or major parasites.

Beyond infectious pathogens

Importantly, in the last decade, vaccine applications have extended way beyond infectious diseases. Therapeutic cancer vaccines can now be designed thanks to the identification of tumor-associated antigens, that is molecules expressed at the surface, or intracellularly by cancer cells, but not, or at a lower extend by normal cellular counterparts (Moingeon, 2001). As for vaccines against chronic viral diseases, it is generally admitted that an optimal vaccine against cancer should elicit broad immune responses, both humoral and cellular, against target antigen(s) (Rosenberg, 1997; Moingeon, 2001; Klein, 2001). In all cases, the cellular arm of the response should ideally include a strong class I-restricted CTL response, as well as a Th1 component. Some of these vaccines are based on autologous tumor cells (either intact or lysed cells) or, alternatively, on well-characterized tumor-associated molecules expressed as recombinant proteins. A variety of such vaccines are being tested in humans with promising results (i.e. induction of tumor-specific immune responses, tumor regression in some patients, or disease stabilization) and a few candidates have now reached large-scale efficacy trials.

Selected autoimmune diseases emerged as potential targets for vaccination as well. A rationale is to design a vaccine based on well-characterized autoantigens (such as collagen in rheumatoid arthritis, glutamic acid decarboxylase and insulin in diabetes, or myelin basic protein in multiple sclerosis) and to formulate the antigen(s) in order to induce regulatory or suppressive immune responses. One approach of therapeutic vaccination against autoimmune diseases relies upon induction of oral tolerance. Several studies have been conducted in humans, against diseases such as multiple sclerosis, rheumatoid arthritis or diabetes, with in some cases, evidence for clinical improvement at least in small series of patients (Steinman, 2001; Bach, 2001). Similarly, therapeutic vaccination based on complex desensitization protocols is being successfully used in patients allergic to either house dust mite, tree or grass pollens, animal epithelia or insect venom. In most allergic patients with type I hypersensitivity, symptoms are linked to the existence of an inappropriate Th2 immune responses following exposure to allergens, leading eventually to allergen-specific IgE production and the involvement of proinflammatory cells such as eosinophils and mast cells. Thus, redirecting the immune response in an allergen-specific manner, from a Th2 to Th1, or possibly a T Reg response, is likely to be beneficial in allergic situations (Rolland *et al.*, 1998; Tian *et al.*, 1999; Harrison *et al.*, 2000). To date, therapeutic vaccination against allergies is being performed using aqueous extracts from natural allergen sources. Current efforts in this field are linked to the development of well-characterized recombinant vaccines based on major allergens (such as the Bet v1 molecule to treat birch pollen allergies). Although the subcutaneous route has been predominantly used in the past, new desensitization strategies against allergies are based on sublingual immunization, which appears to offer a better safety profile, while efficacy is maintained.

In this approach, the vaccine in the form of drops or tablets is kept under the tongue for 1 or 2 minutes prior to being swallowed, thereby achieving some form of oral tolerance.

Although not discussed further, new targets are also considered for vaccination, including a variety of diseases for which the immune system likely plays a role. This includes for example neurodegenerative diseases (Alzheimer disease, prion-associated diseases), metabolic diseases (hypertension, atherosclerosis), or addiction (e.g. nicotine addiction) (see Table 1.2).

THE DEVELOPMENT FRONTIER

Cost and complexity of vaccine development

Innovation as it applies to the development of new vaccines can be defined as a capacity to design, develop, manufacture and commercialize new vaccines. Importantly, all these activities have to comply with an ever more stringent regulatory environment. Thus, cost of development as well as access to intellectual property (for both antigens, vectors, adjuvants), are representing growing challenges. Also, new vaccines have eventually to be made available to developing countries, as part of extended immunization programs. In this regard, from the time a vaccine is commercialized in a developed country, it takes up to 15 to 20 additional years to have it made available to the developing world (Mahoney et al., 1999).

It is now becoming extremely difficult for a single organization to assemble internally the breadth of expertise and the resources to develop a complex molecular vaccine. Thus, alliances and networks, rather than single institutions, are emerging as a solution to tackle innovation complexity: public–private sector partnerships are being put in place in order to deal with a complex environment and with global health problems (Jha et al., 2002; Frenkel et al., 2003). As an example, a Global Alliance for Vaccines and Immunization (GAVI) and a global fund for vaccination have been set up in 2000 and 2002, respectively, to control AIDS, malaria and tuberculosis (Brugha et al., 2002; Attaran et al., 2004). These consortia aim to strengthen health systems and infrastructure in developing countries, to accelerate vaccine research and expand the use of existing vaccines. Such partnerships assemble WHO, the Gates Foundation, the vaccine industry, the World Bank as well as several national governments. A first assessment of results obtained by the GAVI network brought a message of hope, on the basis of a significant involvement of numerous national governments from African countries. It also helped to understand some of the difficulties faced in improving health systems and building up sustainable infrastructure in developing countries (Brugha et al., 2002).

Vaccinogenomics and customized vaccination

Despite the undisputable success of generic vaccination, it may occur that a small proportion of human beings is poorly or even non-responsive to otherwise efficient vaccines. For example, non-responders for the hepatitis B vaccine have been observed. Variability in terms of vaccination responsiveness can obviously be linked, at least in part, with a well-known polymorphism in the development of immune responses. While most vaccines are being developed for healthy children or adults, selected subpopulations, including young infants, the elderly or pregnant women are known to exhibit significant physiological differences in their capacity to mount immune responses. Also, vaccines are now being used therapeutically against chronic infectious diseases, cancer or metabolic diseases, implying that the potential impact of the disease on the immune system should be taken into account. Interestingly, vaccines eliciting strong T cell responses are being designed specifically for human subpopulations bearing particular HLA haplotypes.

For these reasons combined, it is likely that, in the future, at least some new vaccines will be tailored to the needs of individuals or small groups of patients. An important potential outcome of 'vaccinogenomics' would be to identify individuals with a risk of developing adverse effects as a consequence of vaccination. A much-needed vaccine against rotavirus has been withdrawn from the market on the basis that it induces severe but rare adverse events, namely an intestinal inflammation syndrome called intussusception (Bernstein et al., 1999). The identification of those few patients in whom the vaccine could cause some harm would still allow the vast majority of people to benefit from it. In addition, population selection during the clinical development of the vaccine would allow its biological activity to be tested within the most appropriate human subpopulations to maximize its chances of success. As of today, personalized immunotherapies are already being successfully used to treat allergies. Similarly, cancer vaccines based on whole cells, lysates or protein extracts (e.g. heat shock proteins) obtained from the patient's own tumor are being evaluated in humans.

Societal acceptance

At a societal level, the widespread use of vaccines has been a major success in the twentieth century, as seen with pediatric combination vaccines against diphtheria, tetanus, pertussis, hepatitis B or conjugate vaccines against *Streptococcus pneumoniae or Hemophilus influenzae* type B (Olin et al., 1997; Mills et al., 1998; Ulmer et al., 2002). Surprisingly, societal acceptance has been shaken and antivaccine movements have made their voice heard (Balinska, 2003). These groups have contributed to promote the idea of an association between hepatitis B vaccination and multiple sclerosis, or measles/ mumps/rubella vaccination and autism, respectively. In both cases, these associations have been conclusively disproved (Ascherio et al., 2001; Madsen et al., 2002). However on the basis of possible liability issues and given the limited profitability associated with vaccine commercialization relative to drug, the number of companies engaged in vaccine development and production has declined dramatically in the last 20 years. As a consequence, shortages are frequently being observed, even in developed countries, for pediatric vaccines against measles and whopping cough, or adult flu vaccines (Rappuoli et al., 2002).

CONCLUSIONS

A convergence in the development of new technologies and the availability of new scientific knowledge provides significant opportunities to develop modern 'molecular vaccines'. Such vaccines should represent safe and efficient means to cope, in a demanding regulatory environment, with old as well as emerging infectious diseases. New innovative vaccines are also considered as prophylactic or therapeutic means to control a variety of chronic diseases including cancers, neurodegenerative or metabolic diseases to name a few. For a number of such targets (e.g. chronic infectious diseases, cancer), vaccines should induce cellular (Th1) responses and long-term memory. For other targets, such as autoimmune disease and allergies, regulatory T lymphocytes should rather be elicited. Collectively, vaccine development will benefit from new strategies based on the rational design of new antigen presentation platforms and adjuvants. A recurrent challenge faced on a general ground by all new vaccines is the cost of development. This is a serious concern given that a number of these vaccines are needed for developing countries. Facilitating worldwide access to innovative vaccines in order to deal with global health problems will constitute a formidable challenge for the international community in the years to come.

References

Arntzen, C.J. 1997. High-tech herbal medicine: plant-based vaccines. Nature Biotechnol. 15: 221–225.

Ascherio, A., Zhang, S.M., Hernan, M.A., Olek, M.J., Coplan, P.M., Brodovicz, K., and Walker, A.M. 2001. Hepatitis B vaccination and the risk of multiple sclerosis. N. Engl. J. Med. 344: 327–332.

Attaran, A., Barnes, K.I., Curtis, C., d'Alessandro, U., Fanello, C.I., Galinski, M.R., Kokwar, G., Looareesuwan, S., Makanga, M., Mutabingwa, T.K., Talisuna, A., Trape, J.F., and Watkins, W.M. 2004. WHO, the Global Fund, and medical malpractice in malaria treatment. Lancet 363: 237–240.

Bach, J.F. 2001. Immunotherapy of insulin-dependent diabetes mellitus. Curr. Opin. Microbiol. 13: 601–605.

Balinska, M.A. 2003. Vaccination in tomorrow's society. Lancet Infect. Dis. 3: 443–447.

Bernstein, D.I., Sack, D.A., Rothstein, E., Reisinger, K., Smith Vicki, E., O'Sullivan, D., Spriggs, D.R., and Ward, R.L. 1999. Efficacy of live, attenuated, human rotavirus vaccine 89-12 in infants: a randomised placebo-controlled trial. Lancet 354: 287–293.

Bluestone, JA, and Abbas, AK. 2003. Natural versus adaptive regulatory T cells. Nature Rev. Immunol. 3: 253–257.

Bonnet, M.C., Tartaglia, J., Verdier, F., Kourilsky, P., Lindberg, A., Klein, M., and Moingeon, P. 2000. Recombinant viruses as a tool for therapeutic vaccination against human cancers. Immunol. Lett. 74: 11–25.

Bronze, M.S., and Greenfield, R.A. 2003. Therapeutic options for diseases due to potential viral agents bioterrorism. Curr. Opin. Invest. Drugs 2: 172–178.

Brugha, R., Starling, M., and Walt, G. 2002. GAVI, the first steps: lessons for the Global Fund. Lancet 359: 435–438.

Calarota, S., Bratt, G., Nordlund, S., Hinkula, J., Leandersson, A.-C., Sandström, E., and Wahren, B. 1998. Cellular cytotoxic responses induced by DNA vaccination in HIV-1-infected patients. Lancet 351: 1320–1325.

Carding, S.R, and Egan, P.J. 2002. Gamma delta T cells: functional plasticity and heterogeneity. Nature Rev. Immunol. 2: 336–345.

Clark, MA, Blair, H., and Liang, L et al. 2001. Targeting polymerised liposome vaccine carriers to intestinal M cells. Vaccine 20: 208–217.

Csencsits, KL, Jutila, M.A, and Pascual, D.W. 2002. Mucosal addressin expression and binding-interactions with naive lymphocytes vary among the cranial, oral, and nasal-associated lymphoid tissues. Eur. J. Immunol. 32: 3029–3039.

D'Amore, J., Houbiers, J.G., Drijfhout, J.W., Brandt, R.M., Schipper, R., Bavinck, J.N., Melief, C.J., and Kast, W.M. 1995. A computer program for predicting possible cytotoxic T lymphocyte epitopes based on HLA class I peptide-binding motifs. Hum. Immunol. 43: 13–18.

Delves, P.J., Lund, T., and Roitt, I.M. 2002. Antifertility vaccines. Trends Immunol. 23: 213–219.

Eldridge, JH., Staas, JK, Meulbroek, et al. 1991. Biodegradable microspheres as a vaccine delivery system. Mol. Immunol. 28: 287–294.

Eo, S.K., Gierynska, M., Kamer, A.A., and Rouse, B.T. 2001. Prime-boost immunization with DNA vaccine: mucosal route of administration changes the rules. J. Immunol. 166: 5473–5479.

Ferguson, N.M., Galvani, A.P., and Bush, R.M. 2003. Ecological and immunological determinants of influenza evolution. Nature 422: 428–429.

Ferrarini, M., Ferrero, E., and Dagna, L., et al. 2002. Human gamma delta T cells: a nonredundant system in the immune-surveillance against cancer. Trends Immunol. 23: 14–18.

Francois BJ. 2003. Regulatory T cells under scrutiny. Nature Rev. Immunol. 3(3): 189–198.

Frenkel, L.D., and Nielsen, K. 2003. Immunization issues for the 21st century. Ann. Allerg. Asthma Immunol. 90: 45–52.

Fukui, Y., Oono, T., Cabaniols, J.-P., Nakao, K., Hirokawa, K., Inayoshi, A., Sanui, T., Kanellopoulos, J., Iwata, E., Noda, M., Katsuki, M., Kourilsky P., and Sasazuki, T. 2000. Diversity of T cell repertoire shaped by a single peptide ligand is critically affected by its amino acid residue at a T cell receptor contact. Proc. Natl. Acad. Sci. USA 97: 13760–13765.

Giaccone, G, Punt, CJ, Ando, Y, et al. 2002. A phase I study of the natural killer T-cell ligand alpha-galactosylceramide (KRN7000) in patients with solid tumors. Clin. Cancer Res. 8: 3702–3709.

Green, B.A., and Baker, S.M. 2002. Recent advances and novel strategies in vaccine development. Curr. Opin. Microbiol. 5: 483–488.

Grifantini, R., Bartolini, E., Muzzi, A., Draghi, M., Frigimelica, E., Berger, J., Ratti, G., Petracca, R., Galli, G, Agnusdei, M., Giuliani, M.M., Santini, L., Brunelli, B., Tettelin, H., Randazzo, F., and Grandi, G. 2002. Previously unrecognized vaccine candidates against group B meningococcus identified by DNA microarrays. Nature Biotechnol. 20: 914.

Hall, W. 2002. The prospects for immunotherapy in smoking cessation. Lancet 360: 1089–1091.

Hammond, S.A., Walwender, D., Alving, C.R., and Glenn G. 2001. Transcutaneous immunization: T cell responses and boosting of existing immunity. Vaccine 19: 2701–2707.

Harrisson, L.C., and Hafler, D.A. 2000. Antigen-specific therapy for autoimmune disease. Curr. Opin. Immunol. 12: 704–711.

Hodge, J.W., McLaughlin, J.P., Kantor, J.A., and Schlom, J. 1997. Diversified prime and boost protocols using recombinant vaccinia virus and recombinant non-replicating avian pox virus to enhance T-cell immunity and antitumor responses. Vaccine 15: 759–768.

Holmes, K.V., and Enjuanes, L. 2003. The SARS Coronavirus: a postgenomic era. Science 300: 1377–1378.

Janeway, C.A., Jr., and Medzhitov, R. 2002. Innate immune recognition. Annu. Rev. Immunol. 20: 197–216.

Jha, P., Mills, A, Hanson, K, Kumaranayake, L, Conteh, L, Kurowki, C, Nguyen, S.N., Cruz, O.V., Ranson, K, Vaz, L.M.E., Yu, S., Morton, O., and Sachs, J.D. 2002. Improving the health of the global poor. Science 295: 2036–2039.

Jodar, L, Feavers, I.M., Salisbury, D., and Granoff, D.M. 2002. Development of vaccines against meningococcal disease. Lancet 359: 1499–1503.

Klein, M. 2001. Current progress in the development of human immunodeficiency virus vaccines: research and clinical trials. Vaccine 19: 2210–2215.

Klinguer, C., David, D., Kouach, M., Wieruszeski, J.M., Tartar, A., Marzin, D., Levy, J.P., and Gras-Masse, H. 1999. Characterization of a multi-lipopeptides mixture used as an HIV-1 vaccine candidate. Vaccine 18: 259–67.

Kronenberg, M., and Gapin, L. 2002. The unconventional lifestyle of NKT cells. Nature Rev. Immunol. 2: 557–568.

Lanzavecchia, A., and Sallusto, F. 2002. Progressive differentiation and selection of the fittest in the immune response. Nature Rev. Immunol. 2: 982–987.

Levine, M.M. 2003. Can needle-free administration of vaccines become the norm in global immunization? Nature Med. 9: 99–103.

Livingston, B.D., Crimi, C., Grey, H., Ishioka, G., Chisari, F.V., Fikes, J., Grey, H., Chesnut, R.W., and Sette, A. 1997. The hepatitis B virus-specific CTL responses induced in humans by lipopeptide vaccination are comparable to those elicited by acute viral infection. J. Immunol. 159: 1382–92.

Lodge, P.A., Jones, L.A., Bader, R.A., Murphy, G.P., and Salsaller, M.L. 2000. Dendritic cell-based immunotherapy of prostate cancer: immune monitoring of a phase II clinical trial. Cancer Res. 60: 829–833.

Madsen, K.M., Hviid, A., Vestergaard, M., Schendel, D., Wohlfahrt, J., Thorsen, P., Olsen, J., and Melbye, M. 2002. A population-based study of measles, mumps, and rubella vaccination and autism. N. Engl. J. Med. 347: 1477–1482.

Mahoney, R.T., and Maynard, J.E. 1999. The introduction of new vaccines into developing countries. Vaccine 646–652.

Manz, R.A., Arce, S., Cassese, G. et al. 2002. Humoral immunity and long-lived plasma cells. Curr. Opin. Immunol. 114: 517–521.

Marshall, J.L., Hoyer, R.J., Toomey, M.A., Faraguna, K, Chang, P., Richmond, E., Pedicano, J.E., Gehan, E., Peck, R.A., Arlen, P., Tsang, K.Y., and Schlom, J. 2000. Phase I study in advanced cancer patients of a diversified prime-boost vaccination protocol using recombinant vaccinia virus and recombinant non replicating avipox virus to elicit anti carcinoembryonic antigen immune responses. J. Clin. Oncol. 18: 3964–3973.

Mettens, P., and Monteyne, P. 2002. Life-style vaccines. Br. Med. Bull. 62: 175–186.

Mills, E., Gold, R., Thipphawong, J., Barreto, L., Guasparini, R., Meekison, W., Cunning, L., Russell, M., Harrison, D., Boyd, M., and Xie, F. 1998. Safety and immunogenicity of a combined five-component pertussis–diphtheria–tetanus–inactivated poliomyelitis–Haemophilus b conjugate vaccine administered to infants at two, four and six months of age. Vaccine 16: 576–582.

Moingeon, P. 2001. Cancer vaccines. Vaccine 19: 1305–1326.

Moingeon P., Haensler J., and Lindberg A. 2001. Towards the rational design of Th1 adjuvants. Vaccine 19: 4363–4372.

Moingeon, P. 2002. Strategies for designing vaccines eliciting Th1 responses in human. J. Biotech. 98: 189–1998.

Moingeon, P., De Taisne, C., and Almond, J. 2002. Delivery technologies for human vaccines. Br. Med. Bull. 62: 29–44.

Moingeon, P, Almond, J. and De Wilde, M. 2003. Therapeutic vaccines against infectious diseases. Curr. Opin. Microbiol. 6: 462–471.

Moorthy, V.S., Good, M.F., and Hill, A.V. 2004. Malaria vaccine developments. Lancet 363: 150–156.

Mosmann, T.R., and Sad, S. 1996. The expanding universe of T cell subsets: Th1, Th2 and more. Immunol. Today 17: 138–146.

Nestle, F.O., Alijagic, S., Gilliet, M., Sun, Y., Grabbe, S., Dummer, R., Burg, G., and Schadendorf, D. 1998. Vaccination of melanoma patients with peptide or tumor lysate-pulsed dendritic cells. Nature Med. 4: 328–332.

Ochsenbein, A.F., Karrer, U., Klenerman, P. et al. 1999. A comparison of T cell memory against the same antigen induced by virus versus intracellular bacteria. Proc. Natl. Acad. Sci. USA 96: 9293–9298.

Olin, P., Rasmussen, F., Gustafsson, L., Hallander, H.O., and Heijbel, H. 1997. Randomised controlled trial of two-component, three-component, and five-component acellular pertussis vaccines compared with whole-cell pertussis vaccine. Lancet 350: 1569–1574.

Parkhurst, M.R., Salgaller, M.L., Southwood, S., Robbins, P.F., Sette, A., Rosenberg, S.A., and Kawakami, Y. 1996. Improved induction of melanoma-reactive CTL with peptides from the melanoma antigen gp100 modified at HLA-A*0201-binding residues. J. Immunol. 157: 2539–2548.

Pardoll, D.M. 2002. Spinning Molecular Immunology into successful immunotherapy. Nature Rev. Immunol. 2: 227–238.

Rammensee, H.G., Bachman, J., and Stevanovic, S. (eds) 1997. MHC Ligands and Peptide Motifs. Landes Bioscience, Austin, TX.

Ramshaw, I.A., and Ramsay, A.J. 2000. The prime-boost strategy: exciting prospects for improved vaccination. Immunol. Today 21: 163–165.

Rappuoli, R., Pizza, M., and Douce, G., et al. 1999. Structure and mucosal adjuvanticity of cholera and Escherichia coli heat-labile enterotoxins. Immunol. Today 20: 493–500.

Rappuoli, R., Miller, H.I., and Falkow, S. 2002. The intangible value of vaccination. Science 297: 937–939.

Reinherz, E.L., Tan, K., Tang, L., Kern, P., Liu, J.-H., Xiong, Y., Hussey, R.E., Smolyar, A., Hare, B., Zhang, R., Joachimiak, A., Chang, H-C, Wagner, G., and Wang, J.-H. 1999. The crystal structure of a T cell receptor in complex with peptide and MHC class II. Science 286: 1913–1917.

Rolland, J., and O'Hehir, R. 1998. Immunotherapy of allergy: anergy, deletion, and immune deviation. Curr. Opin. Immunol. 10: 640–5.

Rosenberg S.A. 1997. Cancer vaccines based on the identification of genes encoding cancer regression antigens. Immunol. Today 18: 175–82.

Rosenberg, S.A., Yang, J.C., Schwartzentruber, D.J., Hwu, P., Maringola, F.M., Topalian, S.L., Restifo, N.P., Dudley, P.E., Schwarz, S.L., Spiess, P.J., Wunderlich, J.R., Parkhurst, M.R., Kawakami, Y., Seipp, C.A., Einhorn, J.H., and White, D.E. 1998. Immunologic and therapeutic evaluation of a synthetic peptide vaccine for the treatment of patients with metastatic melanoma. Nature Med. 4: 1–7.

Sasada, T., Ghendler, Y., Wang, J.-H., and Reinherz, E.L. 2000. Thymic selection is influenced by subtle structural variation involving the p4 residue of an MHC class 1-bound peptide. Eur. J. Immunol. 30: 1281–1289.

Schenk, D. 2002. Amyloid-β immunotherapy for Alzheimer's disease: the end of the beginning. Nature 3: 824–828.

Schijns, V. 2000. Immunological concepts of vaccine adjuvant activity. Curr. Opin. Immunol. 12: 456–463.

Schuler, G., Schuler-Thurer, B., and Steinman R.M. 2003. The use of dendritic cells in cancer immunotherapy. Curr. Opin. Immunol.15: 138–147.

Seder, R.A., and Hill A.V.S. 2000. Vaccines against intracellular infections requiring cellular immunity. Nature 406: 793–797.

Shinefield, H., Black, S., Fattom, A., Horwith, G., Rasgon, S., Ordonez, J., Yeoh, H., Law, D., Robbins, J.B., Schneerson, R., Muenz, L., and Naso, R. 2002. Use of staphylococcus aureus conjugate vaccine in patients receiving hemodialysis. N. Engl. J. Med. 346: 491–496.

Sireci, G, Espinosa, E., Di Sano, C, et al. 2001. Differential activation of human gamma delta cells by nonpeptide phosphoantigens. Eur. J. Immunol. 31: 1628–1635.

Sodoyer, R. 2004. Expression systems for the production of recombinant pharmaceuticals. Biodrugs 18: 51–62.

Stanberry, L.R., Spruance, S.L., Cunningham, A.L., Bernstein, D.I., Mindel, A., Sacks, S., Tyring, S., Aoki, F.Y., Slaoui, M., Denis, M., Vandepapeliere, P., and Dubin, G. 2002. Glycoprotein-D-adjuvant vaccine to prevent genital herpes. N. Engl. J. Med. 21: 1652–1661.

Steinman, L. 2001. Immunotherapy of multiple sclerosis: the end of the beginning. Curr. Opin. Microbiol. 13: 597–600.

Takeda, K, Kaisho, T., and Akira S. 2003. Toll-like receptors. Annu. Rev. Immunol. 21: 335–376.

Tangri, S., Ishioka, G.Y., Huang, X., Sidney, J., Southwood, S., Fikes, J., and Sette, A. 2001. Structural features of peptide analogs of human histocompatibility leukocyte antigen class I epitopes that are more potent and immunogenic than wild-type peptide. J. Exp. Med. 194: 833–846.

Tian, J., Olcott, A., Hanssen, L., Zekzer, D., and Kaufman, D.L. 1999. Antigen-based immunotherapy for autoimmune disease: from animal models to humans? Immunol. Today 20: 190–195.

Tyler, K.L. 2001. West Nile virus encephalitis in America. N. Engl. J. Med. 24: 1858–1859.

Ulmer, J.B., and Liu, M.A. 2002. Ethical issues for vaccines and immunization. Nature Rev. Immunol. 2: 291–296.

Walker, RI. 1994. New strategies for using mucosal vaccination to achieve more effective immunisation. Vaccine 12: 87–93.

Wang, R., Doolan, D.L., Le Thong, P., Hedstrom, R.C., Coonan, K.M., Charoenvit, Y., Jones, T.R., Hobart, P., Margalith, M., Ng, J., Weiss, W.R., Sedegah, M., de Taisne, C., Norman, J.A., and Hoffman, S.L. 1998. Induction of antigen-specific cytotoxic T lymphocytes in humans by a malaria DNA. Vaccine Sci. 282: 476–480.

Wu, Y, Wang, X, Csencsits, KL., Haddad, A et al. 2001. M cell-targeted DNA vaccination. Proc. Natl. Acad. Sci. USA 98: 9318–9323.

Zaremba, S., Barzaga, E., Zhu, M., Soares, N., Tsang, K-Y., and Schlom, J. 1997. Identification of an enhancer agonist cytotoxic T lymphocyte peptide from human carcinoembryonic antigen. Cancer Res. 57: 4570–4577.

Zhou, F., Kraehenbuhl, J.P., and Neutra, M. 1995. Mucosal IgA response to rectally administered antigen formulated in IgA-coated liposomes. Vaccine 13: 637–644.

Zitvogel, L., Regnault, A., Lozier, A,. and Amigorena, S. 1998. Eradication of established murine tumors using a novel cell-free vaccine: dendritic cell-derived exosomes. Nature Med. 4: 594–600.

Chapter 2

Immunological Basis for the Rational Design of New Vaccines

Laleh Majlessi and Claude Leclerc

Abstract

Vaccines constitute highly powerful tools for preventing infectious diseases. Smallpox eradication and the remarkable decrease in poliomyelitis or measles throughout the world represent the most significant successes of vaccination. However, infectious diseases remain the leading cause of death in both industrialized and developing countries. Thus, both the development of new vaccines to prevent diseases for which no vaccine is available and the improvement in terms of efficacy and safety of existing vaccines remain a priority. An efficient vaccine against a pathogen has to (i) generate protective immune responses in a large proportion of individuals, against all pathogen serotypes, (ii) establish immunological memory, (iii) be effective in newborns, adults and the elderly, (iv) be safe and stable, and (v) be economically feasible. To fulfill these criteria, strong modifications will be required in the methods that have been used so far to design vaccine candidates. In particular, modern vaccinology can strongly benefit from the latest progress in molecular biology, microbiology and immunology. In this review, we discuss some essential features of the immune system and potential implications of our increasing knowledge of pathogen genomes and the physiology of immune system for the development of new strategies for vaccination.

INTRODUCTION

Numerous cell types and molecules, with specialized biological functions, are involved in the host defense against invading pathogens or cancer cells. These components belong to two arms of the immune system, establishing innate and adaptive immunity, respectively. Innate immunity is induced early (within few minutes) following exposure to microorganisms. Cells involved in the innate system comprise natural killer cells (NK), granulocytes, macrophages and dendritic cells (DCs). Macrophages and DC sample their environment by phagocytosis or pinocytosis, process pathogen-derived antigens and create a proinflammatory context in which antigens are efficiently presented to T cells to activate them. The adaptive arm of immune system requires several days or weeks to develop and leads to B, CD4$^+$ or CD8$^+$ T lymphocyte responses to the antigen. Such antigen-specific lymphocytes are able to recognize antigen due to the tremendous diversity of their respective antigen-specific receptors, i.e. immunoglobulin (Ig) or T-cell receptor (TCR). B and T lymphocytes respond much more rapidly and more efficiently upon secondary exposure to the same antigen, a phenomenon referred to as 'immunological memory' which constitutes the basis for protective vaccines. To generate a long-lasting protective immunity, a vaccine has not only to trigger efficiently lymphocytes specific for protective immunogens, but also to stimulate cells of the innate immune system which determine the type of the adaptive immune responses.

MAJOR FEATURES OF INNATE AND ADAPTIVE IMMUNITY

Cells of the innate immune system

Granulocytes and monocytes represent major cells of the innate immune system and are able to migrate into the tissues without returning to the blood. Neutrophil granulocytes are attracted massively to sites of infection and play a significant role in inflammation. Eosinophils are involved in the control of parasites while basophils contribute to many allergic reactions. Monocytes constitute 2% to 5% of leukocytes and circulate in the blood for 1 to 2 days before migrating to the tissues, where they differentiate as macrophages or DCs. Macrophages are highly specialized in the capture of antigens in the periphery and play a critical role in controlling intracellular bacteria and fungal infections. DCs, in addition to their capacity to capture antigen, display unique features in both delivering antigen to secondary lymphoid organs, in antigen processing/presentation and in activating T cells (Steinman, 2003). Because of the crucial role of DCs in the generation of primary immunity and thus in vaccination, we will focus on this subset of potent antigen-presenting leukocytes.

Dendritic cells

Among antigen-presenting cells (APCs), dendritic cells (DCs) are the most potent in initiating and amplifying primary as well as recall immune responses to antigens. DCs are defined by their morphology, the expression of specific surface markers and their unique ability to attract and interact with naive T cells. DCs reside in most peripheral tissues and in particular at potential pathogen entry sites such as skin and mucosal surfaces (Banchereau et al., 2000; Guermonprez et al., 2002). Several subsets of DCs have been described based on their cell surface markers and functions. In mouse spleen, four major DC populations have been identified: (i) $CD11c^+$ $CD11b^-$ $DC205^+$ $CD4^-$ $CD8^+$, (ii) $CD11c^+$ $CD11b^+$ $DC205^-$ $CD4^+$ $CD8^-$, (iii) $CD11c^+$ $CD4^-$ $CD8^-$, and (iv) $CD11c^+$ $B220^+$, the latter referred to as plasmacytoid DCs, given their resemblance to antibody-producing plasma cells (Shortman and Liu, 2002; Steinman, 2003). Although $CD11c^+$ $CD11b^-$ $CD8^+$ or $CD11c^+$ $CD11b^+$ $CD8^-$ DCs have been initially considered to originate from either lymphoid or myeloid stem cells, respectively, more recently these different DC subsets have been shown to derive from the same bone marrow progenitor (Traver et al., 2000). In addition to these major DC subsets, some $CD11c^+$ DCs develop during infection, which migrate from blood into infected tissues. These various DC subsets produce distinct cytokines and chemokines, express different receptors for antigen uptake and for microbial ligands and display different patterns of migration in vivo. For instance, the $CD11b^-$ $CD8^+$ DCs produce IL-12 and low levels of type I interferons (IFN) and IL-12. $CD4^-$ $CD8^-$ DCs essentially produce type II IFN, while plasmacytoid DCs are strong producers of type I IFN and IL-6 (Shortman and Liu, 2002).

Immature DCs express high levels of CCR1, CCR5 and CCR6 chemokine receptors which enable them, in response to corresponding ligands, to migrate from bone marrow, and through the blood, to peripheral tissues. Immature DCs are specialized in antigen capture by phagocytosis, micropinocytosis or receptor-mediated endocytosis. DCs subsequently process captured antigens into peptides and present them in association with major histocompatibility complex (MHC) class I or class II molecules to T cells. The recognition and uptake of pathogens by DCs induces their activation/maturation, thereby creating an inflammatory and costimulatory context for antigen presentation to specific T cells. Activated DCs migrate via afferent lymphatics to draining lymph nodes. Adaptive immunity is then initiated, resulting in elimination of the pathogen and establishment of immune memory. DC maturation is characterized by a loss of endocytic capacity, upregulation of MHC I and II molecules, production of proinflammatory cytokines such as IL-1β, IL-6, tumor necrosis factor (TNF) α, secretion of chemokines (e.g. macrophage inflammatory protein (MIP-1α, MIP-1β), and upregulation of costimulatory molecules (e.g. CD40, CD80, CD86, OX40L, CD70). In parallel, following the downregulation of chemokines receptors like CCR1, CCR5 and CCR6 and upregulation of CCR7, DCs migrate to lymphoid tissues in response to CCR7 ligand. After maturation, DCs become competent for priming both CD4[+] T helper and CD8[+] cytotoxic T cells, leading to stimulation of both humoral and cell-mediated immune responses.

Pathogen-associated molecule patterns and Toll-like receptors

Recently, pathogen-associated molecules have been shown to interact with specific receptors expressed by cells mediating innate immunity. Highly conserved pathogen-associated molecule patterns (PAMPs), absent from evolved multicellular organisms, constitute potent inducers of DC maturation via distinct members of the Toll-like receptor (TLR) family, principal sensors of the innate immune system (Beutler, 2003). PAMPs are perceived as molecular signatures of infection and trigger innate immune responses.

The TLR were initially identified based on their similarity with Toll, a plasma membrane protein involved in development and innate immunity in *Drosophila melanogaster*. During the 1990s, the gene regulating sensitivity to lipopolysaccharide (LPS) was cloned and shown to encode TLR4 (Poltorak *et al.*, 1998a,b). TLR4 was found to belong to a family of mammalian proteins (with at least 10 members described in human). The fact that TLR4 was highly specific in mediating responses to LPS suggested that other members of the family might also recognize distinct microbial products. Indeed, it is now well established that viral double-stranded RNA interacts with TLR3, lipopeptides and mycobacterial extracts with TLR2 and TLR4, flagellin with TLR5, bacterial hypomethylated DNA with TLR9. Microbial ligands for TLR1, 6, 7, 8 and 10 have not yet been identified. Importantly, several synthetic components have also been identified with the capacity to interact with TLR. Indeed, poly-IC interacts with TLR3, imidazoquinolines with TLR7 and unmethylated cytosine-phosphorothiolated guanine (CpG) oligonucleotide motifs with TLR9 (Aderem and Ulevitch, 2000; Medzhitov, 2001; Medzhitov and Janeway Jr, 2002).

All TLRs possess a conserved cytoplasmic domain referred to as TIR (Toll/IL-1 receptor/resistance). Activation of TLR induces recruitment of the adapter MyD88 and subsequently to the translocation of NF-κB to the cell nucleus for activation of transcription of genes involved in inflammatory responses (Medzhitov *et al.*, 1998). TLR signaling triggers the DC maturation program with upregulation of costimulatory molecules and MHC I and II molecules as well as the production of various cytokines and chemokines, critical to prime naive T cells and to regulate adaptive T helper Th1 and Th2 responses. Development of TLR-deficient mice allows to investigate the role of TLRs and components of their signaling pathways in the generation of T-cell responses and on their use as adjuvants in vaccines.

Other DC maturation stimuli are mediated through non-TLR receptors, such as CD14 (interacting with LPS), CD91 (interacting with heat shock proteins), FasL or CD40L. Moreover, DC interaction with NK, NKT or TCRγδ T cells can also induce DC maturation via unidentified mechanisms. For instance, presentation of α-galactosylceramide by DCs to NKT cells induces, upregulation of CD40L and production of IL-4 and IFN-γ by the latter (Smyth *et al.*, 2002). Inflammatory signals like type I or II IFN, granulocyte–macrophage colony-stimulating factor (GM-CSF), IL-4 and members of the TNF family represent also endogenous inducers of DC maturation. Moreover, necrotic cells or danger signals provided by molecules released from injured cells, such as uric acid, can trigger DC maturation as well (Shi *et al.*, 2003).

CELLS OF ADAPTIVE IMMUNE SYSTEM

B lymphocytes

The Ig receptor of B cells as well as secreted antibodies directly recognize antigen. Antibodies mediate several effector mechanisms to clear invading microorganisms:

1 Neutralization, mediated by IgG or IgA, preventing the binding of bacteria to their receptors on epithelial cells and blocking toxins and enzymes degrading the extracellular matrix. Neutralization of infectious virions constitutes also a main protector mechanism. A broad range of antibody specificities is usually generated by viral infection but only neutralizing antibodies – against surface viral antigen – are protective. Many currently available vaccines, including those against diphterial tetanus, measles, poliomyelitis and smallpox protect hosts via neutralizing antibodies (Zinkernagel, 2003).

2 Opsonization, which consists in coating microbes or microbial products with specific antibodies, thereby promoting the uptake of pathogens by Fc-receptors bearing phagocytes (macrophages, DCs or neutrophils). Phagocytes are several hundred-fold more efficient at ingesting opsonized microorganisms when compared with their free counterparts.

3 Activation of the complement system. At an early stage of inflammation, the enzymatic cascade of the complement system is directly triggered by microbial products (through the alternative pathway of complement activation). After binding to microorganisms or infected cells, antibodies activate the complement system via the classical pathway, contributing to the elimination of pathogens or infected cells.

T lymphocytes

Cell-mediated immunity involves direct action of helper (CD4[+]) or cytotoxic (CD8[+]) T cells. T cells recognize short antigenic peptides presented by MHC molecules. The nature of cell-mediated immune response is variable and is essentially characterized by the patterns of cytokines secreted by Th cells. The differentiation of naive CD4[+] T cells into subsets of Th cells has major implications for host defense. Indeed, the effectiveness of CD4[+] T cells, elicited by infection or immunization, depends both on their specificity and their effector functions, linked to their Th1/Th2 phenotype (Mosmann *et al.*, 1986). Th1 lymphocytes essentially produce IL-2, IFN-γ and lymphotoxin-α. This type of response promotes cellular immunity and leads generally to intense phagocytic activity which is critical to control intracellular pathogens such as *Mycobacterium tuberculosis*. Successful vaccination against intracellular pathogens causing chronic infection generally correlates with induction of Th1-type responses. The production of IFN-γ stimulates oxidative burst and intracellular killing of microbes and upregulates the expression of MHC molecules. IFN-γ and lymphotoxin-α induce the secretion of proinflammatory chemokines and cytokines like TNFα (Spellberg and Edwards, 2001). IL-12, IL-23 and IL-27, which all belong to the same family of proteins, as well as type I and type II IFN produced by APCs, activate key transcription factors that promote Th1 polarization. Numerous ligands of TLR are strong inducers of IL-12. Interaction of IL-12 with its receptor on CD4[+] T cells activates the transcription factor STAT4 (signal transducer and activator transcription 4) which then stimulates another transcription factor; namely T-box protein expressed in T cells (T-bet). The latter induces chromatine remodeling following methylation of histone proteins, and thus increases the accessibility of the IFN-γ – but not IL-4 – locus to the transcription machinery (Agnello *et al.*, 2003). Th2 responses in contrast promote allergic reactions to environmental antigens, as well as resistance to helminthic infections. They also help resolving diseases due to cell-mediated inflammation.

Th2 cells produce IL-4, IL-5, IL-9, IL-10 and IL-13. Th2 responses are usually associated with strong antibody responses, with a switch to IgE production and suppression of phagocytic activity. IL-4 is the key cytokine for Th2 polarization. IL-5 stimulates the IgG to IgE switch and activates eosinophils and basophils while IL-9 stimulates mastocytes. In contrast to numerous pro-Th1 cytokines produced by APCs, only few mediators are produced by APCs in response to pathogens driving Th2 responses. Chemokines attracting Th2 cells produced by APCs include CCL17 and CCL22 (Agnello *et al.*, 2003). IL-4 itself is the main promoter of Th2 differentiation. Binding of IL-4 to its receptor activates the transcription factor STAT6, which promotes activation of the transcription factor GATA-3, involved in chromatine remodeling and in increasing accessibility of IL-4/IL-13 locus to the transcription machinery. In addition to distinct cytokine profile produced by Th1 or Th2 cells, several surface markers can distinguish these two cell populations. IL-12Rβ2 and the chemokine receptors CXCR3 and CCR5 are preferentially expressed by Th1 cells, whereas CCR3, CCR4 and CCR8 are preferentially expressed by Th2 cells (Bonecchi *et al.*, 1998; D'Ambrosio *et al.*, 1998; Sallusto *et al.*, 1998). IFN-γ and IL-12 antagonize Th2 differentiation by inhibiting the production of IL-4, IL-5 and IL-13, while IL-4 inhibits secretion of IL-12 and IFN-γ and thus, decreases polarization towards the Th1 type (Spellberg and Edwards, 2001). Importantly, IL-10, is capable of inhibiting the synthesis of several Th1 cytokines by peripheral blood mononuclear cells at the transcriptional and translational level. In macrophages and DCs, IL-10 inhibits the production of proinflammatory cytokines such as TNFα, IL-6 and IL-12. Accordingly, in mice genetically deficient for IL-10, overproduction of inflammatory cytokines and development of chronic inflammatory diseases have been demonstrated (Conti *et al.*, 2003).

Parameters of immunization, such as the dose of antigen, route of immunization and adjuvant, determine the Th1/Th2 phenotype of the immune response generated. Indeed, severe systemic stress, immunosuppression or overwhelming microbial inoculation favor Th2 T cell responses. In contrast, the induction of a primary predominant Th1 response, using a low dose of antigen and Th1 adjuvants (for instance, natural or synthetic ligands of TLRs), favors the induction of a marked Th1 response subsequent to antigenic recall even with high doses of antigen or natural infection (Bretscher *et al.*, 2002). In addition, host genetic factors can modulate the type of the Th response induced. An interesting example is the influence of the Nramp1 (natural resistance-associated macrophage protein) allele on T helper responses generated. Indeed, infection by *Salmonella typhimurium* of mice carrying the resistance Nramp1 allele induces a Th1-biased response while infection of animals carrying the susceptibility Nramp1 allele induces Th2-dominant responses (Soo *et al.*, 1998).

RATIONAL DESIGN OF NEW VACCINES

Although vaccination has dramatically reduced the mortality and morbidity due to infectious diseases, technologies used to develop vaccines remained relatively unchanged since many decades. Indeed, so far, empirical research strategies have been used to develop very successful vaccines with only a minimal understanding of immunological mechanisms responsible for the immune protection. Until recently, immunogens used for vaccination purposes were classified in three main categories: live attenuated microorganisms, whole killed microorganisms and subunit vaccines such as purified toxoids. However, these strategies have clearly shown their limits for the development of vaccines against pathogens such as *Plasmodium falciparum* or the human immunodeficiency virus (HIV). Moreover, it should also be noticed that until recently, vaccines were exclusively used to prevent infectious diseases. Many efforts are currently focused on developing vaccines against chronic infections such as AIDS or against cancer, both for primary prevention (e.g. cancers associated with papillomavirus) or for the treatment of established tumors. Also, autoimmune and allergic diseases represent another challenge for new vaccine development. The development of such vaccines requires a large variety of technologies in order to stimulate memory, regulatory or effector immune responses against target antigens. Fortunately, recent advances in the understanding of host–pathogen interaction as well as our increasing knowledge of how immune responses are triggered and regulated have opened significant opportunities to develop new immunization strategies based on recombinant microorganisms, recombinant polypeptides, as well as bacterial or viral vectors, synthetic peptides, natural or synthetic polysaccharides or plasmid DNA. Thus, it now becomes possible to design safer and more efficacious vaccines based on a rational approach.

New strategies for the identification of protective immunogens

Over 60% of commercially available vaccines are constituted of attenuated or killed microorganisms. Replicating microorganisms of vaccinal interest present the risk of reversion to virulence and may cause clinical symptoms, most particularly in immunocompromised individuals. Therefore, new approaches under development are based on the identification of protective immunogens for the design of subunit vaccines. The identification of new target antigens benefit from genomic and proteomic technologies. Indeed, genomes of most important pathogens have been sequenced or will be deciphered shortly (Sodoyer *et al.*, 2002). Currently, the identification of protective antigens relies on animal models, thereby limiting dramatically the number of antigens that can be tested. A difficulty in defining new antigenic targets based on genomics relates to which criteria should be used to select amongst thousands of genes, those of potential interest for vaccination purposes. Indeed, the capacity of an antigen to induce protective immune responses is not necessarily linked to its immunogenicity. Moreover, immune protection against various pathogen depends upon different effector mechanisms, leading to the selection of a large variety of target antigens. Thus, it can be predicted that antigen discovery will in the future be based on a variety of methods mixing computing, analysis of proteome and classical preclinical studies.

Exploiting knowledge of the whole genome sequence of microorganisms

In conventional vaccinology, the identification of protective antigens is based on purification of the molecules produced by a pathogen and analysis of their recognition by antibodies or T cells. Alternatively, each antigen can also be tested for its ability to induce protective immunity in animal models. However, this approach suffers from many practical limitations. In particular, it relies on the identification of abundant or immunodominant antigens, which may not be the best target for induction of protection against the pathogen. Also, it is also limited to genes that are expressed upon *in vitro* culture of the pathogen. The availability of whole genome sequences for most important pathogens has dramatically changed the approach to identify target antigens for vaccines. Computer analysis is now used to predict antigens that could be potential vaccine candidates. Although this approach focuses on proteins and does not encompass polysaccharides or glycolipids, it has the advantage of not being limited to structural components of the pathogens. Methods based on antigen prediction depend on the capacity to express hundred of genes, to purify the coded antigens and to analyze their immunogenicity and protective properties in a relevant animal model. Clearly, this represents a strong limitation for these approaches. Moreover, a main problem is linked to immunization protocols used to test *in vivo* the immunogenicity of these antigens. Indeed, the choice of adjuvant and/or delivery system can dramatically biase immune responses induced by these proteins. Genome-based strategies have been successful in identifying target antigens for a vaccine against meningococcal meningitis caused by *Neisseria meningitidis* group B.

The meningococcus B genome was analyzed to identify open reading frames (ORFs) encoding surface-exposed or exported proteins using various computer programs. This investigation yielded 570 ORFs, which were then analyzed for conservation amongst several sero-groups (Pizza *et al.*, 2000). All these putative ORFs were cloned and expressed and finally 370 antigens were successfully expressed, purified and used to immunize mice. A total of 91 novel surface-exposed proteins were identified and 28 of these proteins were shown to elicit antibody responses with bactericidal activity (Pizza *et al.*, 2000). Amongst these new antigens, the protein NadA was shown to be present in 52 out of 53 strains of hypervirulent meningococcus B. This antigen was recently demonstrated to be protective in the infant rat model and represents a promising target for vaccine development (Comanducci *et al.*, 2002). Identification of new immunogens of interest for vaccination purposes against meningococcus B has also been investigated from transcriptome analysis of bacteria interacting with host cells. In this original approach, the DNA microarray technology was used to detect changes in gene expression profiles of *Neisseria meningitidis* subsequent to its adhesion to human epithelial cells (Grifantini *et al.*, 2002; Grandi, 2003). The expression of up to 190 genes has been found to be upregulated, notably genes involved in adhesion, host–pathogen interaction, DNA biosynthesis and metabolism. Among them, 12 were essential in adhesion to host epithelial cells or were upregulated after host–pathogen contact. The corresponding recombinant proteins were produced, purified and used to immunize mice. Using murine antisera, the effective upregulation of corresponding proteins at the surface of *N. meningitidis* following contact with host cells was demonstrated. Antibodies specific for 5 out of 12 of these antigens displayed substantial bactericidal activity against *N. meningitidis*, strongly suggesting the efficiency of specific antibodies in the control of this infection.

T cell expression cloning

Another new strategy allowing identification of candidate antigen consists of 'T-cell expression cloning'. The goal of this sensitive technique is to identify protective immunodominant T-cell antigens. To this aim, a DNA library of a pathogen is cloned into *E. coli* and monocyte-derived DCs are used for the uptake of the resulting recombinant *E. coli* clones, leading to processing and presentation of the heterologous antigens. T cells from appropriate donors, possessing a protective T-cell repertoire, i.e. controlling the infection, are then used to screen this antigen library presented by DCs. Clones of *E. coli* able to stimulate cytokine production in Th1 cells are then selected and their DNA inserts are sequenced for identification of the protein immunogens. This elegant approach has been used to identify several *Mycobacterium tuberculosis* immunogens. When used as part of a subunit vaccine, some of these identified immunogens elicited both CD4[+] Th1 and CD8[+] T cell responses and induced protection comparable to that induced by BCG in animal model (Skeiky *et al.*, 2000).

Genetic complementation of live attenuated vaccines with strong immunogens

The BCG vaccine has been obtained by repeated laboratory passage of an isolate of *Mycobacterium bovis* until it had lost the ability to cause disease in animals and was then used as a human vaccine. BCG is the only antituberculosis vaccine in routine use and has been shown to be effective in decreasing the incidence of pulmonary tuberculosis in children in non-endemic areas. Its efficacy in adults and in endemic areas is highly variable. The genetic basis of BCG attenuation is now elucidated and is attributed to the loss of specific chromosomic regions. Indeed, comparative genomic studies have identified 14 chromosomic regions (RD: region of difference) that are present in *Mycobacterium tuberculosis* but missing in *Mycobacterium bovis* BCG (Brosch *et al.*, 2000). Of particular interest is RD1, a region which is absent from all avirulent strains and which encodes for strongly immunogenic mycobacterial antigen. An original approach to improve the BCG vaccine consists in reintroducing RD1 into the BCG genome by genetic manipulation (Pym *et al.*, 2002). Compared to the parental BCG strain, BCG stably complemented with the complete RD1 region (BCG:RD1) displays a certain increased level of virulence and persistence in immunocompetent mice and notably elicits potent Th1 responses specific to RD1-specific mycobacterial antigen in vaccinated mice. Such immunogenicity, together with the enhancement of persistence of BCG:RD1 correlate with the better protective efficacy of BCG:RD1 against challenge with *Mycobacterium tuberculosis* in mice and guinea pigs (Pym *et al.*, 2003).

Molecular population genetics

Molecular population genetic approaches can also be used to identify pathogen genes under selection. Indeed, it can be assumed that highly polymorphic region(s) of an antigen likely indicate that this region is playing a major role in protective immunity. Such hypothesis has been used for instance to identify a region of the merozoite surface protein 1 (Msp 1) of *Plasmodium falciparum* thought to be under strong selection pressure (Conway *et al.*, 2000).

Identification of T cell epitopes by bioinformatics
In the last years, our understanding of the antigenic structure recognized by CD4+ and CD8+ T cell receptors has evolved very rapidly. The demonstration that T cells recognize short peptidic sequences bound to MHC I or II molecules has opened new exciting perspectives in the field of therapeutic and prophylactic vaccines. Indeed, sequencing of peptides eluted from MHC molecules showed that peptides which can bind to MHC molecules share common motifs (Falk *et al.*, 1991), which can be identified using appropriate algorithms (Rotzschke *et al.*, 1991). Importantly, other algorithms have been developed to identify sequences of homology with known proteins. Using such combined approaches, De Groot *et al.* were able to identify hundred of novel, conserved T cell epitopes from HIV and *Mycobacterium tuberculosis* (De Groot *et al.*, 2001).

Additional approaches are being developed based on the combination of bioinformatics, DNA microarrays and virtual HLA class II matrices. It is possible to cluster the pockets in the HLA-DR groove based on the identification of polymorphic residues and to generate databases of profiles that represent the majority of human HLA-DR peptide-binding specificities (Sturniolo *et al.*, 1999). The TEPITOPE algorithm was designed to identify within a protein the subset of peptides that bind to HLA class II. This approach can be coupled to DNA microarrays to identify genes that are specifically expressed or upregulated during a disease.

IMMUNIZATION STRATEGIES

Immunogenicity of vaccines based on proteins or synthetic peptides
The identification of new antigenic targets is only a first step in the design and development of new vaccines. Historically, most vaccines were based on live attenuated pathogens or on whole killed bacteria. However replicating microorganisms of vaccinal interest present the risk of reversion to virulence and may cause clinical symptoms, most particularly in immunocompromised individuals. New approaches under development are based on purified recombinant proteins, synthetic peptides or plasmid DNA that are usually poorly immunogenic when injected alone. Therefore, an adjuvant is usually required to improve the immunogenicity of these subunit vaccines. An adjuvant could be also required to increase the duration of the immune responses and to promote mucosal immunity.

Adjuvants
Although a number of adjuvants of various origins have been evaluated, aluminum salts are currently the only adjuvant broadly used in human. The development of new vaccines is strongly dependent upon our capacity to identify new substances able to promote and selectively stimulate appropriate immune responses. This requires a precise understanding of how immune responses are triggered and regulated.

A large variety of new adjuvants are currently under preclinical or clinical evaluation (Aguado *et al.*, 1999; Singh and O'Hagan, 1999; Moingeon *et al.*, 2001). Many of these adjuvants are based on emulsions such as IFA (incomplete Freund adjuvant), with or without the addition of immunostimulatory compounds. Montanide adjuvants such as

ISA51 and ISA720, formulated as water-in-oil, or oil-in-water, based either on mineral or non-mineral oil are being tested with various immunogens (Moingeon *et al.*, 2001). MF59 (a squalene-in-water emulsion with Span 85 and Tween 80) was recently registered in Italy. This adjuvant was shown in clinical trials to be safe and well tolerated, and to improve antibody responses to an influenza virus vaccine. MF59 is currently tested with various other antigens from human immunodeficiency (HIV), hepatitis C (HCV) or hepatitis B (HBV) viruses, respectively (Aguado *et al.*, 1999). SBAS2, an oil-in water emulsion containing QS21 and monophosphoryl lipid A (MPL), has been shown to be more potent (but more reactogenic) than SBAS4, a formulation of MPL with aluminum salt. In particular, a vaccine candidate against Malaria based on SBAS2 and the circumsporozoite surface (CS) protein of *Plasmodium falciparum*, fused to HBsAg was recently evaluated in humans and shown to induce both specific T cell proliferative responses, characterized by a Th1 profile, and strong antibody responses in healthy volunteers (Stoute *et al.*, 1997). This was associated with protection against a challenge with the parasite (Lalvani *et al.*, 1999). More recently, the efficacy of these recombinant CS: HBsAg particles was evaluated in Gambia in a randomized trial in semi-immune adult men exposed to natural infection. Results were very encouraging since the vaccine candidate was found to be safe and immunogenic and induced a partial protection against natural *P. falciparum* infection (Stoute *et al.*, 1997; Bojang *et al.*, 2001).

Efforts are currently made to identify adjuvants that can selectively promote mucosal immune responses. Bacterial toxins, such as cholera toxin (CT) or *E. coli* heat-labile toxin (LT) stimulate powerful immune responses when administered by mucosal routes or through the skin. However, a major concern for the use of such enterotoxins is their residual toxicity especially for the central nervous system (Fujihashi *et al.*, 2002). Indeed, CT as well as its B subunit have been recently shown to accumulate in the olfactory nerves/epithelium and olfactory bulbs of mice when given by the nasal route (van Ginkel *et al.*, 2000; Fujihashi *et al.*, 2002). Genetically detoxified mutants of the LT toxin, such as LTR72 or LTK63, with reduced or abolished ADP-ribosylase activity, were obtained and shown to retain their adjuvanticity when administered by nasal but not oral route (Douce *et al.*, 1999; Ryan *et al.*, 1999; Ryan *et al.*, 2000). The safety of these mutants remains to be determined in clinical trials.

So far, the mechanisms of action of adjuvants are still poorly understood. However, recent studies open the way to rational approaches for the identification of safe and efficient new adjuvants. Increasing evidence indicates that many adjuvants exert their effect through one of the TLRs expressed by cells of the innate immune system. Triggering TLRs by microbial adjuvants such as CpG leads to Th1 activation, through the production by DCs of cytokines such as IL-12 (Schnare *et al.*, 2001). These recent discoveries also open new possibilities for the identification of adjuvants capable to selectively interact with the various TLRs, and possibly to elicit specific effector or regulatory immune responses.

Targeting antigens to dendritic cells

A variety of molecules expressed at the surface of DCs can be used to increase the capture and endocytosis of antigens. Complement, scavenger and Fc receptors, as well as C-type lectins, such as DC-SIGN (DC-specific intercellular adhesion molecule-3 grabbing non-integrin), the mannose receptor and CD205, are some examples of molecules which can be used to target antigens to DCs for efficient uptake and endocytosis (Steinman and Pope, 2002). A possibility is to use antibodies specific for such molecules linked to the antigen in order to increase its uptake by facilitating binding to DC cell surface. Another alternative is based on modification of the vaccine with ligands for DC surface molecules (for instance mannose). The capacity of some bacterial molecules to use dendritic cell surface molecules as a receptor for cell entry is also providing attractive alternative strategies. For instance, the specific binding of heat shock proteins to DCs (notably through interaction with CD91) may certainly explain their strong capacity to trigger T cell immune responses (Basu *et al.*, 2001). A bacterial toxin produced by *Bordetella pertussis*, the adenylate cyclase, was recently shown to selectively target the MHC I pathway of DCs through its capacity to bind the CD11b integrin, and subsequently to translocate to the cytosol in these cells (Guermonprez *et al.*, 1999; Guermonprez *et al.*, 2001). When used as a vector, this approach was shown to be highly efficient in stimulating CTL and Th1 responses against a variety of viral and tumoral epitopes (Saron *et al.*, 1997; Fayolle *et al.*, 1999; Fayolle *et al.*, 2001; Dadaglio *et al.*, 2003).

Exploiting the cross-presentation pathway

Emerging evidence indicates that DCs have the capacity to present exogenous antigens into the MHC I pathway. The phenomenon, termed cross-presentation, could open new perspectives in the development of vaccines capable to induce strong CTL responses. Indeed, DCs possess the unique ability to present exogenous or cell-associated antigens such as heat-shock proteins, antibody complexes, exosomes, apoptotic cells, necrotic cells and viral pseudo-particles to CD8[+] T cells in association with MHC I molecules (den Haan and Bevan, 2001; Heath and Carbone, 2001a,b; Moron *et al.*, 2003). This could explain the capacity of some exogenous antigens to induce CTL responses. Indeed, we recently showed that an antigen-delivery system based on non-replicative, recombinant parvovirus-virus-like particles (PPV-VLPs) formed by the self-assembly of the VP2 capsid protein of porcine parvovirus (PPV) induced strong CTL responses in the absence of any adjuvant (Boisgérault *et al.*, 2002). The strong immunogenicity of these inert particles is due to the very high capacity of DCs to capture PPV-VLPs *in vivo* and to deliver them to the MHC I pathway after cytosolic processing (Moron *et al.*, 2002; Moron *et al.*, 2004). Such VLPs could represent a new and promising strategy to deliver epitopes or antigens to the immune system for prophylactic and therapeutic vaccines.

Use of recombinant live attenuated microorganisms as immunization vectors

Attenuated viruses or intracellular bacteria, genetically engineered to express heterologous antigens, can be used as vectors for delivery of immunogens to the immune system. Such immunization vectors have the advantage to be inexpensive to produce, allowing large-scale distribution. The use of attenuated pathogens is also attractive as they may generate both protection against the pathogen itself and immunity to heterologous immunogens. Live attenuated vaccine strains have to present a strictly limited virulence in the host, even if their capacity to persist in the host must be sufficient to induce protective immune responses. The risk of reversion to virulence can be eliminated or significantly reduced by the concomitant inactivation or deletion of several genes involved in virulence.

Bacterial vectors

Live, attenuated bacteria used as potential vectors can be used for oral immunization, and can induce protective immunity following a single immunization, probably due to their ability to replicate *in vivo* (Kochi *et al.*, 2003).

Salmonella. This intracellular Gram-negative bacterium persists within the endosomal compartment of host cells and thus resists to the host defense system. Well-characterized non-reverting mutations of virulence-associated genes generates attenuated strains of *Salmonella typhi* and *Salmonella typhimurium* which can be engineered to express heterologous antigens. Such strains are generally immunogenic, well tolerated, safe and have been used in preclinical trials as vectors to express diverse bacterial, viral or protozoan antigens (Killeen and Dirita, 2000). A *S. typhi*-based vector, expressing an immunodominant peptide from the *Plasmodium falciparum* circumsporozoite protein, has been shown, when administered orally, to generate humoral and CD8$^+$ CTL immune responses in human (Gonzalez *et al.*, 1994). Owing to the phagolysosomal localization of this bacterium following infection, the generation of CD8$^+$ T cell responses against *Salmonella*-derived or heterologous antigens delivered by this vector was unexpected, and suggests the existence of a non-endogenous pathway MHC class I presentation for the antigen.

Listeria. *Listeria monocytogenes* is a Gram-positive intracellular bacterium useful for induction of MHC I-restricted CD8$^+$ T cell responses. Indeed, subsequent to its phagocytosis by the host cells, *L. monocytogenes* escapes from acidified endocytic vesicles and gets access to the cytosol of host cells where it replicates (Kaufmann, 1993). This is due to the expression of a hemolytic protein, listeriolysin, which enables *Listeria* to degrade the membrane of phagolysosomes. The phagolysosomal and cytoplasmic localization of this bacterium allows the entry of its antigens into both the endogenous MHC I and exogenous MHC II antigen-processing and presentation pathways, and thus generation of both CD4$^+$ and CD8$^+$ T-cell responses. Mutations in several virulence-associated genes of *L. monocytogenes* have been well characterized and successfully used for the development of attenuated strains recombinant for heterologous immunogens. Such strains were shown to generate long-term immune memory and CD8$^+$ T-cell-mediated protective immunity in lymphocytic choriomeningitis virus (LCMV) infection as well as in prophylaxis and therapy of tumors in animal models (Goossens *et al.*, 1995; Paterson and Ikonomidis, 1996).

Shigella. Like *L. monocytogenes*, *Shigella flexneri* possesses the ability to escape endocytic vesicles and to reach the host cell cytosol. It thus constitutes an immunization vector to induce CD8$^+$ T cell responses. The main problem of *Shigella* as a bacterial vector is its high immunogenicity. Generation of mutations in multiple loci of *Shigella* allows a better tolerance by the host immune system but decreases its immunogenicity (Kochi *et al.*, 2003).

Vaccination with DNA encoding protective immunogens is another promising strategy for induction of immunity. As many attenuated bacterial vectors are targeted to APCs, they provide potential vehicles for delivery of heterologous antigen-encoding plasmid DNA to host APC cytoplasm. In this context, the heterologous gene is under the control of eukaryotic promoter and therefore is not expressed by the bacterial vector but is delivered to the host transcription machinery. Bacteria with the capacity to access to the cytoplasm of infected cells, such *Listeria* and *Shigella*, have been successfully used for the delivery of such DNA constructs (Medina and Guzman, 2001). Evidence of direct transfer of functional DNA from invasive bacteria to mammalian cells has been provided in a bacterial model of *E. coli*, made invasive by cloning the invasin gene from *Yersinia* pseudotuberculosis. Moreover, in this model the efficiency of DNA transfer from *E. coli* to the host cells was enhanced by coexpression of the listeriolysin gene (Grillot-Courvalin *et al.*, 1998).

BCG. Live, attenuated *Mycobacterium bovis* bacille Calmette–Guerin (BCG), used as an antituberculosis vaccine, displays strong adjuvanticity and can persist and replicate within the APCs of infected host including DCs. BCG delivers its antigens mainly to the MHC II presentation pathway and thus generates essentially CD4$^+$ T-cell immunity. This bacillus provides an interesting vector for delivery of heterologous antigens in a highly safe manner. Indeed, BCG is the world's most widely used vaccine with over 3 billion doses administered, without major side-effect reported. The genes encoding for heterologous immunogens can be introduced in BCG either with episomal replicating vectors (often rapidly lost in the absence of antibiotic selection) or with vectors integrating into the BCG chromosome (achieved with high stability). Heterologous antigens can be differentially displayed, i.e. expressed in the cytoplasm, bound on the surface or be secreted. Secreted antigen are the most efficient in inducing immune responses. However, the main factor controlling immunogenicity is the level of antigen expression (Himmelrich *et al.*, 2000). Recombinant BCG harboring antigens from bacteria (*Bordetella pertussis*, *Corynebacterium diphtheriae*) or parasites (*Leishmania major*, *Plasmodium falciparum*) have been shown to generate both humoral and cellular immune responses. Of note is the observation that the generation of prominent Th1 T-cell immunity is characterized by production of high levels of IFN-γ, which correlates with protective immunity. Importantly, pre-existing immunity to BCG does not constitute a limit to the induction of immune responses to heterologous antigen delivered by BCG vectors (Gheorghiu *et al.*, 1994). Immunization of mice with recombinant BCG-expressing viral antigens (simian or human immunodeficiency viruses) (Lagranderie *et al.*, 1998), has also been shown to induce MHC I-restricted CD8$^+$ T-cell responses. However, the molecular mechanisms by which mycobacterial antigens gain access to the MHC I presentation pathway remain poorly understood. Evidence has been provided that live and slow-growing mycobacteria reside in immature and nonacidified phagosomes and, in contrast to *Listeria*, do not escape into the cytosol of infected cells. Coincubation of macrophages with soluble ovalbumin and live *Mycobacterium tuberculosis* facilitates the delivery of this model antigen to the MHC I presentation pathway (Mazzaccaro *et al.*, 1996). Further analysis using confocal microscopy led to the hypothesis that live mycobacteria can permeabilize phagosomal membrane by formation of still uncharacterized-pores. The latter allow translocation of relatively low-molecular-mass mycobacterial macromolecules (<70 kDa) to the host cell cytosol (Teitelbaum *et al.*, 1999). Interestingly, a recombinant BCG strain expressing the lysteriolysin of *L. monocytogenes*, becomes able to perforate the membrane of phagolysosomes, and to facilitate the presentation of antigen by the MHC I pathway. It may thus constitute a vector for the induction of both CTL responses and Th CD4$^+$ responses (Hess *et al.*, 1998).

More recently, it has been shown that mycobacteria induce apoptosis in macrophages and thereby the release of apoptotic vesicles carrying mycobacterial antigen. By-stander uninfected DCs can engulf such apoptotic bodies and cross-present mycobacterial antigens to specific CD8$^+$ T cells (Schaible *et al.*, 2003).

Viral vectors

Viral infection leads to efficient host cell penetration and to presentation of virus-derived antigens by MHC I or II molecules. Therefore, viruses in which DNA encoding for heterologous immunogens is genetically inserted can constitute prominent immunization vectors. The safety of a potential viral vector is based on: (i) its natural host restriction and (ii) its attenuation profile due to serial passages or genetic manipulation. For optimal immunogenicity, a vector must be able to infect professional APCs. Recent evidence however indicates that viruses prime strong CTL responses by cross-presentation of infected cells. Optimal viral vectors have to generate limited antivirus immunogenicity to avoid its rapid elimination by the host immune responses (Bonnet *et al.*, 2000). Retroviruses, poxviruses, alphaviruses, herpes simplex virus, adenoviruses and adeno-associated viruses constitute main immunization viral vectors.

Retroviruses. These vectors are able to infect APCs and allow a sustained heterologous gene expression. The major inconvenient of retroviral vectors is the potential risk of insertional mutagenesis in the host genome. Indeed, the genetic material of retroviruses consists of diploid RNA strand and virus replication requires a DNA intermediate which can be transferred to the host genome. To circumvent this problem, retroviral vectors have been engineered to be replication defective (Jolly, 1994; Hodge and Schlom, 1999)

Poxviruses. Poxvirus-derived vectors are able to efficiently infect APCs but express only transiently the heterologous proteins. The high safety of these double-stranded DNA-containing viruses is due to their replication limited to the cytoplasm of infected cells. The main advantage of poxviruses is the possibility to insert large DNA fragments, (up to 30 kb) allowing simultaneous expression of several heterologous immunogens (Perkus *et al.*, 1995; Gonin *et al.*, 1996; Roth *et al.*, 1996). Among poxvirus vectors, attenuated vaccinia strains are of particular interest. Indeed, vaccinia viruses possess a large genome, 14% of which is non-essential for viral replication and thus can be replaced by heterologous genes under the control of vaccinia promoters. The main limit concerning the use of recombinant vaccinia virus is related to their residual capacity to replicate and to present some risk in immunocompromised individuals. Moreover, because of the pre-existing antivaccine immunity in the general population, the use of recombinant vaccinia virus is limited to non-immune populations. The vaccinia strain modified vaccinia virus ankara (MVA) presents a markedly attenuated replication and is under extensive study in preclinical and clinical trials. It has recently shown marked efficacy in the generation of protective immunity against HIV (Amara *et al.*, 2001). NYVAC, a highly attenuated vaccinia virus strain, was derived from a plaque-cloned isolate of the Copenhagen vaccine strain by the precise deletion of 18 open reading frames involving in pathogenicity. This vector exhibits a good safety profile. The canarypox virus-based vector ALVAC presents the strong advantage to be non-replicative in non-avian species. Compared with vaccinia-derived viruses, canarypox and fowlpox viruses present the advantage to induce a limited immune response against the vector itself.

Adenovirus. Adenoviruses enter the host organism via mucosal surfaces and replicate in respiratory or gastrointestinal tracts. Adenoviruses are thus prominent vectors for delivering vaccines to mucosal surfaces (Babiuk and Tikoo, 2000). Adenoviral vectors are able to efficiently infect epithelial cells, myoblasts, glial cells, macrophages and hepatocytes and are powerful stimulators of cellular immune responses. Following entry into the cells, adenoviruses escape endosomal lysis and enters the nucleus. Their high degree of safety is due to their double-stranded linear DNA, which replicates within the nucleus of infected cells without integration to the host genome. Replication-competent or -incompetent adenoviral vectors have been constructed and genomic regions which can be deleted for subsequent insertion of heterologous genes have been well characterized (Randrianarison-Jewtoukoff and Perricaudet, 1995; Chen *et al.*, 1996; Warnier *et al.*, 1996).

Adenoviral vectors have been largely used as vaccine vectors against infectious diseases, cancers or for gene therapy. Yet their great disadvantage is their strong immunogenicity, and the barrier of pre-existing neutralizing antibodies and cellular responses against these viruses. Deletion of genes involved in replication increased their safety and allowed to reduce the production of viral proteins, thereby decreasing immunogenicity. Immunity and protection have been demonstrated in numerous preclinical models despite pre-existing anti-adenoviral humoral immune responses.

Bacterial or viral vector expressing immunomodulatory molecules

Immunogenicity of live attenuated vaccines is usually proportional to their virulence/replication in the host organism, and attenuation leads to a decrease in their immunogenicity. Live attenuated vaccines, genetically engineered to express immunomodulatory molecules, like cytokines, represent a promising approach as they can influence antigen presentation, T-cell triggering or production of other cytokines (Bukreyev and Belyakov, 2002).

The choice of immunomodulatory molecules may allow stimulation of antigen presentation, enhancement or suppression of CD4[+], CTL, NK, cells antibody responses, production of other cytokines or Th1-Th2 polarization. When expressed by live attenuated vaccines (i) IL-2 has been shown to stimulate NK cells and to enhance production of IFN-γ, (ii) IFN-γ can increase production of IL-12, (iii) IL-7 stimulates NK and CTL activity, and increases production of IL-2 or IL-6, as well as specific IgG antibodies, (iv) IL-4 or IL-10 reduce NK and CTL activity, IL-4 further suppresses IL-2, IL-12 and IFN-γ, (v) GM-CSF reduces CTL activity, increases numbers of IFN-γ^+ and IL-4[+] CD4[+] T cells, enhances IFN-γ and IL-12 production and significantly stimulate APCs (Bukreyev and Belyakov, 2002).

The prime-boost strategy

Vaccination is commonly based on single or repeated administration of the same vaccine preparation. Recently, a novel strategy involving priming and boosting with different immunogens has resulted in the generation of unprecedented levels of cell-mediated immunity (CMI). Indeed, several new vector delivery systems, such as plasmid DNA vector, recombinant MVA or replication-incompetent adenovirus type (Ad5) expressing the same antigens have been compared for their capacity to induce immune responses, including CMI. Although, these vectors are capable to induce excellent CMI and high level of antibody responses, they have generally been insufficient to afford protection against challenge with highly pathogenic microorganisms. Interestingly enough, the consecutive use of DNA vaccines and attenuated poxvirus vectors encoding similar heterologous antigens was shown to induce much stronger immune responses than the same vectors given alone. Complete, long-lasting protection against malaria have been achieved in mice primed with a replication-defective adenovirus expressing the circumsporozoite protein of *Plasmodium yoelli*, followed by a boost with an attenuated recombinant vaccinia virus expressing the same antigen (Bruna-Romero *et al.*, 2001). This protection correlated with increased numbers of CD4$^+$ and CD8$^+$ T cells. In a model where DNA and MVA expressed multiple immunodeficiency proteins, DNA priming followed by a recombinant MVA boost protected against challenge with a highly pathogenic immunodeficiency virus in a rhesus macaque model (Amara *et al.*, 2001). This heterologous prime-boost generated high frequencies of virus-specific T cells and efficiently protected against an intrarectal challenge administered 7 months after the boost (Amara *et al.*, 2002). In a study comparing several combinations of vectors expressing the SIV gag protein, Shiver *et al.* demonstrated that the most effective responses were induced by the Ad5 vector, used either alone or as a booster following priming with DNA. After challenge with a pathogenic SIV-HIV hybrid virus, animals immunized with Ad5 vector exhibited the lowest levels of infection (Shiver *et al.*, 2002). It should be mentioned that the efficacy of prime-boost immunization requires an initial priming with DNA followed by boosting with attenuated viruses. Reversing the order in using those vectors dramatically reduces the efficacy of vaccination (Ramshaw and Ramsay, 2000).

Clinical trials based on the prime-boost strategy have already started. In a phase I dose–response, an AIDS vaccine based on a recombinant adenovirus expressing HIV-gag induced CD8$^+$ T cells responses in seven out of nine of the volunteers who received the highest dose (10^{11} viral particles). It should be mentioned that macaques boosted with 10^7 Ad5-gag particles after a DNA-gag vaccine responded as strongly than those who received only 10^{11} particles. A prime-boost study of DNA-gag plus Ad5-gag in HIV-infected people has been initiated (Jefferys, 2002). Prime-boost trials are also conducted both in England and in Kenya based on DNA and MVA. Both vaccines contain most of the HIV-gag gene fused to a string of 25 partially overlapping CTL epitopes from *gag*, *pol*, *nef* and *env*. These vaccines have been already tested in 26 HIV-negative volunteers (Hanke and McMichael, 2000, Jefferys, 2002).

IMPROVING THE IMMUNOLOGICAL MEMORY INDUCED BY VACCINES

The understanding of the mechanisms underlying the generation, maintenance and function of memory T cells have enormous implications for the design of more efficient immunization procedures. Indeed, in most cases, the analysis of vaccine efficacy in preclinical models is based on the determination of effector responses (antibodies, CTL responses) shortly after immunization. However, the efficacy of most vaccines relies on their capacity to generate responses still able to protect against infections encountered years after immunization. Clearly, our knowledge of how immune responses are induced by vaccines is often limited to the early steps of activation of naive T cells. The mechanisms responsible for the persistence of a pool of memory cells remain to be elucidated. Very recently, several studies have highlighted the role of certain cytokines in the generation and survival of memory T cells. Indeed, it is now well established that antigen is not required to maintain memory CD8$^+$ T cells (Kennedy *et al.*, 2000; Sprent and Surh, 2001) and several groups are searching for factors other than antigen that are responsible for memory persistence. The leading candidate is cytokine IL-15. Indeed, knockout mice lacking IL-15 or the high affinity IL-15Rα have reduced numbers of memory CD8$^+$ CD44high T cells, apparently due to a decreased proliferation rate. Moreover, transgenic mice overexpressing IL-15 contain increased numbers of memory CD8$^+$ T cells (Fehniger *et al.*, 2001). Recently, it was shown that mice deficient in IL-15 or in IL-15Rα made potent primary CTL responses in response to infection with LCMV and generated a pool of memory CD8$^+$ T cells similar to memory T cells induced in normal mice (Becker *et al.*, 2002). However, this study showed that virus-specific memory CD8$^+$ T cells gradually declined in numbers in the absence of IL-15. This was due to a defect in the proliferation of these cells, demonstrating that IL-15 is required for homeostatic proliferation of memory CD8$^+$ T cells (Becker *et al.*, 2002; Goldrath *et al.*, 2002). The dependency of memory CD8$^+$ cells on IL-15 can be overcome by overexpression of IL-7 (Kieper *et al.*, 2002). Interestingly, unlike memory CD8$^+$ T cells, homeostatic proliferation of memory CD4$^+$ T cells is independent of IL-7 and IL-15 (Tan *et al.*, 2002). These findings strongly support the idea that coadministration of cytokines such as IL-7 or IL-15 could be useful in vaccination and could increase the potency of vaccines through their capacity to maintain the proliferation of a memory pool for CD8$^+$ T lymphocytes.

CONCLUSIONS

During the last decade, considerable advances have been made in our understanding of the interactions between pathogens and the host immune system, as well as in development of new vaccines technologies. We are therefore entering a new era in which our capacity to induce and manipulate immune responses in more sophisticated and specific manners will find applications in several fields of medicine. These progresses are now leading to the rational design and development of novel immunization strategies to prevent or to treat infectious diseases and cancers. So far, successful vaccines have been in most cases based on the induction of neutralizing antibody responses against pathogens. One of the challenges is now to generate T-cell-mediated immunity against persisting intracellular microorganisms. Although it is difficult to predict exactly how long the implementation of such new strategies will take, it is already clear that new families of vaccines will be emerging in the following years.

References

Aderem, A., and Ulevitch, R.J. (2000). Toll-like receptors in the induction of the innate immune response. Nature 406: 782–787.

Agnello, D., Lankford, C.S., Bream, J., Morinobu, A., Gadina, M., O'Shea, J.J., and Frucht, D.M. 2003. Cytokines and transcription factors that regulate T helper cell differentiation: new players and new insights. J. Clin. Immunol. 23: 147–161.

Aguado, T., Engers, H., Pang, T., and Pink, R. 1999. Novel adjuvants currently in clinical testing November 2–4, 1998, Fondation Mérieux, Annecy, France: A meeting sponsored by the World Health Organization. Vaccine 17: 2321–2328.

Amara, R.R., Villinger, F., Altman, J.D., Lydy, S.L., O'Neil, S.P., Staprans, S.I., Montefiori, D.C., Xu, Y., Herndon, J.F., Wyatt, L.S., *et al.* 2001. Control of a mucosal challenge and prevention of AIDS by a multiprotein DNA/MVA vaccine. Science 292: 69–74.

Amara, R.R., Villinger, F., Altman, J.D., Lydy, S.L., O'Neil, S.P., Staprans, S.I., Montefiori, D.C., Xu, Y., Herndon, J.G., Wyatt, L.S., *et al.* 2002. Control of a mucosal challenge and prevention of AIDS by a multiprotein DNA/MVA vaccine. Vaccine 20: 1949–1955.

Babiuk, L.A., and Tikoo, S.K. 2000. Adenoviruses as vectors for delivering vaccines to mucosal surfaces. J. Biotechnol. 83: 105–113.

Banchereau, J., Briere, F., Caux, C., Davoust, J., Lebecque, S., Liu, Y.-J., Pulendran, B., and Palucka, K. 2000. Immunobiology of dendritic cells. Annu. Rev. Immunol. 18: 767–811.

Basu, S., Binder, R.J., Ramalingam, T., and Srivastava, P.K. 2001. CD91 Is a common receptor for heat shock proteins gp96, hsp90, hsp70, and Calreticulin. Immunity 14: 303–313.

Becker, T.C., Wherry, E.J., Boone, D., Murali-Krishna, K., Antia, R., Ma, A., and Ahmed, R. 2002. Interleukin 15 is required for proliferative renewal of virus-specific memory CD8 T cells. J. Exp. Med. 195: 1541–1548.

Beutler, B. 2003. Innate immune responses to microbial poisons: discovery and function of the Toll-like receptors. Annu. Rev. Pharmacol Toxicol. 43: 609–628.

Boisgérault, F., Moron, G., and Leclerc, C. 2002. Virus-like particles: a new family of delivery systems. Expert Rev. Vaccines 1: 101–109.

Bojang, K.A., Milligan, P.J., Pinder, M., Vigneron, L., Alloueche, A., Kester, K.E., Ballou, W.R., Conway, D.J., Reece, W.H., Gothard, P., et al. 2001. Efficacy of RTS,S/AS02 malaria vaccine against Plasmodium falciparum infection in semi-immune adult men in The Gambia: a randomised trial. Lancet 358: 1927–1934.

Bonecchi, R., Bianchi, G., Bordignon, P.P., D'Ambrosio, D., Lang, R., Borsatti, A., Sozzani, S., Allavena, P., Gray, P.A., Mantovani, A., and Sinigaglia, F. 1998. Differential expression of chemokine receptors and chemotactic responsiveness of type 1 T helper cells (Th1s) and Th2s. J. Exp. Med. 187: 129–134.

Bonnet, M.C., Tartaglia, J., Verdier, F., Kourilsky, P., Lindberg, A., Klein, M., and Moingeon, P. 2000. Recombinant viruses as a tool for therapeutic vaccination against human cancers. Immunol. Lett. 74: 11–25.

Bretscher, P.A., Hamilton, D., and Ogunremi, O. 2002. What information is needed to design effective vaccination against intracellular pathogens causing chronic disease? Expert Rev. Vaccines 1: 179–192.

Brosch, R., Gordon, S.V., Pym, A., Eiglmeier, K., Garnier, T., and Cole, S.T. 2000. Comparative genomics of the mycobacteria. Int. J. Med. Microbiol. 290: 143–152.

Bruna-Romero, O., Gonzalez-Aseguinolaza, G., Hafalla, J.C.R., Tsuji, M., and Nussenzweig, R.S. 2001. Complete, long-lasting protection against malaria of mice primed and boosted with two distinct viral vectors expressing the same plasmodial antigen. Proc. Natl. Acasd. Sci. USA 98: 11491–11496.

Bukreyev, A., and Belyakov, I.M. 2002. Expression of immunomodulating Mol.ecules by recombinant viruses: can the immunogenicity of live virus vaccines be improved? Expert Rev. Vaccines 1: 233–245.

Chen, P.W., Wang, M., Bronte, V., Zhai, Y., Rosenberg, S.A., and Restifo, N.P. 1996. Therapeutic antitumor response after immunization with a recombinant adenovirus encoding a model tumor-associated antigen. J. Immunol. 156: 224–231.

Comanducci, M., Bambini, S., Brunelli, B., Adu-Bobie, J., Arico, B., Capecchi, B., Giuliani, M.M., Masignani, V., Santini, L., Savino, S., et al. 2002. NadA, a novel vaccine candidate of Neisseria meningitidis. J. Exp. Med. 195: 1445–1454.

Conti, P., Kempuraj, D., Kandere, K., Gioacchino, M.D., Barbacane, R.C., Castellani, M.L., Felaco, M., Boucher, W., Letourneau, R., and Theoharides, T.C. 2003. IL-10, an inflammatory/inhibitory cytokine, but not always. Immunol. Lett. 86: 123–129.

Conway, D.J., Cavanagh, D.R., Tanabe, K., Roper, C., Mikes, Z.S., Sakihama, K., Bojang, A., Oduola, A.M.J., Kremsner, P.G., Arnot, D.E., et al. 2000. A principal target of human immunity to malaria identified by Molecular population genetic and Immunological analyses. Nature Med. 6: 689–692.

D'Ambrosio, D., Iellem, A., Bonecchi, R., Mazzeo, D., Sozzani, S., Mantovani, A., and Sinigaglia, F. 1998. Selective up-regulation of chemokine receptors CCR4 and CCR8 upon activation of polarized human type 2 Th cells. J. Immunol. 161: 5111–5115.

Dadaglio, G., Morel, S., Bauche, C., Moukrim, Z., Lemonnier, F., Van Den Eynde, B., Ladant, D., and Leclerc, C. 2003. Recombinant adenylate cyclase toxin of Bordetella pertussis induces cytotoxic T lymphocyte responses against HLA*0201-restricted melanoma epitopes. Int. Immunol. 15: 1423–1430.

De Groot, A.S., Bosma, A., Chinai, N., Frost, J., Jesdale, B.M., Gonzalez, M.A., Martin, W., and Saint-Aubin, C. 2001. From genome to vaccine: in silico predictions, ex vivo verification. Vaccine 19: 4385–4395.

den Haan, J.M.M., and Bevan, M.J. 2001. Antigen presentation to CD8[+] T cells: cross-priming in infectious diseases. Curr. Opin. Immunol. 13: 437–441.

Douce, G., Giannelli, V., Pizza, M., Lewis, D., Everest, P., Rappuoli, R., and Dougan, G. 1999. Genetically detoxified mutants of heat-labile toxin from Escherichia coli are able to act as oral adjuvants. Infect. Immun. 67: 4400–4406.

Falk, K., Rötzschke, O., Stevanovic, S., Jung, G., and Rammensee, H.-G. 1991. Allele-specific motifs revealed by sequencing of self-eptides eluted from MHC Mol.ecules. Nature 351: 290–296.

Fayolle, C., Ladant, C., Karimova, G., Ullmann, G., and Leclerc, C. 1999. Therapy of murine tumors with recombinant Bordetella pertussis adenylate cyclase carrying a cytotoxic T cell epitope. J. Immunol. 162: 4157–4162.

Fayolle, C., Osickova, A., Osicka, R., Henry, T., Rojas, M.J., Saron, M.F., Sebo, P., and Leclerc, C. 2001. Delivery of multiple epitopes by recombinant detoxified adenylate cyclase of Bordetella pertussis induces protective antiviral immunity. J. Virol. 75: 7330–7338.

Fehniger, T.A., Suzuki, K., Ponnappan, A., VanDeusen, J.B., Cooper, M.A., Florea, S.M., Freud, A.G., Robinson, M.L., Durbin, J., and Caligiuri, M.A. 2001. Fatal leukemia in interleukin 15 transgenic mice follows early expansions in natural killer and memory phenotype CD8[+] T cells. J. Exp. Med. 193.

Fujihashi, K., Koga, T., van Ginkel, F.W., Hagiwara, Y., and McGhee, J.R. 2002. A dilemma for mucosal vaccination: efficacy versus toxicity using enterotoxin-based adjuvants. Vaccine 20: 2431–2438.

Gheorghiu, M., Lagranderie, M R., Gicquel, B.M., and Leclerc, C.D. 1994. *Mycobacterium bovis* BCG priming induces a strong potentiation of the antibody response induced by recombinant BCG expressing a foreign antigen. Infect. Immun. 62: 4287–4295.

Goldrath, A.W., Sivakumar, P.V., Glaccum, M., Kennedy, M.K., Bevan, M.J., Benoist, C., Mathis, D., and Butz, E.A. 2002. Cytokine requirements for acute and basal homeostatic proliferation of naive and memory CD8[+] T cells. J. Exp. Med. 195: 1515–1522.

Gonin, P., Oualikene, W., Fournier, A., and Eloit, M. 1996. Comparison of the efficacy of replication-defective adenovirus and Nyvac poxvirus as vaccine vectors in mice. Vaccine 14: 1083–1087.

Gonzalez, C., Hone, D., Noriega, F.R., Tacket, C.O., Davis, J.R., Losonsky, G., Nataro, J.P., Hoffman, S., Malik, A., Nardin, E., and *et al.* 1994. Salmonella typhi vaccine strain CVD 908 expressing the circumsporozoite protein of *Plasmodium falciparum*: strain construction and safety and immunogenicity in humans. J. Infect. Dis. 169: 927–931.

Goossens, P.L., Milon, G., Cossart, P., and Saron, M.F. 1995. Attenuated *Listeria monocytogenes* as a live vector for induction of CD8[+] T cells in vivo: a study with the nucleoprotein of the lymphocytic choriomeningitis virus. Int. Immunol. 7: 797–805.

Grandi, G. 2003. Rational antibacterial vaccine design through genomic technologies. Int. J. Parasitol. 33: 615–620.

Grifantini, R., Bartolini, E., Muzzi, A., Draghi, M., Frigimelica, E., Berger, J., Ratti, G., Petracca, R., Galli, G., Agnusdei, M., *et al.* 2002. Previously unrecognized vaccine candidates against group B meningococcus identified by DNA microarrays. Nature Biotechnol. 20: 914–921.

Grillot-Courvalin, C., Goussard, S., Huetz, F., Ojcius, D.M., and Courvalin, P. 1998. Functional gene transfer from intracellular bacteria to mammalian cells. Nature Biotechnol. 16: 862–866.

Guermonprez, P., Khelef, N., Blouin, E., Rieu, P., Ricciardi-Castagnoli, P., Guiso, N., Ladant, D., and Leclerc, C. 2001. The adenylate cyclase toxin of *Bordetella pertussis* binds to target cells via the alpha(M)beta(2) integrin (CD11b/CD18. J. Exp. Med. 193: 1035–1044.

Guermonprez, P., Ladant, D., Karimova, G., Ullmann, A., and Leclerc, C. 1999. Direct delivery of the *Bordetella pertussis* adenylate cyclase toxin to the MHC class I antigen presentation pathway. J. Immunol. 162: 1910–1916.

Guermonprez, P., Valladeau, J., Zitvogel, L., Théry, C., and Amigorena, S. 2002. Antigen presentation and T cell stimulation by dendritic cells. Annu. Rev. Immunol. 20: 621–667.

Hanke, T., and McMichael, A.J. 2000. Design and construction of an experimental HIV-1 vaccine for a year-2000 clinical trial in Kenya. Nature Med. 6: 951–955.

Heath, W.R., and Carbone, F.R. 2001a. Cross-presentation, dendritic cells, tolerance and immunity. Annu. Rev. Immunol. 19: 47–64.

Heath, W.R., and Carbone, R. 2001b. Cross-presentation in viral immunity and self-tolerance. Nature 116: 126–135.

Hess, J., Miko, D., Catic, A., Lehmensiek, V., Russell, D.G., and Kaufmann, S.H. 1998. *Mycobacterium bovis* Bacille Calmette–Guerin strains secreting listeriolysin of *Listeria monocytogenes*. Proc. Natl. Acad. Sci. USA 95: 5299–5304.

Himmelrich, H., Lo-Man, R., Winter, N., Guermonprez, P., Sedlik, C., Rojas, M., Monnaie, D., Gheorghiu, M., Lagranderie, M., Hofnung, M., *et al.* 2000. Immune responses induced by recombinant BCG strains according to level of production of a foreign antigen: malE. Vaccine 18: 2636–2647.

Hodge, J.W., and Schlom, J. 1999. Comparative studies of a retrovirus versus a poxvirus vector in whole tumor-cell vaccines. Cancer Res. 59: 5106–5111.

Jefferys, R. 2002. Expanded DNA-MVA prime-boost trial begins in UK. IAVI Report 6: 1–15.

Jolly, D. 1994. Viral vector systems for gene therapy. Cancer Gene Ther. 1: 51–64.

Kaufmann, S.H. 1993. Immunity to intracellular bacteria. Annu. Rev. Immunol. 11: 129–163.

Kennedy, M.K., Glaccum, M., Brown, S.N., Butz, E.A., Viney, J.L., Embers, M., Matsuki, N., Charrier, K., Sedger, L., Willis, C.R., *et al.* 2000. Reversible defects in natural killer and memory CD8 T cell lineages in interleukin 15-deficient mice. J. Exp. Med. 191: 771–780.

Kieper, W.C., Tan, J.T., Bondi-Boyd, B., Gapin, L., Sprent, J., Ceredig, R., and Surh, C.D. 2002. Overexpression of Interleukin (IL)-7 leads to IL-15-independent generation of memory phenotype CD8[+] T cells. J. Exp. Med. 195: 1533–1539.

Killeen, K., and DiRita, V. 2000. Live attenuated bacterial vaccines. In: New Vaccine Technologies Ellis, R. (ed.). Landes Bioscience, Georgetown, TX.

Kochi, S.K., Killeen, K.P., and Ryan, U.S. 2003. Advances in the development of bacterial vector technology. Expert Rev. Vaccines 2: 31–43.

Lagranderie, M., Winter, N., Balazuc, A.M., Gicquel, B., and Gheorghiu, M. 1998. A cocktail of *Mycobacterium bovis* BCG recombinants expressing the SIV Nef, Env, and Gag antigens induces antibody and cytotoxic responses in mice vaccinated by different mucosal routes. AIDS Res. Hum. Retroviruses 14: 1625–1633.

Lalvani, A., Moris, P., Voss, G., Pathan, A.A., Kester, K.E., Brookes, R., Lee, E., Koutsoukos, M., Plebanski, M., Delchambre, M., *et al.* 1999. Potent induction of focused Th1-type cellular and humoral immune responses by RTS,S/SBAS2, a recombinant *Plasmodium falciparum* malaria vaccine. J. Infect Dis. 180: 1656–1664.

Mazzaccaro, R.J., Gedde, M., Jensen, E.R., van Santen, H.M., Ploegh, H.L., Rock, K.L., and Bloom, B.R. 1996. Major histocompatibility class I presentation of soluble antigen facilitated by *Mycobacterium tuberculosis* infection. Proc. Natl. Acad. Sci. USA 93: 11786–11791.

Medina, E., and Guzman, C.A. 2001. Use of live bacterial vaccine vectors for antigen delivery: potential and limitations. Vaccine 19: 1573–1580.

Medzhitov, R. 2001. Toll-like receptors and innate immunity. Nature Rev. 1: 135–145.

Medzhitov, R., and Janeway Jr, C.A. 2002. Decoding the patterns of self and nonself by the innate immune system. Science 296: 298–300.

Medzhitov, R., Preston-Hurlburt, P., Kopp, E., Stadlen, A., Chen, C., Ghosh, S., and Janeway, C.A., Jr. 1998. MyD88 is an adaptor protein in the hToll/IL-1 receptor family signaling pathways. Mol. Cell 2: 253–258.

Moingeon, P., Haensler, J., and Lindberg, A. 2001. Towards the rational design of Th1 adjuvants. Vaccine 19: 4363–4372.

Moron, G., Rueda, P., Casal, I., and Leclerc, C. 2002. CD8α-CD11b⁺ Dendritic cells present exogenous virus-like particles to CD8⁺ T cells and subsequently express CD8α and CD205 molecules. J. Exp. Med. 195: 1233–1245.

Moron, V.G., Rueda, P., Sedlik, C., and Leclerc, C. 2003. In vivo, dendritic cells can cross-present virus-like particles using an endosome-to-cytosol pathway. J. Immunol. 171: 2242–2250.

Moron, V., Dadaglio, G., and Leclerc, C. 2004. New tools for antigen delivery to the MHC class I pathway. Trends Immunol. 25: 97.

Mosmann, T., Cherwinski, H., Bond, M., Giedlin, M., and Coffman, R. 1986. Two types of murine helper T cell clone. I. Definition according to profiles of lymphokine activities and secreted proteins. J. Immunol. 136: 2348–2357.

Paterson, Y., and Ikonomidis, G. 1996. Recombinant *Listeria monocytogenes* cancer vaccines. Curr. Opin. Immunol. 8: 664–669.

Perkus, M.E., Tartaglia, J., and Paoletti, E. 1995. Poxvirus-based vaccine candidates for cancer, AIDS, and other infectious diseases. J. Leukoc. Biol. 58: 1–13.

Pizza, M., Scarlato, V., Masignani, V., Giuliani, M.M., Arico, B., Comanducci, M., Jennings, G.T., Baldi, L., Bartolini, E., Capecchi, B., *et al.* 2000. Identification of vaccine candidates against serogroup b meningococcus by whole-genome sequencing. Science 287: 1816–1820.

Poltorak, A., He, X., Smirnova, I., Liu, M.Y., Van Huffel, C., Du, X., Birdwell, D., Alejos, E., Silva, M., Galanos, C., *et al.* 1998a. Defective LPS signaling in C3H/HeJ and C57BL/10ScCr mice: mutations in Tlr4 gene. Science 282: 2085–2088.

Poltorak, A., Smirnova, I., He, X., Liu, M.Y., Van Huffel, C., McNally, O., Birdwell, D., Alejos, E., Silva, M., Du, X., *et al.* 1998b. Genetic and physical mapping of the Lps locus: identification of the toll-4 receptor as a candidate gene in the critical region. Blood Cells Mol. Dis. 24: 340–355.

Pym, A.S., Brodin, P., Brosch, R., Huerre, M., and Cole, S.T. 2002. Loss of RD1 contributed to the attenuation of the live tuberculosis vaccines *Mycobacterium bovis* BCG and *Mycobacterium microti*. Mol. Microbiol. 46: 709–717.

Pym, A.S., Brodin, P., Majlessi, L., Brosch, R., Demangel, C., Williams, A., Griffiths, K.E., Marchal, G., Leclerc, C., and Cole, S.T. 2003. Recombinant BCG exporting ESAT-6 confers enhanced protection against tuberculosis. Nature Med. 9: 533–539.

Ramshaw, I.A., and Ramsay, A.J. 2000. The prime-boost strategy: exciting prospects for improved vaccination. Immunol. Today 21: 163–165.

Randrianarison-Jewtoukoff, V., and Perricaudet, M. 1995. Recombinant adenoviruses as vaccines. Biologicals 23: 145–157.

Roth, J., Dittmer, D., Rea, D., Tartaglia, J., Paoletti, E., and Levine, A.J. 1996. p53 as a target for cancer vaccines: recombinant canarypox virus vectors expressing p53 protect mice against lethal tumor cell challenge. Proc. Natl. Acad. Sci. USA 93: 4781–4786.

Rotzschke, O., Falk, K., Stevanovic, S., Jung, G., Walden, P., and Rammensee, H.G. 1991. Exact prediction of a natural T cell epitope. Eur. J. Immunol. 21: 2891–2894.

Ryan, E.J., McNeela, E., Murphy, G.A., Stewart, H., O'Hagan, D., Pizza, M., Rappuoli, R., and Mills, K.H. 1999. Mutants of *Escherichia coli* heat-labile toxin act as effective mucosal adjuvants for nasal delivery of an acellular pertussis vaccine: differential effects of the nontoxic AB complex and enzyme activity on Th1 and Th2 cells. Infect. Immun. 67: 6270–6280.

Ryan, E.J., McNeela, E., Pizza, M., Rappuoli, R., O'Neill, L., and Mills, K.H. 2000. Modulation of innate and acquired immune responses by *Escherichia coli* heat-labile toxin: distinct pro- and anti-inflammatory effects of the nontoxic AB complex and the enzyme activity. J. Immunol. 165: 5750–5759.

Sallusto, F., Lenig, D., Mackay, C.R., and Lanzavecchia, A. 1998. Flexible programs of chemokine receptor expression on human polarized T helper 1 and 2 lymphocytes. J. Exp. Med. 187: 875–883.

Saron, M.F., Fayolle, C., Sebo, P., Ladant, D., Ullmann, A., and Leclerc, C. 1997. Anti-viral protection conferred by recombinant adenylate cyclase toxins from *Bordetella pertussis* carrying a CD8[+] T cell epitope from lymphocytic choriomeningitis virus. Proc. Natl. Acad. Sci. USA 94: 3314–3319.

Schaible, U.E., Winau, F., Sieling, P.A., Fischer, K., Collins, H.L., Hagens, K., Modlin, R.L., Brinkmann, V., and Kaufmann, S.H. 2003. Apoptosis facilitates antigen presentation to T lymphocytes through MHC-I and CD1 in tuberculosis. Nature Med. 9: 1039–1046.

Schnare, M., Barton, G.M., Holt, A.C., Takeda, K., Akira, S., and Medzhitov, R. 2001. Toll-like receptors control activation of adaptive immune responses. Nature Immunol. 2: 947–950.

Shi, Y., Evans, J.E., and Rock, K.L. 2003. Molecular identification of a danger signal that alerts the immune system to dying cells. Nature 425: 516–521.

Shiver, J.W., Fu, T.M., Chen, L., Casimiro, D.R., Davies, M.-E., Evans, R.K., Zhang, Z.Q., Simon, A.J., Trigona, W.L., Dubey, S.A., *et al.* 2002. Replication-incompetent adenoviral vaccine vector elicits effective anti-immunodeficiency-virus immunity. Nature 415: 331–335.

Shortman, K., and Liu, Y.J. 2002. Mouse and human dendritic cell subtypes. Nature Rev. Immunol. 2: 151–161.

Singh, M., and O'Hagan, D. 1999. Advances in vaccine adjuvants. Nature Biotechnol. 17: 1075–1081.

Skeiky, Y.A., Ovendale, P.J., Jen, S., Alderson, M.R., Dillon, D.C., Smith, S., Wilson, C.B., Orme, I.M., Reed, S.G., and Campos-Neto, A. 2000. T cell expression cloning of a *Mycobacterium tuberculosis* gene encoding a protective antigen associated with the early control of infection. J. Immunol. 165: 7140–7149.

Smyth, M.J., Crowe, N.Y., Hayakawa, Y., Takeda, K., Yagita, H., and Godfrey, D.I. 2002. NKT cells – conductors of tumor immunity? Curr. Opin. Immunol. 14: 165–171.

Sodoyer, R., Guy, B., Burdin, N., Lissolo, L., Oomen, R., Aujame, L., and Moingeon, P. 2002. Nouveaux vaccins à l'ère post-génomique. Annales Institut Pasteur Actualités, pp. 119–133.

Soo, S.S., Villarreal-Ramos, B., Anjam Khan, C.M., Hormaeche, C.E., and Blackwell, J.M. 1998. Genetic control of immune response to recombinant antigens carried by an attenuated Salmonella typhimurium vaccine strain: Nramp1 influences T-helper subset responses and protection against leishmanial challenge. Infect. Immun. 66: 1910–1917.

Spellberg, B., and Edwards, J.E., Jr. 2001. Type 1/Type 2 immunity in infectious diseases. Clin. Infect. Dis. 32: 76–102.

Sprent, J., and Surh, C.D. 2001. Generation and maintenance of memory T cells. Curr. Opin. Immunol. 13: 248–254.

Steinman, R.M. 2003. Some interfaces of dendritic cell biology. Apmis 111: 675–697.

Steinman, R.M., and Pope, M. 2002. Exploiting dendritic cells to improve vaccine efficacy. J. Clin. Invest. 109: 1519–1526.

Stoute, J.A., Slaoui, M., Heppner, D.G., Momin, P., Kester, K.E., Desmons, P., Wellde, B.T., Garcon, N., Krzych, U., and Marchand, M. 1997. A preliminary evaluation of a recombinant circumsporozoite protein vaccine against *Plasmodium falciparum* malaria. RTS,S Malaria Vaccine Evaluation Group. N. Engl. J. Med. 336: 86–91.

Sturniolo, T., Bono, E., Ding, J., Raddrizzani, L., Tuereci, O., Sahin, U., Braxenthaler, M., Gallazzi, F., Protti, M.P., Sinigaglia, F., and Hammer, J. 1999. Generation of tissue-specific and promiscuous HLA ligand databases using DNA microarrays and virtual HLA class II matrices. Nature Biotechnol. 17: 555–561.

Tan, J.T., Ernst, B., Kieper, W.C., LeRoy, E., Sprent, J., and Surh, C.D. 2002. Interleukin (IL)-15 and IL-7 jointly regulate homeostatic proliferation of memory phenotype CD4[+] cells. J. Exp. Med. 195: 1523–1532.

Teitelbaum, R., Cammer, M., Maitland, M.L., Freitag, N.E., Condeelis, J., and Bloom, B.R. 1999. Mycobacterial infection of macrophages results in membrane-permeable phagosomes. Proc. Natl. Acad. Sci. USA 96: 15190–15195.

Traver, D., Akashi, K., Manz, M., Merad, M., Miyamoto, T., Engleman, E.G., and Weissman, I.L. 2000. Development of CD8alpha-positive dendritic cells from a common myeloid progenitor. Science 290: 2152–2154.

van Ginkel, F.W., Jackson, R.J., Yuki, Y., and McGhee, J.R. 2000. Cutting edge: the mucosal adjuvant cholera toxin redirects vaccine proteins into olfactory tissues. J. Immunol. 165: 4778–4782.

Warnier, G., Duffour, M.T., Uyttenhove, C., Gajewski, T.F., Lurquin, C., Haddada, H., Perricaudet, M., and Boon, T. 1996. Induction of a cytolytic T-cell response in mice with a recombinant adenovirus coding for tumor antigen P815A. Int. J. Cancer 67: 303–310.

Zinkernagel, R.M. 2003. On natural and artificial vaccinations. Annu. Rev. Immunol. 21: 515–546.

Chapter 3

Targeting Innate Immunity With Adjuvants: Can Accurate Danger Signals Drive More Protective Immune Responses?

Nicolas Burdin

Abstract

Innate immunity was largely ignored for decades as it was thought to be a simplistic first line of defense providing non-specific microbicidal activity and acute inflammation signals to delay the growth of infectious agents, while giving more time for antigen-specific lymphocytes (adaptive immunity) to develop and then eradicate pathogens. It is now clear that the level of protection conferred by B and T cells in response to pathogen insults largely depends on the quality and accuracy of the initial 'danger' signals perceived by innate immune cells at the site of entry of infectious agents. Pathogen-derived compounds capable of activating innate immune cells are being characterized at the molecular level and their mechanisms of action deciphered. Synthetic homologues of these microbial agents are currently being evaluated and developed for clinical applications as vaccine adjuvants or therapeutic agents. This chapter reviews the immunostimulatory properties of some of these molecules, including antimicrobial peptides, Toll-like receptor agonists, synthetic ligands for non-conventional T cells and the possible opportunity of targeting regulatory T cells with some of the above adjuvants. Benefits and expected limitations of using these novel pathogen-mimicking adjuvants are also discussed.

INNATE IMMUNITY: IDENTIFYING THE DANGER TO DRIVE AN APPROPRIATE ADAPTIVE RESPONSE

The vast majority of host invading pathogens do not cause disease. Physical barriers (skin, mucosa), secreted proteins or hydrolytic enzymes (lactoferrin, transferrin, fibronectin, complement, antimicrobial peptides) form an effective 'shield' sufficient to eliminate microbes and protect the host in most cases. Rarely, however, some pathogens escape this first line of defense and trigger an immune response. Cells of the innate immune system such as phagocytic cells, granulocytes, NK cells, dendritic cells (DCs) are the first to be recruited to the inflamed site of pathogen entry. The main function of such cells is to reduce the microbial burden through phagocytosis or direct lysis. It is now established that they also play a key role in orchestrating downstream immune effector phases. In particular, cells of the innate immune system are critical to deliver appropriate signals to T and B lymphocytes in order to drive a protective adaptive immunity. The main features (similarity and specificities) of innate and adaptive immune responses are shown in Table 3.1.

Table 3.1 Features of the innate and adaptive immune responses

Innate immunity	Adaptive immunity
Multicellular organisms	Vertebrates
Immediate response	Delayed and adapted response (5–7 days)
Constitutive effector functions upon pathogen encounter (inflammation, phagocytosis)	Inducible effector functions (phases of proliferation, activation, maturation, differentiation)
Polynuclear cells, NK cells, monocytes/macrophages, dendritic cells	T lymphocytes and B lymphocytes
PRR (pathogen recognition receptors): hundreds of non-polymorphic specific receptors recognizing invariant molecular structures shared by families of pathogens	TCR and Ig: polymorphic antigen-specific receptors with a large stochastic repertoire (10^{14} to 10^{18}) generated by somatic rearrangement
No memory	Memory
No affinity maturation	Affinity maturation
Recognition and identification of danger (no selection)	Self versus non-self discrimination (clonal selections: positive and negative)

ANTIMICROBIAL PEPTIDES

General properties of antimicrobial peptides

Antimicrobial peptides (aMPs) are evolutionarily conserved effector molecules of the innate immune system. Initially described in the early 1960s, more than 500 of these natural aMPs have been isolated from multiple plant and animal species (extensive list on http://www.bbcm.univ.trieste.it/~tossi/antimic.html). They are amphipathic peptides of 20 to 50 amino acids that are enriched in basic or hydrophobic residues (for general reviews see Lehrer and Ganz, 1999; Scott and Hancock, 2000; Hancock and Diamond, 2000; Zasloff, 2002; Gallo et al., 2002). aMPs are classified in four different families based on their tertiary structure: β-sheet peptides, α-helix peptides, extended peptides, and loop peptides. Other peptides, such as lactoferrin and cathepsin G, produced by proteolysis of cationic proteins, form a fifth family of small size proteins. aMPs are produced constitutively or upon activation by a variety of cells including epithelial cells, keratinocytes, Paneth cells, leukocytes (NK and γδ T cells), neutrophils and myeloid cells and are present in high concentrations at the host–pathogen interfaces: mucosa, skin (Yang et al., 2002). As expected, even higher concentrations of aMPs are found in biological fluids of infected patients/animals (Raj and Dentino, 2002; Gallo et al., 2002). The interaction of these peptides with the cell wall of bacteria causes permeabilization of the membrane through the formation of 'barrel-stave' or 'torroidal' pores and thus leads to the lysis of invading microbes. aMP-sensitive pathogens include not only bacteria, but also parasites, fungi and viruses (Zasloff, 2002; Ganz, 2003).

aMPs have been conserved throughout the evolution of plant and animal kingdoms, even in species that have developed more sophisticated adaptive immune systems. This is in accordance with the fact that aMPs are crucial mediators of immunity not only through their direct antimicrobial functions but also through their ability to regulate and influence other critical downstream immune processes such as cell activation/maturation/proliferation, cytokine release, chemotaxis. Deficiencies in aMPs result in increased susceptibility to infections in mice (Wilson et al., 1999; Nizet et al., 2001) and humans

(Hancock and Diamond, 2000; Raj and Dentino, 2002). aMPs are not only able to regulate other mechanisms of the innate immune response (upregulation of phagocytosis, mast cell degranulation, wound healing, inhibition of fibrinolysis), but they also participate in the activation of cells involved in the adaptive responses: APCs and T or B lymphocytes (for general reviews see Zasloff, 2002; Gallo *et al.*, 2002).

Adjuvant effects of antimicrobial peptides

Such an activity has been shown recently for two subgroups of the β-sheet superfamily, the so-called α- and β-defensins (Yang *et al.*, 2002; Ganz, 2003) and Figure 3.1. Defensins can regulate and interact with the classical pathway of the complement through their ability to bind to the C1q component (Prohaszka *et al.*, 1997; Prohaszka and Fust, 1998; van den Berg *et al.*, 1998).Various defensins have been reported to exhibit chemotactic activity for monocytes, T cells and DCs (Chertov *et al.*, 1996; Yang *et al.*, 1999; Yang *et al.*, 2000). Human neutrophil peptides 1–3 (HNP1–3 α-defensins) are chemotactic factor for monocytes, naïve T cells and immature DCs, but their specific receptor has not been identified yet. On the contrary, human β-defensin-1 (HBD1) and HBD2 attract memory T cells and immature DCs through their interaction with the known CCR6 chemokine receptor (Yang *et al.*, 1999). HBD1 and HBD2 have a lower affinity for CCR6 than its natural ligand CC chemokine ligand 20 (CCL20/MIP3α) but it is possible that in inflamed tissues where concentrations of HBD are high, it can compete with CCL20 for CCR6 binding. Interestingly, CCL20 can also act as an antimicrobial agent (Yang *et al.*, 2003), a property shared by many others chemokines (Durr and Peschel, 2002; Yang *et al.*, 2003), thus indicating a close functional relationship between both family of molecules.

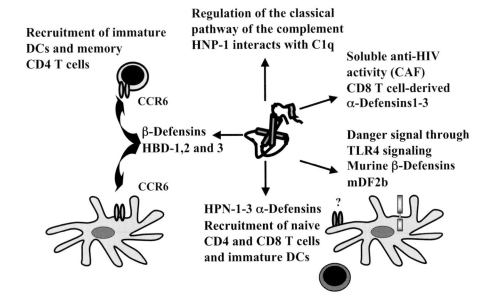

Figure 3.1 Immunoregulatory functions displayed by mouse and human defensins. Defensins are not only lytic antimicriobial peptides, but they can also modulate some effector phases of innate immunity such as the conventional pathway of complement or the recruitment of immunocompetent cells such as DCs and T cells. They may act as danger signals through Toll-like receptor-4 and some of them may also possess some anti-HIV activities. This figure is also reproduced in colour in the colour section at the end of the book.

In addition to acting through CCR6 like its human counterpart, mouse β-defensin 2 (MDF2β) has been reported to bind and signal through Toll-like receptor 4, TLR4 (Biragyn *et al.*, 2002), a key receptor for the host response to bacterial lipopolysaccharides (LPS), as described below. MDF2β induces a fully functional maturation of bone marrow DCs *in vitro*. Moreover, injections of non-immunogenic tumor antigens fused to MDF2β elicit a polarized Th1, protective, and therapeutic immunity against two different syngenic lymphomas (Biragyn *et al.*, 2001; Biragyn *et al.*, 2002). It should be emphasized, however, that it still remains to be formally proven that MDF2β is not a 'fake' ligand for TLR4, which would only act as a potentiator of suboptimal amounts of LPS tightly bound to it (Biragyn *et al.*, 2002).

Immunopotentiation and adjuvant effects have been identified for other defensins. Antigen-specific proliferation and induction of Th1- and Th2-type cytokine secretion by spleen- and mucosa-derived CD4 T cells are enhanced by the addition in the vaccine of peptide defensins purified from human neutrophils (Lillard *et al.*, 1999). Additional reports reinforce the potential of neutrophil defensins to act as potent immune adjuvants by inducing the production of lymphokines, which promote T cell-dependent cellular immunity and antigen-specific Ig production (Tani *et al.*, 2000; Brogden *et al.*, 2003). Interestingly, α-defensins 1, 2 and 3 could collectively account for part of the soluble, CD8 T cell-derived activity (called CAF) known to suppress HIV replication (Zhang *et al.*, 2002), the other part being assigned to β-chemokines. This latter observation deserves further investigation in order to consider the potential of including such aMPs in HIV vaccine candidates.

Therefore, aMPs can qualify as prototypes of innovative therapeutic drugs. They represent a new generation of antibiotic candidates that could help facing the growing issue of antibiotic resistance. Although it is too early to conclude what their actual potential is, it is tempting to propose these molecules as vaccine adjuvant candidates. They offer an appealing novel approach, because (1) they are small peptides, easy to manufacture as pure, synthetic and stable products and (2) they are immunoregulatory compounds capable of recruiting/activating dendritic cells and T cells. In addition, the amphipathic property of aMPs allows them to cross not only bacterial walls but also eukaryote lipidic membranes (Lichtenstein, 1991). Like other previously described amphiphatic proteins, they can possibly be considered as peptide transducers (transfer to the cytosol) for a covalently linked antigen. They then could support antigen cross-priming and act as an adjuvant for CD8 cytotoxic T cell responses.

A lot of work remains to be achieved to further refine the actual immunostimulatory properties of aMPs and to assess their potential use as vaccine adjuvants. Some aMPs are already in commercial use, including ambicin (nisin), polymyxin B, gramicidin and several others are currently being tested in human clinical trials to evaluate their value as natural antibiotics in different infectious diseases (Zasloff, 2002; Hancock and Patrzykat, 2002; Bradshaw, 2003). Results from *in vivo* toxicity and pharmacokinetic studies (in particular resistance to proteolysis) of such aMPs will be critical for the future of their clinical applications.

TOLL-LIKE RECEPTORS (TLRS)

TLR-mediated pathogen recognition

Invading pathogens are rapidly detected by multiple innate immune cell subsets, especially professional antigen-presenting cells (APCs), including the highly specialized 'sentinels' that are DCs. Infectious agents are then identified by DCs – and other host cells – because they express specific members of a family of pathogen-associated molecular patterns (PAMPs). PAMPs are structural supramolecular entities shared by phylogenetically related microbes: Lipopolysaccharides (LPS) or peptidoglycans from Gram-negative and Gram-positive bacteria, respectively, bacterial DNA, viral RNA, flagellin. PAMPs represent danger signals recognized by innate cells through non-polymorphic but specific pathogen-recognition receptors (PRRs). This PRR family includes various scavenger receptors or C-type lectins, but is mainly well known for a particular subgroup of molecules: the Toll-like receptors (TLRs) that have been the focus of a lot of interest in the past few years (for recent general reviews see Akira *et al.*, 2001; Medzhitov, 2001; Barton and Medzhitov, 2002; Takeda *et al.*, 2003). These TLRs specifically bind to pathogen-derived ligands (PAMPs) or host-derived compounds that are induced by inflammation or other stress stimuli. Although non-polymorphic, this identification system via single or combinations of TLRs creates a repertoire for pattern recognition of pathogens (Ozinsky *et al.*, 2000; Underhill and Ozinsky, 2002). For example, double-stranded RNA (TLR3) would identify viral infections, simultaneous signals through LPS (TLR4) and bacterial DNA (TLR9) would be a signature for Gram-negative bacteria, whereas peptidoglycans (TLR2/6) and bacterial DNA (TLR9) would alert for the presence of Gram-positive bacteria.

TLR agonists as vaccine adjuvants: what do we know?

Signaling through any of the TLRs was initially thought to transduce almost identical transactivation and phosphorylation pathways because all TLRs (except TLR3) share a common adaptor protein: MyD88. This pathway leads to the activation of the NFκB transcription factor and of JNK and p38 MAP kinases (Medzhitov, 2001). This signaling cascade appears to be critical for the development of antigen specific T helper type 1 (Th1) biased responses, as observed in MyD88 deficient mice (Schnare *et al.*, 2001). This is consistent with the fact that some of the TLR ligands were previously known and are still developed as promising Th1 adjuvant candidates for vaccines (see below and Figure 3.2). Recent reports however clearly state that signal transduction through TLRs is more complicated than initially anticipated and that most TLRs have, in addition to this core MyD88 pathway, other specific signaling components conferring specific properties to each member of the family (Wasserman, 2000; Martin and Wesche, 2002; O'Neill, 2002a). TIRAP or MyD88 adapter like (Mal) has initially been described as another intracellular component of TLR signaling downstream of TLR4 (O'Neill, 2002b) and TLR2 (Horng *et al.*, 2001; Yamamoto *et al.*, 2002a) but is also shared by TLR1 and 6 (Horng *et al.*, 2002). TICAM-1 is an adaptor molecule that participates in TLR3-mediated interferon beta (IFN-β) induction (Yamamoto *et al.*, 2002b; Imler and Hoffmann, 2003; Oshiumi *et al.*, 2003). Similarly, TRIF is essential for TLR3- and TLR4-mediated signaling pathways and facilitates mammalian antiviral host defense (Yamamoto *et al.*, 2003). In addition, negative regulators of the TLR pathways are progressively being identified, i.e. IRAK-M or Tollip, that probably help keeping inflammation under control (Mak and Yeh, 2002). One can speculate that several other adaptors or components of the TLR signaling cascade will be identified in the upcoming months and will further add to the complexicity of the system (Kobayashi *et al.*, 2002; Zhang and Ghosh, 2002), especially because some of the transducer molecules of TLR signaling may be cell specific (Hoebe *et al.*, 2003).

These multicomponent pathways of signal transduction through TLRs are the molecular basis underlying the overlapping but distinct sets of biological effects mediated

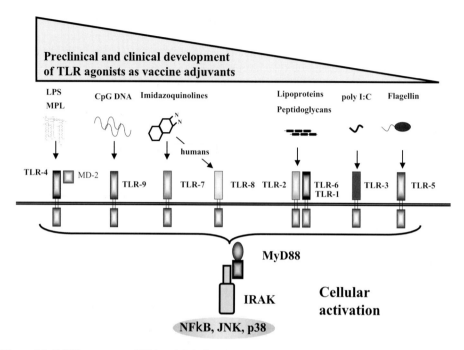

Figure 3.2 Toll-like receptors (TLR) and their ligands. TLR specifically recognize pathogen-derived ligands (PAMPS) or host-derived compounds that are induced by inflammation or other stress stimuli. The triggering of single or combinations of TLRs create a repertoire for pathogen recognition. Several natural or synthetic ligands for TLRs are being evaluated and developed as vaccine adjuvants. This includes (from the most to the least developmentally advanced for vaccine application): monophosphoryl lipid A analogues (TLR4), CpG sequences (TLR9), imidazoquinolines (TLR7), lipopeptides (TLR1/2/6), polyI:C like compounds (TLR3) and flagellin (TLR5). All TLRs share a common core MyD88/NFκB activation pathway but additional and more specific signaling components have been identified for most of them. This figure is also reproduced in colour in the colour section at the end of the book.

by TLR ligands. In addition, microbial recognition by TLRs is not solely determined by single TLR molecules. Homo or heterodimerizations and additional soluble or membrane coreceptors (such as MD2, LBP and CD14 for TLR4 mediated signaling of LPS) can be required (Wasserman, 2000; Martin and Wesche, 2002; O'Neill, 2002a). Therefore, TLR agonists not only act as immunostimulatory agents with a generalized Th1 polarizing effect (Kaisho and Akira, 2002), but also each TLR is likely to have some specialized properties:

1   TLR3 and TLR4, for example, have evolutionarily diverged from other TLRs to activate an interferon regulatory element (IRF3 for IFN regulatory factor 3), which triggers a specific gene program responsible for innate antiviral responses (Doyle *et al.*, 2002).

2   Instead of driving Th1 responses, signaling through TLR4 with low doses of inhaled LPS or allergen would rather favor Th2 polarization (Eisenbarth *et al.*, 2002; Dabbagh *et al.*, 2002).

3   TLR5 activates defense responses induced by many different species of flagellated bacteria both systemically and at epithelial surfaces (Smith and Ozinsky, 2002).

TLR agonists as vaccine adjuvants: the 'most clinically advanced' examples

The main feature shared by all TLR agonists described below is their ability to deliver a potent activation signal to APCs (Figure 3.3). This so-called signal 0 rapidly licences APCs to become optimal stimulatory cells for antigen specific T cells. TLR ligand-activated APCs can then provide an accessory activation signal (signal 2) in addition to the antigen derived specific signal 1 (peptide presented in MHC molecules). This signal 1 + signal 2 costimulation is required to obtain fully functional activation and differentiation of antigen specific T cells, while signal 1 alone usually results in anergy.

CpG sequences

CpG sequences are TLR9 agonists: A long list of papers have demonstrated the potent immunostimulatory properties of CpG oligodeoxynucleotide (ODN) in multiple preclinical models in mice and primates, *in vitro* as well as *in vivo* (for recent reviews, see McCluskie *et al.*, 2001; Krieg, 2002a; Krieg, 2003; Klinman, 2003; Ashkar and Rosenthal, 2002). CpG ODN are potent adjuvants of both humoral and cell-mediated immunity, with a strong Th1 polarizing ability: IFNγ production by CD4 T cells and induction of IgG2a titers. Many CpG sequences are highly active on human cells, although the optimal motifs are slightly different from those in mice (Krieg, 2003; Leifer *et al.*, 2003; Bauer *et al.*, 2001).

No PAMPS: no danger: no TLR mediated activation

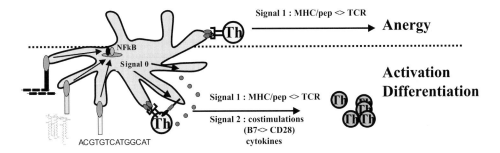

PAMPS = danger signal → activation through TLRs (specific combinations → accurately tuned effectors)

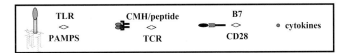

Figure 3.3 TLR ligand-conditioned APCs can then deliver potent costimulatory signals to cognate antigen-specific T cells. Antigen presentation to T cells by APCs that have not previously been accurately conditioned usually leads to anergy. Ligands of TLRs deliver potent activation signals to APCs (signal 0) that induce the up regulation of costimulatory molecules and the production of cytokines. APCs are then licensed to present antigen derived peptides (signal 1) in an accurate costimulation context (signal 2) that will lead to the induction of a fully functional immune response. Delivery of various pathogen-derived signals through specific TLRs and combinations thereof (molecular pattern) constitutes a first level of identification of the nature of the invading microbe. This might allow for a more adapted conditioning of APCs in order to optimize the activation of the cognate T cells. This figure is also reproduced in colour in the colour section at the end of the book.

Chemical modifications of the ODN backbone (Kandimalla *et al.*, 2002; Agrawal and Kandimalla, 2002) or different formulations of CpG ODN have been developed to further potentiate their activity. For example, CpG ODNs are more powerful Th1 adjuvants if they are covalently linked to the antigens: up to 100-fold superior compared with the corresponding mix. In particular, such CpG ODN–antigen conjugates induce a stronger Th1 bias (Shirota *et al.*, 2000) with a more robust CD8 cytotoxic T cell response (Cho *et al.*, 2000; Heit *et al.*, 2003). CpG ODN are currently being evaluated in human clinical trials (Krieg, 2002b). The addition of a CpG ODN to the hepatitis B vaccine causes a noticeable increase in seroconversion and protective titers in the majority of subjects by two weeks after the prime. CpG used as a stand-alone therapeutic molecule is also being evaluated in oncology. Preliminary data in patients suffering from carcinoma or melanoma show that intralesional injections of CpG ODN lead to significant tumor regression (Krieg, 2002b). Although some toxicity problems can be expected with the strong Th1, proinflammatory burst induced by CpG ODN (Schwartz *et al.*, 1997; Sacher *et al.*, 2002), clinical trials have revealed that some active and well-tolerated doses can be defined. Additional trials with CpG ODN are in progress and will be required to confirm their potential as human vaccine adjuvants.

Monophosphoryl lipid A (MPL) compounds

Monophosphoryl lipid A (MPL) compounds are TLR4 agonists. Similarly to CpG ODN with TLR9, MPL and their related derivatives were evaluated as vaccine adjuvants before being identified as TLR4 ligands. The ability of purified MPL or its synthetic analogues to act as Th1 adjuvants on antibody and T cell responses has been documented in various animal models following systemic or mucosal delivery (Baldridge and Crane, 1999; Childers *et al.*, 2000; De Becker *et al.*, 2000; Persing *et al.*, 2002; Pajak *et al.*,2003). MPL compounds might be less potent than CpG in their ability to induce CD8 cytotoxic T cells (Schwarz *et al.*, 2003), although such responses have been observed with MPL for some antigens (Zhou and Huang, 1993; Mbawuike *et al.*, 1996). MPL derivatives stimulate cells of the innate immune system, including professional APCs such as myeloid DCs (Martin *et al.*, 2003), but they can also directly activate T cells (Ismaili *et al.*, 2002). MPL share some of the advantages of CpG: they can be formulated in liposomes, emulsions or mixed with aluminum salts (Persing *et al.*, 2002; Thoelen *et al.*, 2001; Liao *et al.*, 2002). Preclinical safety data obtained with MPL are satisfactory (Baldrick *et al.*, 2002; Thoelen *et al.*, 2001). Consistent with this, purified MPL or its synthetic analogues are well tolerated in human clinical trials (McCormack *et al.*, 2000; Vernacchio *et al.*, 2002; Jacques *et al.*, 2002; Desombere *et al.*, 2002). Immunogenicity results have shown that MPL compounds can potentiate humoral responses for some vaccines such as hepatitis B (Jacques *et al.*, 2002; Desombere *et al.*, 2002) but not for others such as pneumococcal glycoconjugates (Vernacchio *et al.*, 2002). Characterization and selection of 'lead' MPL analogues and optimization of formulations remain to be continued to further improve the adjuvanticity of these TLR4 agonists.

Imidazoquinolines

Imidazoquinolines are TLR7/8 agonists. These antiviral heterocyclic amine-based compounds are known to be potent immune modifiers (Syed, 2001; Dockrell and Kinghorn, 2001; Garland, 2003). They have been recently identified as ligands for mouse TLR7

(Hemmi *et al.*, 2002) and human TLR7 and/or TLR8 (Jurk *et al.*, 2002). Imidazoquinolines can stimulate various cell types, including B cells (Bishop *et al.*, 2000; Tomai *et al.*, 2000) and DCs (Burns, Jr. *et al.*, 2000; Fogel *et al.*, 2002). In contrast to CpG sequences or MPL analogues that can only specifically induce the maturation of either plasmacytoid DCs (TLR9[+]) or myeloid DCs (TLR4[+]) respectively, imidazoquinolines have the advantage of being capable of stimulating both DC subsets (Jarrossay *et al.*, 2001; Ito *et al.*, 2002). This leads to the secretion of two complementary Th1 polarizing cytokines: IFNα (by plasmacytoid DCs) and IL-12 (by myeloid DCs) that probably synergize and contribute to the potent adjuvant effect of imidazoquinolines on both humoral and cell-mediated immune responses (Vasilakos *et al.*, 2000; Dockrell and Kinghorn, 2001). Imiquimod, the lead compound of this family of molecules, exhibits antiviral, antitumour and immunoregulatory activities and was first approved in 1997 in human clinics for the topical treatment of viral-induced (HPV, HSV) external genital and perianal warts (Cutler *et al.*, 2000; Gruber and Wilkinson, 2001; Syed, 2001). It is incorporated (1–5% by weight) in an oil-in-water cream emulsion and is reported to be well-tolerated with only mild-to-moderate drug-related side-effects (itching, erythema). Further investigations are mandatory to explore the real potential of imiquimod and other imidazoquinoline compounds, not only as 'stand alone' immunotherapeutic agents but also as vaccine adjuvants.

Other TLR agonists

Poly I:C is also a potent immunostimulatory molecule (Jiang *et al.*, 2003) with well-known IFN-mediated antitumor and antiviral activity (Pyo *et al.*, 1993; Hendrix *et al.*, 1993; Hirabayashi *et al.*, 1999; Adams *et al.*, 2003). It has recently been described as a TLR3 agonist, which can enhance antigen-specific immune responses (Alexopoulou *et al.*, 2001; Lore *et al.*, 2003). The originally identified poly I:C compounds had prohibitive toxicity but we might expect that new analogues with improved activity and acceptable toxicity may be developed in the upcoming years.

Microbial or synthetic lipopeptides/lipoproteins are recognized by homodimers of TLR2 (Lien *et al.*, 1999) or heterodimers of TLR2 associated with either TLR1 (Takeuchi *et al.*, 2002) or TLR6 (Takeuchi *et al.*, 2001; Morr *et al.*, 2002). TLR1 and TLR6 are in fact responsible for the discrimination of subtle differences between triacyl and diacyl lipopeptides through interaction with TLR2 (Takeda *et al.*, 2002). Such lipopeptide mediated signaling through the TLR1/2/6 pathway also results in the activation of innate immune cells (Takeuchi *et al.*, 2000; Kurt-Jones *et al.*, 2002), including DCs (Hertz *et al.*, 2001). The adjuvant potential of lipopeptides has been studied for more than a decade (Bessler and Jung, 1992) and is still under evaluation (Bessler *et al.*, 1997; Mittenbuhler *et al.*, 1997; BenMohamed *et al.*, 1997; BenMohamed *et al.*, 2002c; Zeng *et al.*, 2002; Mittenbuhler *et al.*, 2003). In particular, lipopeptides are described as potent self-adjuvanted immunogens for mucosal vaccinations (Rharbaoui *et al.*, 2002; BenMohamed *et al.*, 2002a; BenMohamed *et al.*, 2002b). Lipopeptide-based vaccines have been tested in human clinical trials and proven to be safe and immunogenic in various models: HIV (Pialoux *et al.*, 2001), hepatitis B (Vitiello *et al.*, 1995; Livingston *et al.*, 1997) and human papillomavirus type16 E7 (Steller *et al.*, 1998). Although some encouraging results have been obtained with lipopeptides, remaining challenges include the need for sequence optimization, synthesis, formulation, delivery and toxicity.

TLR agonists as vaccine adjuvants: what remains to be resolved?

A large panel of TLRs agonists have been proven to efficiently activate APCs and other immune cells, and therefore to strongly potentiate humoral as well as cell-mediated immune responses (Kaisho and Akira, 2002; Sieling and Modlin, 2002; Takeda et al., 2003). However, several areas remain to be studied to improve our knowledge of these immunostimulatory compounds and their possible clinical applications. Additional investigations are required to further explore the distribution of TLR expression on immune cells as well as in other tissues (mucosa, skin) in order to map the potential cellular targets of each TLR agonist adjuvant candidates. This could be helpful for the choice of the appropriate TLR agonist to be selected for a particular vaccine depending on its delivery route.

Additional work remains to be performed to determine what are the most accurate signals 0 to be provided to APCs in order to induce a protective adaptive immunity against each specific pathogen. It is tempting to speculate that specific TLR ligands or combinations of them could be more appropriate than others to respectively 'fight' Gram-negative or Gram-positive bacteria, viruses or parasites. This needs to be taken into account when selecting the most accurate TLR agonist adjuvant for a defined vaccine.

More importantly, an extensive and comparative analysis of the potential adverse effects (local or systemic reactogenicity, pyrogenicity and toxicity) of TLR agonist adjuvants must be carried out in animal models and in in vitro systems with human cells. Safety of such adjuvants is obviously critical and represents a key parameter to document in preclinical and clinical studies. Side-effects in animal models have already been reported for CpG sequences, one of the most advanced TLR agonist adjuvant: arthritis (Deng et al., 1999; Miyata et al., 2000; Ronaghy et al., 2002) and inflammation of the lungs (Schwartz et al., 1997). This excessive immunostimulatory activity of TLR agonists could threaten their use as vaccine adjuvants in humans. There is hope however that dose titrations and formulations of these TLR ligands can be found that will minimize local inflammation and systemic pyrogenicity, thus providing a compromise solution between adjuvanticity and reactogenicity. For example, MPL compounds (TLR4 agonists) have proven to be safe in humans in several clinical trials (Drachenberg et al., 2001; Thoelen et al., 2001; Vernacchio et al., 2002). In keeping with this, further investigation is required to uncouple TLR-mediated adjuvanticity from pyrogenicity/exacerbated inflammation. For this, libraries of synthetic analogues of TLR agonists could be screened and compared in vivo and in vitro for both of the above parameters. Such structure–function analysis, combined with an extended dissection of the signal transduction pathways of TLRs, will be helpful for the design of synthetic TLR agonists with potent adjuvant properties but limited adverse effects.

NON-CONVENTIONAL NATURAL T LYMPHOCYTES

In addition to conventional innate immune cells such as NK cells, granulocytes, macrophages and DCs, some subsets of T lymphocytes are capable of rapidly responding to infections and contribute to the development of a protective adaptive immunity. These innate/natural T lymphocytes reside mainly in tissues (specific organs such as the liver or mucosa). They usually express recurrent families of germ-line encoded T cell receptors (TCR) and are specific for a restricted set of conserved ligands, mainly non-peptidic microbial and/or self-derived antigens (Bendelac et al., 2001).

Natural killer T lymphocytes (NK T cells)

This T cell subset expresses an invariant TCR (Vα24/Vβ11 in humans) and displays an activated/memory phenotype. NK T cells share some common features with both NK cells and conventional T cells (for general review see Godfrey *et al.*, 2000; Biron and Brossay, 2001; Kronenberg and Gapin, 2002; MacDonald, 2002). Because they are lytic and capable of secreting high levels of cytokines, NK T cells have potent antitumor properties and are also thought to contribute to the control of the balance between tolerance and autoimmunity (reviewed in Godfrey *et al.*, 2000; Smyth *et al.*, 2002; Sharif *et al.*, 2002). The role of NK T cells in anti-infectious responses against bacteria, viruses and parasites is also largely documented (reviewed in Schaible and Kaufmann, 2000; Biron and Brossay, 2001; Gumperz and Brenner, 2001).

NK T cells are specifically activated by a synthetic glycolipid compound called α-galactosylceramide, α-GalCer (Kawano *et al.*, 1997; Brossay *et al.*, 1998; Burdin *et al.*, 1998; Burdin and Kronenberg, 1999). α-GalCer activated NKT cells can in turn stimulate other immune cells such as B cells, CD4 and CD8 memory T cells, NK cells and DCs (Kronenberg and Gapin, 2002). This compound could also be used to bias the Th1/Th2 balance of antigen-specific responses depending on the dose and/or number of administrations (Cui *et al.*, 1999; Hayakawa *et al.*, 2001; Miyamoto *et al.*, 2001). Therefore, α-GalCer can be considered as a synthetic immunostimulatory/modulatory compound. α-GalCer has been shown to act as a potent adjuvant in mice, as its coadministration with suboptimal doses of irradiated sporozoites or recombinant viruses expressing a malaria antigen greatly enhances the level of protective anti-malaria immunity (Gonzalez-Aseguinolaza *et al.*, 2000; Gonzalez-Aseguinolaza *et al.*, 2002). In fact, a single dose of α-GalCer rapidly stimulates DCs to mature *in situ*, and therefore activates both Th1 CD4$^+$ and CD8$^+$ T cell immunity to the coadministered antigen (Fujii *et al.*, 2003). However, much more investigation is required to fully understand and master the concept of adjuvantation through α-GalCer-mediated activation of NK T cells. For example, α-GalCer does not improve a DNA-based vaccine against *Trypanosma cruzii* (Miyahira *et al.*, 2003), although it increases protection against the very same pathogen, when it is used as a stand-alone molecule. Regarding clinical safety, α-GalCer was well-tolerated over a wide range of doses in a phase I study in cancer patients (Giaccone *et al.*, 2002), indicating future potential vaccine applications for this highly specific synthetic adjuvant. The use of α-GalCer as a therapeutic immunomodulator for the treatment of several autoimmune diseases is also being carefully considered (Shi *et al.*, 2001; Hammond and Godfrey, 2002; Wilson *et al.*, 2002).

Gamma/delta T lymphocytes ($\gamma\delta$ T cells)

Up to 5% of circulating T lymphocytes do not express classical alpha and beta TCRs, but rather bear less conventional TCRs that are heterodimers of gamma and delta chains. These $\gamma\delta$ T cells are even more represented in epithelium-rich tissues such as the skin, gut and reproductive tracts. Similarly to NK T cells, $\gamma\delta$ T cells are cytolytic and produce high levels of cytokines and chemokines. This probably underlies the ability of $\gamma\delta$ T cells to contribute to immune surveillance against cancer (Ferrarini *et al.*, 2002) and to regulate autoimmunity/tolerance (Hayday and Geng, 1997; Yin and Craft, 2000; Hanninen and Harrison, 2000). Their location in mucosa, at the host/environment interface, is consistent with the involvement of $\gamma\delta$ T cells in anti-infectious immunity (for review, see Carding and Egan, 2000; Boismenu, 2000; Carding and Egan, 2002). Human $\gamma9\delta2$ T cells are specifically activated by small antigens, such as organic phosphoesters, alkylamines and nucleotide-conjugates. Interestingly, these γ9δ2 T cells are strongly reactive against intracellular pathogens and have potent anti viral activities. They can lyse human immunodeficiency virus (HIV) infected cells, and release cytokines capable of controlling HIV replication. The γ9δ2 T cell subset substantially declines in HIV-infected patients (Lehner *et al.*, 2000; Poccia *et al.*, 2002; Martini *et al.*, 2002). Targeting such γδ T cell subsets with synthetic ligands such as phosphonucleotide antigens is likely to be of potential interest (Sireci *et al.*, 2001; Espinosa *et al.*, 2001).

TARGETING REGULATORY T CELLS TO ENHANCE IMMUNE RESPONSES

Regulatory T cells and infections

In addition to γδ and NK T cells mentioned above, other specific T lymphocyte subpopulations exhibit some crucial immunomodulatory properties on ongoing immune responses. Regulatory T cells, initially referred to as suppressor cells in the early 1970s, are currently the focus of a lot of interest. Different subsets of regulatory T cells with immunomodulatory and suppressive properties have been identified: CD4+ CD25+ T reg, Tr, Th3 and CD8Tr cells. Such regulatory T cells represent 5 to 10% of peripheral CD4 T cells in rodents and humans. They specifically regulate the balance between tolerance and immune responses for both T and B lymphocytes, either through direct cell–cell contact or through the production of immunosuppressive cytokines: mainly TGFβ and IL-10 (for general review see Sakaguchi, 2000; Coutinho *et al.*, 2001; Sakaguchi *et al.*, 2001; Read and Powrie, 2001; Groux, 2001; Mason, 2001; Maloy and Powrie, 2001; Bluestone and Abbas, 2003; Francois, 2003). The main function of these cells is to inhibit harmful immunopathological responses directed against self and foreign antigens. The existence of such regulatory T cells explain why adoptive transfer of CD4 cells can prevent or cure autoimmune diseases in several animal models (Shevach, 2002), a phenomenon which could not be explained by other tolerance mechanisms such as anergy or clonal deletion. They express typical markers such as CD25 (Treg) and the inhibitory molecule CD152 (CTLA-4), are usually anergic cells (with a low proliferation rate and dependence on exogenous IL-2) and produce high amounts of TGFβ alone (Th3 cells) or together with IL-10 (Tr1 cells). These latter features at least partly explain why such cells can inhibit the proliferation of surrounding cells. The immunomodulatory role of regulatory T cells has been studied in autoimmune diseases (Shevach, 2000; Tung *et al.*, 2001; von Herrath and Harrison, 2003), transplantation tolerance (Karim *et al.*, 2002; Wood and Sakaguchi, 2003) and cancer (Sakaguchi *et al.*, 2001; Seo *et al.*, 2002).

In addition to contributing to the regulation of peripheral tolerance and homeostasis (self antigens), recent reports show that regulatory T cells also play a role in the activation of pathogen-specific immune responses (virus, bacteria and parasite), in mice (McGuirk *et al.*, 2002a; Belkaid *et al.*, 2002; Aseffa *et al.*, 2002; Kullberg *et al.*, 2002; Xu *et al.*, 2003) as well as in humans (Doetze *et al.*, 2000; MacDonald *et al.*, 2002; Lundgren *et al.*, 2003). Regulatory T cells are in fact capable of inhibiting or enhancing the activation of both Th1 and/or Th2 responses induced by infections (McGuirk and Mills, 2002b). In the course of an infection, regulatory T cells may be induced to serve several purposes that are beneficial either to the host or to the pathogen. Regulatory T cells have been shown to prevent pathological immune responses by controlling excessive inflammation or deleterious effect of cytopathic T cells (Belkaid *et al.*, 2002; Kullberg *et al.*, 2002), thus protecting the host. Regulatory T cells can also contribute to the establishment of an overall immunosuppressive state or a strongly biased Th1 or Th2 response, thus facilitating pathogen survival or escape, by subverting protective responses and favouring the development of a chronic infection (Doetze *et al.*, 2000; McGuirk and Mills, 2002b; McGuirk *et al.*, 2002a; Belkaid *et al.*, 2002; MacDonald *et al.*, 2002). In keeping with this, regulatory T cells also control the activation of effector CD8 T cells (Piccirillo and Shevach, 2001) and limit the development of both CD8$^+$ (Murakami *et al.*, 2002; Suvas *et al.*, 2003) and CD4$^+$ (Lundgren *et al.*, 2003) T cell memory.

Together, regulatory T cells not only deal with the control of peripheral tolerance and homeostasis, but they also actively participate in the 'surveillance' of pathogen-specific immune responses.

Signals that can control regulatory T cell functions in order to improve vaccine efficacy

The biochemical nature and diversity of pathogen-derived entities or infection-induced, host-derived compounds that induce and support the differentiation and activation of such regulatory T cells remain to be determined (McGuirk and Mills, 2002b), but it seems that, for example, bacterial proteins such as filamentous hemagglutinin (FHA) of *Bordetella pertussis* can induce Tr1 cells in mice (McGuirk *et al.*, 2002a) and Purified Protein Derivative (PPD) from *Mycobacterium tuberculosis* can induce anergic IL-10-producing T cells in humans (Boussiotis *et al.*, 2000). Such 'immunomodulatory' compounds could support the generation of regulatory T cells (1) because they trigger the production of IL-10 by antigen-presenting cells during T cell priming (McGuirk and Mills, 2002b), (2) because they target specific dendritic cell subsets or maturation stages (Jonuleit *et al.*, 2001), (3) because they trigger specific ligand-receptor pair such as ICOS/ICOSL (Akbari *et al.*, 2002), or (4) through other yet unidentified mechanisms.

Much more research work is required to improve our understanding of the physiology and function of regulatory T cells. The ability to inhibit or induce regulatory T cells, to control their functions in an antigen-specific manner, and to elicit a memory pool of this regulatory subpopulation, opens new avenues in the vaccine field, not only for the therapy of autoimmune or allergic diseases or for preventing allograft rejections, but also for the development of more potent anti-infectious vaccines. In particular, as regulatory T cells seem to play important roles in the transitional process from acute to chronic infections they could be attractive vaccine target for pathogens that have a propensity to establish such a latent state (McGuirk *et al.*, 2002a,b). Regulatory T cells control the intensity of elicited immune responses to a degree sufficient to contain the infection and induce memory cells but not strong enough to eradicate the microbes, which then persist latently (Belkaid *et al.*, 2002).

It could be important to identify compounds (synthetic 'T reg' adjuvants) or pathogen-specific antigenic determinants (natural 'T reg' adjuvants) that will be capable of controlling regulatory T cell subsets *in vivo*, thus preventing inappropriate responses by specifically suppressing non-protective or cytopathic Th1 or Th2 responses. The addition of these 'T reg adjuvants' to vaccine containing 'conventional' pathogen specific antigens, known to trigger effector cells, will be helpful for a fine tuning of the response and for the induction of a long-term protective immunity (Sakaguchi, 2003b).

Very recently it has been reported that the immunosuppressive effects of regulatory T cells can also be regulated through the triggering of TLRs (Sakaguchi, 2003a). LPS directly acts on TLR4 expressing regulatory T cells to increase their suppressor property to control inflammation and limit overactivation of T cells (Caramalho *et al.*, 2003). Surprisingly TLR ligands can have an opposite indirect effect as TLR-induced APC-derived IL-6 blocks the suppressive activity of regulatory T cells allowing full-activation of T cells (Pasare and Medzhitov, 2003). These recent reports illustrate how TLR agonist-like adjuvants, such as CpG or monophosphoryl lipid A, could potentially be used, to manipulate regulatory T cells (Figure 3.4). But the apparent controversy of the above findings also indicates that a lot of research work remains to be achieved to consider potential clinical applications.

CONCLUSIONS

Conventional adjuvants such as aluminum salts or emulsions have proven to be efficient and useful in human vaccinology. Such adjuvants are thought to provoke long-term persistence of the antigen at the site of injection ('depot' effect). These compounds strongly improve the immunogenicity and efficacy of many vaccine targets for which high titers of functionally active antibodies are sufficient to mediate protection. It is however well accepted that for many pathogens vaccine-induced humoral immunity alone

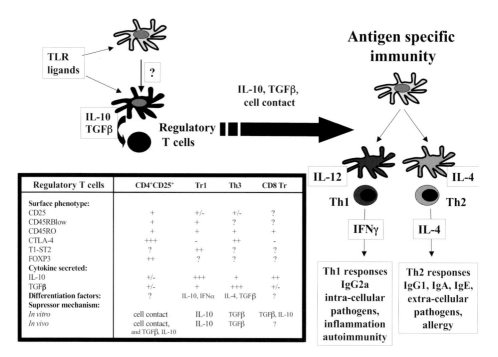

Figure 3.4 Vaccine adjuvants to manipulate regulatory T cells? Considering their role in the regulation of the balance between tolerance and immunity against self as well as foreign antigens, it is tempting to speculate that it will be useful to target subsets of regulatory T cells with vaccine adjuvants. This may allow better control over vaccine-induced immunity against infectious pathogens (intensity, diversity and Th1 versus Th2 polarization) but also the prevention of harmful immunopathological situations associated with exacerbated or inappropriate responses. Specific TLR ligands or any other adjuvants that can trigger the production of IL-10, TGFβ or engage ICOSL should be tested for their ability to control the function of regulatory T cells in the context of an antigen-specific immune response. This figure is also reproduced in colour in the colour section at the end of the book.

will not provide satisfactory protection or cure. Fighting viruses (especially those that efficiently produce escape mutants such as HIV, hepatitis C), eradicating intracellular parasites or bacteria that can hide from circulating antibodies (*Plasmodium falciparum, Mycobacterium tuberculosis*) and preventing tumor growth require appropriately polarized CD4 responses (usually Th1 biased) associated or not with a strong CD8 T cell-mediated lytic activity. The successful licensing of vaccines against such targets is likely to be at least partly dependent on the discovery and development of novel adjuvants that will elicit broad (systemic and mucosal) and sustained (long-term memory) immunity. In addition, many vaccines under development are based on rationally selected recombinant antigens (purified protein, peptide(s), plasmid DNA or recombinant virus) and no longer on whole inactivated or attenuated pathogens. Adjuvants will be necessary to improve the efficacy of these molecular vaccines of more limited immunogenicity and to allow dose reduction for these recombinant antigens that usually are costly and/or difficult to produce. Finally, novel adjuvants are also likely to be needed to facilitate the development of safer, pain-free, needleless vaccines that will use new routes of administration (e.g. transcutaneous, intradermal, intranasal).

Conventional approaches used in the past to develop vaccine adjuvants have been largely empirical and probably not optimal. Recent advances in our understanding of the immune system can be considered as the main foundations for the design of novel adjuvants. Among these immunological findings, it is worth mentionning our improved knowledge of the induction, regulation and maintenance of anamnestic responses and our understanding of the critical role that the initial innate immune response can play to drive an accurate and protective cell-mediated adaptive immunity. Genomic approaches (microarrays and proteomics) are accelerating this learning process as they produce a precious amount of useful information on the physiology of immune responses, both at the cellular and molecular levels. All this work is progressively leading to the identification of new critical regulatory pathways (TLR signaling), cell types (specific regulatory or unconventional T cells) and several other soluble components of the innate immune system (antimicrobial peptides or chemokines).

The vaccine field is therefore moving into a more 'rational' and accelerated approach for the design of molecularly characterized adjuvants. Some potent biological targets have been validated (e.g. TLRs), and some lead molecules (CpG, MPL) have been identified. More investigations must be conducted to produce libraries of synthetic analogues of such compounds in order to screen, compare and select the best candidates in preclinical models. Gene profilings induced by selected adjuvants on various human cell types might also be useful to better understand their immunostimulatory activity, their mechanism of action, as well as their potential toxicity profile, thereby improving chances of acceptance by regulatory authorities. Considering the complex cascade of events that are necessary for a successful and fully functional protective antigen-specific immune response, one can anticipate that combinations of two or more synthetic adjuvants might be required for some vaccines in order to achieve optimal recruitment, targeting, survival, proliferation, activation and long-term persistence of immune cells.

One of the most important challenges in the vaccine field is to be successful in the development and licensing of such safe and efficient novel adjuvants in humans.

Burdin

Acknowledgments
The author would like to thank Elyzabeth Ryan, Pascal Chaux, Emanuelle Trannoy and Jean Haensler for helpful comments and critical readings of the manuscript and Catherine Rossignol for her technical assistance.

References
Adams, M., Navabi, H., Jasani, B., Man, S., Fiander, A., Evans, A.S., Donninger, C., and Mason, M. 2003. Dendritic cell (DC) based therapy for cervical cancer: use of DC pulsed with tumour lysate and matured with a novel synthetic clinically non-toxic double stranded RNA analogue poly [I]: poly [C(12)U] (Ampligen((R). Vaccine 21: 787–790.

Agrawal, S. and Kandimalla, E.R. 2002. Medicinal chemistry and therapeutic potential of CpG DNA. Trends Mol. Med. 8: 114–121.

Akbari, O., Freeman, G.J., Meyer, E.H., Greenfield, E.A., Chang, T.T., Sharpe, A.H., Berry, G., DeKruyff, R.H., and Umetsu, D.T. 2002. Antigen-specific regulatory T cells develop via the ICOS-ICOS-ligand pathway and inhibit allergen-induced airway hyperreactivity. Nature Med. 8: 1024–1032.

Akira, S., Takeda, K., and Kaisho, T. 2001. Toll-like receptors: critical proteins linking innate and acquired immunity. Nature Immunol. 2: 675–680.

Alexopoulou, L., Holt, A.C., Medzhitov, R., and Flavell, R.A. 2001. Recognition of double-stranded RNA and activation of NF-kappaB by Toll-like receptor 3. Nature 413: 732–738.

Aseffa, A., Gumy, A., Launois, P., MacDonald, H.R., Louis, J.A., and Tacchini-Cottier, F. 2002. The early IL-4 response to *Leishmania major* and the resulting Th2 cell maturation steering progressive disease in BALB/c mice are subject to the control of regulatory $CD4^+CD25^+$ T cells. J. Immunol. 169: 3232–3241.

Ashkar, A.A. and Rosenthal, K.L. 2002. Toll-like receptor 9, CpG DNA and innate immunity. Curr. Mol. Med. 2: 545–556.

Baldrick, P., Richardson, D., Elliott, G., and Wheeler, A.W. 2002. Safety evaluation of monophosphoryl lipid A (MPL): an immunostimulatory adjuvant. Regul. Toxicol. Pharmacol. 35: 398–413.

Baldridge, J.R. and Crane, R.T. 1999. Monophosphoryl lipid A (MPL) formulations for the next generation of vaccines. Methods 19: 103–107.

Barton, G.M. and Medzhitov, R. 2002. Toll-like receptors and their ligands. Curr. Top. Microbiol. Immunol. 270: 81–92.

Bauer, S., Kirschning, C.J., Hacker, H., Redecke, V., Hausmann, S., Akira, S., Wagner, H., and Lipford, G.B. 2001. Human TLR9 confers responsiveness to bacterial DNA via species-specific CpG motif recognition. Proc. Natl. Acad. Sci. USA 98: 9237–9242.

Belkaid, Y., Piccirillo, C.A., Mendez, S., Shevach, E.M., and Sacks, D.L. 2002. $CD4^+CD25^+$ regulatory T cells control *Leishmania major* persistence and immunity. Nature 420: 502–507.

Bendelac, A., Bonneville, M., and Kearney, J.F. 2001. Autoreactivity by design: innate B and T lymphocytes. Nature Rev. Immunol. 1: 177–186.

BenMohamed, L., Belkaid, Y., Loing, E., Brahimi, K., Gras-Masse, H., and Druilhe, P. 2002a. Systemic immune responses induced by mucosal administration of lipopeptides without adjuvant. Eur. J. Immunol. 32: 2274–2281.

BenMohamed, L., Krishnan, R., Auge, C., Primus, J.F., and Diamond, D.J. 2002b. Intranasal administration of a synthetic lipopeptide without adjuvant induces systemic immune responses. Immunology 106: 113–121.

BenMohamed, L., Wechsler, S.L., and Nesburn, A.B. 2002c. Lipopeptide vaccines – yesterday, today, and tomorrow. Lancet Infect. Dis. 2: 425–431.

BenMohamed, L., Gras-Masse, H., Tartar, A., Daubersies, P., Brahimi, K., Bossus, M., Thomas, A., and Druilhe, P. 1997. Lipopeptide immunization without adjuvant induces potent and long-lasting B, T helper, and cytotoxic T lymphocyte responses against a malaria liver stage antigen in mice and chimpanzees. Eur. J. Immunol. 27: 1242–1253.

Bessler, W.G., Heinevetter, L., Wiesmuller, K.H., Jung, G., Baier, W., Huber, M., Lorenz, A.R., Esche, U.V., Mittenbuhler, K., and Hoffmann, P. 1997. Bacterial cell wall components as immunomodulators – I. Lipopeptides as adjuvants for parenteral and oral immunization. Int. J. Immunopharmacol. 19: 547–550.

Bessler, W.G. and Jung, G. 1992. Synthetic lipopeptides as novel adjuvants. Res. Immunol. 143: 548–553.

Biragyn, A., Ruffini, P.A., Leifer, C.A., Klyushnenkova, E., Shakhov, A., Chertov, O., Shirakawa, A.K., Farber, J.M., Segal, D.M., Oppenheim, J.J., and Kwak, L.W. 2002. Toll-like receptor 4-dependent activation of dendritic cells by beta-defensin 2. Science 298: 1025–1029.

Biragyn, A., Surenhu, M., Yang, D., Ruffini, P.A., Haines, B.A., Klyushnenkova, E., Oppenheim, J.J., and Kwak, L.W. 2001. Mediators of innate immunity that target immature, but not mature, dendritic cells induce antitumor immunity when genetically fused with nonimmunogenic tumor antigens. J. Immunol. 167: 6644–6653.

Biron, C.A. and Brossay, L. 2001. NK cells and NKT cells in innate defense against viral infections. Curr. Opin. Immunol. 13: 458–464.

Bishop, G.A., Hsing, Y., Hostager, B.S., Jalukar, S.V., Ramirez, L.M., and Tomai, M.A. 2000. Molecular mechanisms of B lymphocyte activation by the immune response modifier R-848. J. Immunol. 165: 5552–5557.

Bluestone, J.A. and Abbas, A.K. 2003. Natural versus adaptive regulatory T cells. Nature Rev. Immunol. 3: 253–257.

Boismenu, R. 2000. Function of intestinal gammadelta T cells. Immunol. Res. 21: 123–127.

Boussiotis, V.A., Tsai, E.Y., Yunis, E.J., Thim, S., Delgado, J.C., Dascher, C.C., Berezovskaya, A., Rousset, D., Reynes, J.M., and Goldfeld, A.E. 2000. IL-10-producing T cells suppress immune responses in anergic tuberculosis patients. J. Clin. Invest 105: 1317–1325.

Bradshaw, J. 2003. Cationic antimicrobial peptides: issues for potential clinical use. Biodrugs 17: 233–240.

Brogden, K.A., Heidari, M., Sacco, R.E., Palmquist, D., Guthmiller, J.M., Johnson, G.K., Jia, H.P., Tack, B.F., and McCray, P.B. 2003. Defensin-induced adaptive immunity in mice and its potential in preventing periodontal disease. Oral Microbiol. Immunol. 18: 95–99.

Brossay, L., Chioda, M., Burdin, N., Koezuka, Y., Casorati, G., Dellabona, P., and Kronenberg, M. 1998. CD1d-mediated recognition of an alpha-galactosylceramide by natural killer T cells is highly conserved through mammalian evolution. J. Exp. Med. 188: 1521–1528.

Burdin, N. and Kronenberg, M. 1999. CD1-mediated immune responses to glycolipids. Curr. Opin. Immunol. 11: 326–331.

Burdin, N., Brossay, L., Koezuka, Y., Smiley, S.T., Grusby, M.J., Gui, M., Taniguchi, M., Hayakawa, K., and Kronenberg, M. 1998. Selective ability of mouse CD1 to present glycolipids: alpha-galactosylceramide specifically stimulates V alpha 14+ NK T lymphocytes. J. Immunol. 161: 3271–3281.

Burns, R.P., Jr., Ferbel, B., Tomai, M., Miller, R., and Gaspari, A.A. 2000. The imidazoquinolines, imiquimod and R-848, induce functional, but not phenotypic, maturation of human epidermal Langerhans' cells. Clin. Immunol. 94: 13–23.

Caramalho, I., Lopes-Carvalho, T., Ostler, D., Zelenay, S., Haury, M., and Demengeot, J. 2003. Regulatory T cells selectively express toll-like receptors and are activated by lipopolysaccharide. J. Exp. Med. 197: 403–411.

Carding, S.R. and Egan, P.J. 2000. The importance of gamma delta T cells in the resolution of pathogen-induced inflammatory immune responses. Immunol. Rev. 173: 98–108.

Carding, S.R. and Egan, P.J. 2002. Gammadelta T cells: functional plasticity and heterogeneity. Nature Rev. Immunol. 2: 336–345.

Chertov, O., Michiel, D.F., Xu, L., Wang, J.M., Tani, K., Murphy, W.J., Longo, D.L., Taub, D.D., and Oppenheim, J.J. 1996. Identification of defensin-1, defensin-2, and CAP37/azurocidin as T-cell chemoattractant proteins released from interleukin 8-stimulated neutrophils. J. Biol. Chem. 271: 2935–2940.

Childers, N.K., Miller, K.L., Tong, G., Llarena, J.C., Greenway, T., Ulrich, J.T., and Michalek, S.M. 2000. Adjuvant activity of monophosphoryl lipid A for nasal and oral immunization with soluble or liposome-associated antigen. Infect. Immun. 68: 5509–5516.

Cho, H.J., Takabayashi, K., Cheng, P.M., Nguyen, M.D., Corr, M., Tuck, S., and Raz, E. 2000. Immunostimulatory DNA-based vaccines induce cytotoxic lymphocyte activity by a T-helper cell-independent mechanism. Nature Biotechnol. 18: 509–514.

Coutinho, A., Hori, S., Carvalho, T., Caramalho, I., and Demengeot, J. 2001. Regulatory T cells: the physiology of autoreactivity in dominant tolerance and 'quality control' of immune responses. Immunol. Rev. 182: 89–98.

Cui, J., Watanabe, N., Kawano, T., Yamashita, M., Kamata, T., Shimizu, C., Kimura, M., Shimizu, E., Koike, J., Koseki, H., Tanaka, Y., Taniguchi, M., and Nakayama, T. 1999. Inhibition of T helper cell type 2 cell differentiation and immunoglobulin E response by ligand-activated Valpha14 natural killer T cells. J. Exp. Med. 190: 783–792.

Cutler, K., Kagen, M.H., Don, P.C., McAleer, P., and Weinberg, J.M. 2000. Treatment of facial verrucae with topical imiquimod cream in a patient with human immunodeficiency virus. Acta Derm. Venereol. 80: 134–135.

Dabbagh, K., Dahl, M.E., Stepick-Biek, P., and Lewis, D.B. 2002. Toll-like receptor 4 is required for optimal development of Th2 immune responses: role of dendritic cells. J. Immunol. 168: 4524–4530.

De Becker, G., Moulin, V., Pajak, B., Bruck, C., Francotte, M., Thiriart, C., Urbain, J., and Moser, M. 2000. The adjuvant monophosphoryl lipid A increases the function of antigen-presenting cells. Int. Immunol. 12: 807–815.

Deng, G.M., Nilsson, I.M., Verdrengh, M., Collins, L.V., and Tarkowski, A. 1999. Intra-articularly localized bacterial DNA containing CpG motifs induces arthritis. Nature Med. 5: 702–705.

Desombere, I., Van der, W.M., Van Damme, P., Stoffel, M., De Clercq, N., Goilav, C., and Leroux-Roels, G. 2002. Immune response of HLA DQ2 positive subjects, vaccinated with HBsAg/AS04, a hepatitis B vaccine with a novel adjuvant. Vaccine 20: 2597–2602.

Dockrell, D.H. and Kinghorn, G.R. 2001. Imiquimod and resiquimod as novel immunomodulators. J. Antimicrob. Chemother. 48: 751–755.

Doetze, A., Satoguina, J., Burchard, G., Rau, T., Loliger, C., Fleischer, B., and Hoerauf, A. 2000. Antigen-specific cellular hyporesponsiveness in a chronic human helminth infection is mediated by T(h)3/T(r)1-type cytokines IL-10 and transforming growth factor-beta but not by a T(h)1 to T(h)2 shift. Int. Immunol. 12: 623–630.

Doyle, S., Vaidya, S., O'Connell, R., Dadgostar, H., Dempsey, P., Wu, T., Rao, G., Sun, R., Haberland, M., Modlin, R., and Cheng, G. 2002. IRF3 mediates a TLR3/TLR4-specific antiviral gene program. Immunity 17: 251–263.

Drachenberg, K.J., Wheeler, A.W., Stuebner, P., and Horak, F. 2001. A well-tolerated grass pollen-specific allergy vaccine containing a novel adjuvant, monophosphoryl lipid A, reduces allergic symptoms after only four preseasonal injections. Allergy 56: 498–505.

Durr, M. and Peschel, A. 2002. Chemokines meet defensins: the merging concepts of chemoattractants and antimicrobial peptides in host defense. Infect. Immun. 70: 6515–6517.

Eisenbarth, S.C., Piggott, D.A., Huleatt, J.W., Visintin, I., Herrick, C.A., and Bottomly, K. 2002. Lipopolysaccharide-enhanced, toll-like receptor 4-dependent T helper cell type 2 responses to inhaled antigen. J. Exp. Med. 196: 1645–1651.

Espinosa, E., Belmant, C., Pont, F., Luciani, B., Poupot, R., Romagne, F., Brailly, H., Bonneville, M., and Fournie, J.J. 2001. Chemical synthesis and biological activity of bromohydrin pyrophosphate, a potent stimulator of human gamma delta T cells. J. Biol. Chem. 276: 18337–18344.

Ferrarini, M., Ferrero, E., Dagna, L., Poggi, A., and Zocchi, M.R. 2002. Human gammadelta T cells: a nonredundant system in the immune-surveillance against cancer. Trends Immunol. 23: 14–18.

Fogel, M., Long, J.A., Thompson, P.J., and Upham, J.W. 2002. Dendritic cell maturation and IL-12 synthesis induced by the synthetic immune-response modifier S-28463. J. Leukoc. Biol. 72: 932–938.

Francois, B.J. 2003. Regulatory T cells under scrutiny. Nature Rev. Immunol. 3: 189–198.

Fujii, S., Shimizu, K., Smith, C., Bonifaz, L., and Steinman, R.M. 2003. Activation of natural killer T cells by alpha-galactosylceramide rapidly induces the full maturation of dendritic cells in vivo and thereby acts as an adjuvant for combined CD4 and CD8 T cell immunity to a coadministered protein. J. Exp. Med. 198: 267–279.

Gallo, R.L., Murakami, M., Ohtake, T., and Zaiou, M. 2002. Biology and clinical relevance of naturally occurring antimicrobial peptides. J. Allergy Clin. Immunol. 110: 823–831.

Ganz, T. 2003. Defensins: antimicrobial peptides of innate immunity. Nature Rev. Immunol. 3: 710–720.

Garland, S.M. 2003. Imiquimod. Curr. Opin. Infect Dis. 16: 85–89.

Giaccone, G., Punt, C.J., Ando, Y., Ruijter, R., Nishi, N., Peters, M., von Blomberg, B.M., Scheper, R.J., van der Vliet, H.J., van den Eertwegh, A.J., Roelvink, M., Beijnen, J., Zwierzina, H., and Pinedo, H.M. 2002. A phase I study of the natural killer T-cell ligand alpha-galactosylceramide (KRN7000) in patients with solid tumors. Clin. Cancer Res. 8: 3702–3709.

Godfrey, D.I., Hammond, K.J., Poulton, L.D., Smyth, M.J., and Baxter, A.G. 2000. NKT cells: facts, functions and fallacies. Immunol. Today 21: 573–583.

Gonzalez-Aseguinolaza, G., de Oliveira, C., Tomaska, M., Hong, S., Bruna-Romero, O., Nakayama, T., Taniguchi, M., Bendelac, A., Van Kaer, L., Koezuka, Y., and Tsuji, M. 2000. Alpha-galactosylceramide-activated Valpha 14 natural killer T cells mediate protection against murine malaria. Proc. Natl. Acad. Sci. USA 97: 8461–8466.

Gonzalez-Aseguinolaza, G., Van Kaer, L., Bergmann, C.C., Wilson, J.M., Schmieg, J., Kronenberg, M., Nakayama, T., Taniguchi, M., Koezuka, Y., and Tsuji, M. 2002. Natural killer T cell ligand alpha-galactosylceramide enhances protective immunity induced by malaria vaccines. J. Exp. Med. 195: 617–624.

Groux, H. 2001. An overview of regulatory T cells. Microbes Infect. 3: 883–889.

Gruber, P.C. and Wilkinson, J. 2001. Successful treatment of perianal warts in a child with 5% imiquimod cream. J. Dermatol. Treat. 12: 215–217.

Gumperz, J.E. and Brenner, M.B. 2001. CD1-specific T cells in microbial immunity. Curr. Opin. Immunol. 13: 471–478.

Hammond, K.J. and Godfrey, D.I. 2002. NKT cells: potential targets for autoimmune disease therapy? Tissue Antigens 59: 353–363.

Hancock, R.E. and Diamond, G. 2000. The role of cationic antimicrobial peptides in innate host defences. Trends Microbiol. 8(9): 402–410.

Hancock, R.E. and Patrzykat, A. 2002. Clinical development of cationic antimicrobial peptides: from natural to novel antibiotics. Curr. Drug Targets. Infect. Disord. 2: 79–83.

Hanninen, A. and Harrison, L.C. 2000. Gamma delta T cells as mediators of mucosal tolerance: the autoimmune diabetes model. Immunol. Rev. 173: 109–119.

Hayakawa, Y., Takeda, K., Yagita, H., Van Kaer, L., Saiki, I., and Okumura, K. 2001. Differential regulation of Th1 and Th2 functions of NKT cells by CD28 and CD40 costimulatory pathways. J. Immunol. 166: 6012–6018.

Hayday, A. and Geng, L. 1997. Gamma delta cells regulate autoimmunity. Curr. Opin. Immunol. 9: 884–889.

Heit, A., Maurer, T., Hochrein, H., Bauer, S., Huster, K.M., Busch, D.H., and Wagner, H. 2003. Cutting edge: Toll-like receptor 9 expression is not required for CpG DNA-aided cross-presentation of DNA-conjugated antigens but essential for cross-priming of CD8 T cells. J. Immunol. 170: 2802–2805.

Hemmi, H., Kaisho, T., Takeuchi, O., Sato, S., Sanjo, H., Hoshino, K., Horiuchi, T., Tomizawa, H., Takeda, K., and Akira, S. 2002. Small anti-viral compounds activate immune cells via the TLR7 MyD88-dependent signaling pathway. Nature Immunol. 3: 196–200.

Hendrix, C.W., Margolick, J.B., Petty, B.G., Markham, R.B., Nerhood, L., Farzadegan, H., Ts'o, P.O., and Lietman, P.S. 1993. Biologic effects after a single dose of poly(I): poly(C12U) in healthy volunteers. Antimicrob. Agents Chemother. 37: 429–435.

Hertz, C.J., Kiertscher, S.M., Godowski, P.J., Bouis, D.A., Norgard, M.V., Roth, M.D., and Modlin, R.L. 2001. Microbial lipopeptides stimulate dendritic cell maturation via Toll-like receptor 2. J. Immunol. 166: 2444–2450.

Hirabayashi, K., Yano, J., Takesue, H., Fujiwara, N., and Irimura, T. 1999. Inhibition of metastatic carcinoma cell growth in livers by poly(I): poly(C)/cationic liposome complex (LIC). Oncol. Res. 11: 497–504.

Hoebe, K., Du, X., Georgel, P., Janssen, E., Tabeta, K., Kim, S.O., Goode, J., Lin, P., Mann, N., Mudd, S., Crozat, K., Sovath, S., Ha,n J., and Beutler, B. 2003. Identification of Lps2 as a key transducer of MyD88-independent TIR signalling. Nature 424: 743–748.

Horng, T., Barton, G.M., Flavell, R.A., and Medzhitov, R. 2002. The adaptor Mol.ecule TIRAP provides signalling specificity for Toll-like receptors. Nature 420: 329–333.

Horng, T., Barton, G.M., and Medzhitov, R. 2001. TIRAP: an adapter Mol.ecule in the Toll signaling pathway. Nature Immunol. 2: 835–841.

Imler, J.L. and Hoffmann, J.A. 2003. Toll signaling: the TIReless quest for specificity. Nature Immunol. 4: 105–106.

Ismaili, J., Rennesson, J., Aksoy, E., Vekemans, J., Vincart, B., Amraoui, Z., Van Laethem, F., Goldman, M., and Dubois, P.M. 2002. Monophosphoryl lipid A activates both human dendritic cells and T cells. J. Immunol. 168: 926–932.

Ito, T., Amakawa, R., Kaisho, T., Hemmi, H., Tajima, K., Uehira, K., Ozaki, Y., Tomizawa, H., Akira, S., and Fukuhara, S. 2002. Interferon-alpha and interleukin 12 are induced differentially by Toll-like receptor 7 ligands in human blood dendritic cell subsets. J. Exp. Med. 195: 1507–1512.

Jacques, P., Moens, G., Desombere, I., Dewijngaert, J., Leroux-Roels, G., Wettendorff, M., and Thoelen, S. 2002. The immunogenicity and reactogenicity profile of a candidate hepatitis B vaccine in an adult vaccine non-responder population. Vaccine 20: 3644–3649.

Jarrossay, D., Napolitani, G., Colonna, M., Sallusto, F., and Lanzavecchia, A. 2001. Specialization and complementarity in microbial Mol.ecule recognition by human myeloid and plasmacytoid dendritic cells. Eur. J. Immunol. 31: 3388–3393.

Jiang, Z., Zamanian-Daryoush, M., Nie, H., Silva, A.M., Williams, B.R., and Li, X. 2003. Poly (I-C)-induced Toll-like receptor 3 (TLR3)-mediated activation of NFkappa B and MAP kinase is through an interleukin 1 receptor-associated kinase (IRAK)-independent pathway employing the signaling components TLR3-TRAF6-TAK1-TAB2-PKR. J. Biol Chem. 278: 16713–16719.

Jonuleit, H., Schmitt, E., Steinbrink, K., and Enk, A.H. 2001. Dendritic cells as a tool to induce anergic and regulatory T cells. Trends Immunol. 22: 394–400.

Jurk, M., Heil, F., Vollmer, J., Schetter, C., Krieg, A.M., Wagner, H., Lipford, G., and Bauer, S. 2002. Human TLR7 or TLR8 independently confer responsiveness to the antiviral compound R-848. Nature Immunol. 3: 499.

Kaisho, T. and Akira, S. 2002. Toll-like receptors as adjuvant receptors. Biochim. Biophys. Acta 1589: 1–13.

Kandimalla, E.R., Yu, D., and Agrawal, S. 2002. Towards optimal design of second-generation immunomodulatory oligonucleotides. Curr. Opin. Mol. Ther. 4: 122–129.

Karim, M., Bushell, A.R., and Wood, K.J. 2002. Regulatory T cells in transplantation. Curr. Opin. Immunol. 14: 584–591.

Kawano, T., Cui, J., Koezuka, Y., Toura, I., Kaneko, Y., Motoki, K., Ueno, H., Nakagawa, R., Sato, H., Kondo, E., Koseki, H., and Taniguchi, M. 1997. CD1d-restricted and TCR-mediated activation of valpha14 NKT cells by glycosylceramides. Science 278: 1626–1629.

Klinman, D.M. 2003. CpG DNA as a vaccine adjuvant. Expert Rev. Vaccines 2: 305–315.

Kobayashi, K., Hernandez, L.D., Galan, J.E., Janeway, C.A., Jr., Medzhitov, R., and Flavell, R.A. 2002. IRAK-M is a negative regulator of Toll-like receptor signaling. Cell 110: 191–202.

Krieg, A.M. 2002a. CpG motifs in bacterial DNA and their immune effects. Annu. Rev. Immunol. 20: 709–760.

Krieg, A.M. 2002b. From A to Z on CpG. Trends Immunol. 23: 64–65.

Krieg, A.M. 2003. CpG motifs: the active ingredient in bacterial extracts? Nature Med. 9: 831–835.

Kronenberg, M. and Gapin, L. 2002. The unconventional lifestyle of NKT cells. Nature Rev. Immunol. 2: 557–568.

Kullberg, M.C., Jankovic, D., Gorelick, P.L., Caspar, P., Letterio, J.J., Cheever, A.W., and Sher, A. 2002. Bacteria-triggered CD4(+) T regulatory cells suppress Helicobacter hepaticus-induced colitis. J. Exp. Med. 196: 505–515.

Kurt-Jones, E.A., Mandell, L., Whitney, C., Padgett, A., Gosselin, K., Newburger, P.E., and Finberg, R.W. 2002. Role of toll-like receptor 2 (TLR2) in neutrophil activation: GM-CSF enhances TLR2 expression and TLR2-mediated interleukin 8 responses in neutrophils. Blood 100: 1860–1868.

Lehner, T., Mitchell, E., Bergmeier, L., Singh, M., Spallek, R., Cranage, M., Hall, G., Dennis, M., Villinger, F., and Wang, Y. 2000. The role of gammadelta T cells in generating antiviral factors and beta-chemokines in protection against mucosal simian immunodeficiency virus infection. Eur. J. Immunol. 30: 2245–2256.

Lehrer, R.I. and Ganz, T. 1999. Antimicrobial peptides in mammalian and insect host defence. Curr. Opin. Immunol. 11: 23–27.

Leifer, C.A., Verthelyi, D., and Klinman, D.M. 2003. Heterogeneity in the human response to immunostimulatory CpG oligodeoxynucleotides. J. Immunother. 26: 313–319.

Liao, H.X., Cianciolo, G.J., Staats, H.F., Scearce, R.M., Lapple, D.M., Stauffer, S.H., Thomasch, J.R., Pizzo, S.V., Montefiori, D.C., Hagen, M., Eldridge, J., and Haynes, B.F. 2002. Increased immunogenicity of HIV envelope subunit complexed with alpha2-macroglobulin when combined with monophosphoryl lipid A and GM-CSF. Vaccine 20: 2396–2403.

Lichtenstein, A. 1991. Mechanism of mammalian cell lysis mediated by peptide defensins. Evidence for an initial alteration of the plasma membrane. J. Clin. Invest 88: 93–100.

Lien, E., Sellati, T.J., Yoshimura, A., Flo, T.H., Rawadi, G., Finberg, R.W., Carroll, J.D., Espevik, T., Ingalls, R.R., Radolf, J.D., and Golenbock, D.T. 1999. Toll-like receptor 2 functions as a pattern recognition receptor for diverse bacterial products. J. Biol Chem. 274: 33419–33425.

Lillard, J.W.J., Boyaka, P.N., Chertov, O., Oppenheim, J.J., and McGhee, J.R. 1999. Mechanisms for induction of acquired host immunity by neutrophil peptide defensins. Proc. Natl. Acad. Sci. USA 96: 651–656.

Livingston, B.D., Crimi, C., Grey, H., Ishioka, G., Chisari, F.V., Fikes, J., Grey, H., Chesnut, R.W., and Sette, A. 1997. The hepatitis B virus-specific CTL responses induced in humans by lipopeptide vaccination are comparable to those elicited by acute viral infection. J. Immunol. 159: 1383–1392.

Lore, K., Betts, M.R., Brenchley, J.M., Kuruppu, J., Khojasteh, S., Perfetto, S., Roederer, M., Seder, R.A., and Koup, R.A. 2003. Toll-like receptor ligands modulate dendritic cells to augment cytomegalovirus- and HIV-1-Specific T Cell Responses. J. Immunol. 171: 4320–4328.

Lundgren, A., Suri-Payer, E., Enarsson, K., Svennerholm, A.M., and Lundin, B.S. 2003. *Helicobacter pylori*-Specific CD4(+) CD25(high) Regulatory T cells suppress memory T-cell responses to *H. pylori* in infected individuals. Infect. Immun. 71: 1755–1762.

MacDonald, A.J., Duffy, M., Brady, M.T., McKiernan, S., Hall, W., Hegarty, J., Curry, M., and Mills, K.H. 2002. CD4 T helper type 1 and regulatory T cells induced against the same epitopes on the core protein in hepatitis C virus-infected persons. J. Infect. Dis. 185: 720–727.

MacDonald, H.R. 2002. Development and selection of NKT cells. Curr. Opin. Immunol. 14: 250–254.

Mak, T.W. and Yeh, W.C. 2002. Immunology: a block at the toll gate. Nature 418: 835–836.

Maloy, K.J. and Powrie, F. 2001. Regulatory T cells in the control of immune pathology. Nature Immunol. 2: 816–822.

Martin, M., Michalek, S.M., and Katz, J. 2003. Role of innate immune factors in the adjuvant activity of monophosphoryl lipid A. Infect. Immun. 71: 2498–2507.

Martin, M.U. and Wesche, H. 2002. Summary and comparison of the signaling mechanisms of the Toll/interleukin 1 receptor family. Biochim. Biophys. Acta 1592: 265–280.

Martini, F., Poccia, F., Goletti, D., Carrara, S., Vincenti, D., D'Offizi, G., Agrati, C., Ippolito, G., Colizzi, V., Pucillo, L.P., and Montesano, C. 2002. Acute human immunodeficiency virus replication causes a rapid and persistent impairment of Vgamma9Vdelta2 T cells in chronically infected patients undergoing structured treatment interruption. J. Infect. Dis. 186: 847–850.

Mason, D. 2001. Some quantitative aspects of T-cell repertoire selection: the requirement for regulatory T cells. Immunol. Rev. 182: 80–88.

Mbawuike, I.N., Acuna, C., Caballero, D., Pham-Nguyen, K., Gilbert, B., Petribon, P., and Harmon, M. 1996. Reversal of age-related deficient influenza virus-specific CTL responses and IFN-γamma production by monophosphoryl lipid A. Cell Immunol. 173: 64–78.

McCluskie, M.J., Weeratna, R.D., Payette, P.J., and Davis, H.L. 2001. The potential of CpG oligodeoxynucleotides as mucosal adjuvants. Crit Rev. Immunol. 21: 103–120.

McCormack, S., Tilzey, A., Carmichael, A., Gotch, F., Kepple, J., Newberry, A., Jones, G., Lister, S., Beddows, S., Cheingsong, R., Rees, A., Babiker, A., Banatvala, J., Bruck, C., Darbyshire, J., Tyrrell, D., Van Hoecke, C., and Weber, J. 2000. A phase I trial in HIV negative healthy volunteers evaluating the effect of potent adjuvants on immunogenicity of a recombinant gp120W61D derived from dual tropic R5X4 HIV-1ACH320. Vaccine 18: 1166–1177.

McGuirk, P., McCann, C., and Mills, K.H. 2002a. Pathogen-specific T regulatory 1 cells induced in the respiratory tract by a bacterial Mol.ecule that stimulates interleukin 10 production by dendritic cells: a novel strategy for evasion of protective T helper type 1 responses by Bordetella pertussis. J. Exp. Med. 195: 221–231.

McGuirk, P. and Mills, K.H. 2002b. Pathogen-specific regulatory T cells provoke a shift in the Th1/Th2 paradigm in immunity to infectious diseases. Trends Immunol. 23: 450–455.

Medzhitov, R. 2001. Toll-like receptors and innate immunity. Nature Rev. Immunol. 1: 135–145.

Mittenbuhler, K., Esche, U., Heinevetter, L., Bessler, W.G., and Huber, M. 2003. Lipopeptides: adjuvanticity in conventional and genetic immunization. FEMS Immunol. Med. Microbiol. 37: 193–200.

Mittenbuhler, K., Loleit, M., Baier, W., Fischer, B., Sedelmeier, E., Jung, G., Winkelmann, G., Jacobi, C., Weckesser, J., Erhard, M.H., Hofmann, A., Bessler, W., and Hoffmann, P. 1997. Drug specific antibodies: T-cell epitope-lipopeptide conjugates are potent adjuvants for small antigens in vivo and in vitro. Int. J. Immunopharmacol. 19: 277–287.

Miyahira, Y., Katae, M., Takeda, K., Yagita, H., Okumura, K., Kobayashi, S., Takeuchi, T., Kamiyama, T., Fukuchi,Y., and Aoki, T. 2003. Activation of natural killer T cells by alpha-galactosylceramide impairs DNA vaccine-induced protective immunity against Trypanosoma cruzi. Infect. Immun. 71: 1234–1241.

Miyamoto, K., Miyake, S., and Yamamura, T. 2001. A synthetic glycolipid prevents autoimmune encephalomyelitis by inducing TH2 bias of natural killer T cells. Nature 413: 531–534.

Miyata, M., Kobayashi, H., Sasajima, T., Sato, Y., and Kasukawa, R. 2000. Unmethylated oligo-DNA containing CpG motifs aggravates collagen-induced arthritis in mice. Arthritis Rheum. 43: 2578–2582.

Morr, M., Takeuchi, O., Akira, S., Simon, M.M., and Muhlradt, P.F. 2002. Differential recognition of structural details of bacterial lipopeptides by toll-like receptors. Eur. J. Immunol. 32: 3337–3347.

Murakami, M., Sakamoto, A., Bender, J., Kappler, J., Marrack, P. 2002. CD25+CD4+ T cells contribute to the control of memory CD8+ T cells. Proc. Natl. Acad. Sci. USA 25: 8832–88377.

Nizet, V., Ohtake, T., Lauth, X., Trowbridge, J., Rudisill, J., Dorschner, R.A., Pestonjamasp, V., Piraino J., Huttner K., and Gallo R.L. 2001. Innate antimicrobial peptide protects the skin from invasive bacterial infection. Nature 414: 454–457.

O'Neill, L.A. 2002a. Signal transduction pathways activated by the IL-1 receptor/toll-like receptor superfamily. Curr. Top. Microbiol. Immunol. 270: 47–61.

O'Neill, L.A. 2002b. Toll-like receptor signal transduction and the tailoring of innate immunity: a role for Mal? Trends Immunol. 23: 296–300.

Oshiumi, H., Matsumoto, M., Funami, K., Akazawa, T., and Seya, T. 2003. TICAM-1, an adaptor molecule that participates in Toll-like receptor 3-mediated interferon-beta induction. Nature Immunol. 4: 161–167.

Ozinsky, A., Underhill, D.M., Fontenot, J.D., Hajjar, A.M., Smith, K.D., Wilson, C.B., Schroeder, L., and Aderem, A. 2000. The repertoire for pattern recognition of pathogens by the innate immune system is defined by cooperation between toll-like receptors. Proc. Natl. Acad. Sci. USA 97: 13766–13771.

Pajak, B., Garze, V., Davies, G., Bauer, J., Moser, M., and Chiavaroli, C. 2003. The adjuvant OM-174 induces both the migration and maturation of murine dendritic cells in vivo. Vaccine 21: 836–842.

Pasare, C. and Medzhitov, R. 2003. Toll pathway-dependent blockade of CD4+CD25+ T cell-mediated suppression by dendritic cells. Science 299: 1033–1036.

Persing, D.H., Coler, R.N., Lacy, M.J., Johnson, D.A., Baldridge, J.R., Hershberg, R.M., and Reed, S.G. 2002. Taking toll: lipid A mimetics as adjuvants and immunomodulators. Trends Microbiol. 10: S32-S37.

Pialoux, G., Gahery-Segard, H., Sermet, S., Poncelet, H., Fournier, S., Gerard, L., Tartar, A., Gras-Masse, H., Levy, J.P., and Guillet, J.G. 2001. Lipopeptides induce cell-mediated anti-HIV immune responses in seronegative volunteers. AIDS 15: 1239–1249.

Piccirillo, C.A. and Shevach, E.M. 2001. Cutting edge: control of CD8+ T cell activation by CD4+CD25+ immunoregulatory cells. J. Immunol. 167: 1137–1140.

Poccia, F., Gougeon, M.L., Agrati, C., Montesano, C., Martini, F., Pauza, C.D., Fisch, P., Wallace, M., and Malkovsky, M. 2002. Innate T-cell immunity in HIV infection: the role of Vgamma9Vdelta2 T lymphocytes. Curr. Mol. Med. 2: 769–781.

Prohaszka, Z. and Fust, G. 1998. Contribution of complement to defensin action in eye. Lancet 352: 1152.

Prohaszka, Z., Nemet, K., Csermely, P., Hudecz, F., Mezo, G., and Fus, G. 1997. Defensins purified from human granulocytes bind C1q and activate the classical complement pathway like the transmembrane glycoprotein gp41 of HIV-1. Mol. Immunol. 34: 809–816.

Pyo, S., Gangemi, J.D., Ghaffar, A., and Mayer, E.P. 1993. Poly I: C-induced antiviral and cytotoxic activities are mediated by different mechanisms. Int. J. Immunopharmacol. 15: 477–486.

Raj, P.A. and Dentino, A.R. 2002. Current status of defensins and their role in innate and adaptive immunity. FEMS Microbiol. Lett. 206: 9–18.

Read, S. and Powrie, F. 2001. CD4(+) regulatory T cells. Curr. Opin. Immunol. 13: 644–649.

Rharbaoui, F., Drabner, B., Borsutzky, S., Winckler, U., Morr, M., Ensoli, B., Muhlradt, P.F., and Guzman, C.A. 2002. The Mycoplasma-derived lipopeptide MALP-2 is a potent mucosal adjuvant. Eur. J. Immunol. 32: 2857–2865.

Ronaghy, A., Prakken, B.J., Takabayashi, K., Firestein, G.S., Boyle, D., Zvailfler, N.J., Roord, S.T., Albani, S., Carson, D.A., and Raz, E. 2002. Immunostimulatory DNA sequences influence the course of adjuvant arthritis. J. Immunol. 168: 51–56.

Sacher, T., Knolle, P., Nichterlein, T., Arnold, B., Hammerling, G.J., and Limmer, A. 2002. CpG-ODN-induced inflammation is sufficient to cause T-cell-mediated autoaggression against hepatocytes. Eur. J. Immunol. 32: 3628–3637.

Sakaguchi, S. 2000. Regulatory T cells: key controllers of Immunologic self-tolerance. Cell 101: 455–458.

Sakaguchi, S. 2003a. Control of immune responses by naturally arising CD4⁺ regulatory T cells that express toll-like receptors. J. Exp. Med. 197: 397–401.

Sakaguchi, S. 2003b. Regulatory T cells: mediating compromises between host and parasite. Nature Immunol. 4: 10–11.

Sakaguchi, S., Sakaguchi, N., Shimizu, J., Yamazaki, S., Sakihama, T., Itoh, M., Kuniyasu, Y., Nomura, T., Toda, M., and Takahashi, T. 2001. Immunologic tolerance maintained by CD25⁺ CD4⁺ regulatory T cells: their common role in controlling autoimmunity, tumor immunity, and transplantation tolerance. Immunol. Rev. 182: 18–32.

Schaible, U.E. and Kaufmann, S.H. 2000. CD1 Mol.ecules and CD1-dependent T cells in bacterial infections: a link from innate to acquired immunity? Semin. Immunol. 12: 527–535.

Schnare, M., Barton, G.M., Holt, A.C., Takeda, K., Akira, S., and Medzhitov, R. 2001. Toll-like receptors control activation of adaptive immune responses. Nature Immunol. 2: 947–950.

Schwartz, D.A., Quinn, T.J., Thorne, P.S., Sayeed, S., Yi, A.K., and Krieg, A.M. 1997. CpG motifs in bacterial DNA cause inflammation in the lower respiratory tract. J. Clin. Invest 100: 68–73.

Schwarz, K., Storni, T., Manolova, V., Didierlaurent, A., Sirard, J.C., Rothlisberger, P., and Bachmann, M.F. 2003. Role of Toll-like receptors in costimulating cytotoxic T cell responses. Eur. J. Immunol. 33: 1465–1470.

Scott, M.G. and Hancock, R.E. 2000. Cationic antimicrobial peptides and their multifunctional role in the immune system. Crit. Rev. Immunol. 20: 407–431.

Seo, N., Hayakawa, S., and Tokura, Y. 2002. Mechanisms of immune privilege for tumor cells by regulatory cytokines produced by innate and acquired immune cells. Semin. Cancer Biol. 12: 291–300.

Sharif, S., Arreaza, G.A., Zucker, P., Mi, Q.S., and Delovitch, T.L. 2002. Regulation of autoimmune disease by natural killer T cells. J. Mol. Med. 80: 290–300.

Shevach, E.M. 2000. Regulatory T cells in autoimmmunity. Annu. Rev. Immunol. 18: 423–449.

Shevach, E.M. 2002. CD4⁺ CD25⁺ suppressor T cells: more questions than answers. Nature Rev. Immunol. 2: 389–400.

Shi, F., Ljunggren, H.G., and Sarvetnick, N. 2001. Innate immunity and autoimmunity: from self-protection to self-destruction. Trends Immunol. 22: 97–101.

Shirota, H., Sano, K., Kikuchi, T., Tamura, G., and Shirato, K. 2000. Regulation of murine airway eosinophilia and Th2 cells by antigen-conjugated CpG oligodeoxynucleotides as a novel antigen-specific immunomodulator. J. Immunol. 164: 5575–5582.

Sieling, P.A. and Modlin, R.L. 2002. Toll-like receptors: mammalian 'taste receptors' for a smorgasbord of microbial invaders. Curr. Opin. Microbiol. 5: 70–75.

Sireci, G., Espinosa, E., Di Sano, C., Dieli, F., Fournie, J.J., and Salerno, A. 2001. Differential activation of human gammadelta cells by nonpeptide phosphoantigens. Eur. J. Immunol. 31: 1628–1635.

Smith, K.D. and Ozinsky, A. 2002. Toll-like receptor-5 and the innate immune response to bacterial flagellin. Curr. Top. Microbiol. Immunol. 270: 93–108.

Smyth, M.J., Crowe, N.Y., Hayakawa, Y., Takeda, K., Yagita, H., and Godfrey, D.I. 2002. NKT cells – conductors of tumor immunity? Curr. Opin. Immunol. 14: 165–171.

Steller, M.A., Gurski, K.J., Murakami, M., Daniel, R.W., Shah, K.V., Celis, E., Sette, A., Trimble, E.L., Park, R.C., and Marincola, F.M. 1998. Cell-mediated Immunological responses in cervical and vaginal cancer patients immunized with a lipidated epitope of human papillomavirus type 16 E7. Clin. Cancer Res. 4: 2103–2109.

Suvas, S., Kumaraguru, U., Pack, C.D., Lee, S., and Rouse, B.T. 2003. CD4$^+$CD25$^+$ T cells regulate virus-specific primary and memory CD8$^+$ T cell responses. J. Exp. Med. 198: 889–901.

Syed, T.A. 2001. A review of the applications of imiquimod: a novel immune response modifier. Expert Opin. Pharmacother. 2: 877–882.

Takeda, K., Kaisho, T., and Akira, S. 2003. Toll-like receptors. Annu. Rev. Immunol. 21: 335–376.

Takeda, K., Takeuchi, O., and Akira, S. 2002. Recognition of lipopeptides by Toll-like receptors. J. Endotoxin Res. 8: 459–463.

Takeuchi, O., Kaufmann, A., Grote, K., Kawai, T., Hoshino, K., Morr, M., Muhlradt, P.F., and Akira, S. 2000. Cutting edge: preferentially the R-stereoisomer of the mycoplasmal lipopeptide macrophage-activating lipopeptide-2 activates immune cells through a toll-like receptor 2- and MyD88-dependent signaling pathway. J. Immunol. 164: 554–557.

Takeuchi, O., Kawai, T., Muhlradt, P.F., Morr, M., Radolf, J.D., Zychlinsky, A., Takeda, K., and Akira, S. 2001. Discrimination of bacterial lipoproteins by Toll-like receptor 6. Int. Immunol. 13: 933–940.

Takeuchi, O., Sato, S., Horiuchi, T., Hoshino, K., Takeda, K., Dong, Z., Modlin, R.L., and Akira, S. 2002. Cutting edge: role of Toll-like receptor 1 in mediating immune response to microbial lipoproteins. J. Immunol. 169: 10–14.

Tani, K., Murphy, W.J., Chertov, O., Salcedo, R., Koh, C.Y., Utsunomiya, I., Funakoshi, S., Asai, O., Herrmann, S.H., Wang, J.M., Kwak, L.W., and Oppenheim, J.J. 2000. Defensins act as potent adjuvants that promote cellular and humoral immune responses in mice to a lymphoma idiotype and carrier antigens. Int. Immunol. 12: 691–700.

Thoelen, S., De Clercq, N., and Tornieporth, N. 2001. A prophylactic hepatitis B vaccine with a novel adjuvant system. Vaccine 19: 2400–2403.

Tomai, M.A., Imbertson, L.M., Stanczak, T.L., Tygrett, L.T., and Waldschmidt, T.J. 2000. The immune response modifiers imiquimod and R-848 are potent activators of B lymphocytes. Cell Immunol. 203: 55–65.

Tung, K.S., Agersborg, S.S., Alard, P., Garza, K.M., and Lou, Y.H. 2001. Regulatory T-cell, endogenous antigen and neonatal environment in the prevention and induction of autoimmune disease. Immunol. Rev. 182: 135–148.

Underhill, D.M. and Ozinsky, A. 2002. Toll-like receptors: key mediators of microbe detection. Curr. Opin. Immunol. 14: 103–110.

van den Berg, R.H., Faber-Krol, M.C., van Wetering, S., Hiemstra, P.S., and Daha, M.R. 1998. Inhibition of activation of the classical pathway of complement by human neutrophil defensins. Blood 92: 3898–3903.

Vasilakos, J.P., Smith, R.M., Gibson, S.J., Lindh, J.M., Pederson, L.K., Reiter, M.J., Smith, M.H., and Tomai, M.A. 2000. Adjuvant activities of immune response modifier R-848: comparison with CpG ODN. Cell Immunol. 204: 64–74.

Vernacchio, L., Bernstein, H., Pelton, S., Allen, C., MacDonald, K., Dunn, J., Duncan, D.D., Tsao, G., LaPosta, V., Eldridge, J., Laussucq, S., Ambrosino, D.M., and Mol.rine, D.C. 2002. Effect of monophosphoryl lipid A (MPL on T-helper cells when administered as an adjuvant with pneumocococcal-CRM197) conjugate vaccine in healthy toddlers. Vaccine 20: 3658–3667.

Vitiello, A., Ishioka, G., Grey, H.M., Rose, R., Farness, P., LaFond, R., Yuan, L., Chisari, F.V., Furze, J., Bartholomeuz, R. 1995. Development of a lipopeptide-based therapeutic vaccine to treat chronic HBV infection. I. Induction of a primary cytotoxic T lymphocyte response in humans. J. Clin. Invest 95: 341–349.

Von Herrath, M.G. and Harrison, L.C. 2003. Antigen-induced regulatory T cells in autoimmunity. Nature Rev. Immunol. 3: 223–232.

Wasserman, S.A. 2000. Toll signaling: the enigma variations. Curr. Opin. Genet. Dev. 10: 497–502.

Wilson, C.L., Ouellette, A.J., Satchell, D.P., Ayabe, T., Lopez-Boado, Y.S., Stratman, J.L., Hultgren, S.J., Matrisian, L.M., and Parks, W.C. 1999. Regulation of intestinal alpha-defensin activation by the metalloproteinase matrilysin in innate host defense. Science 286: 113–117.

Wilson, M.T., Singh, A.K., and Van Kaer, L. 2002. Immunotherapy with ligands of natural killer T cells. Trends Mol. Med. 8: 225–231.

Wood, K.J. and Sakaguchi, S. 2003. Regulatory T cells in transplantation tolerance. Nature Rev. Immunol. 3: 199–210.

Xu, D., Liu, H., Komai-Koma, M., Campbell, C., McSharry, C., Alexander, J., and Liew, F.Y. 2003. CD4+CD25+ regulatory T cells suppress differentiation and functions of Th1 and Th2 cells, *Leishmania major* infection, and colitis in mice. J. Immunol. 170: 394–399.

Yamamoto, M., Sato, S., Hemmi, H., Hoshino, K., Kaisho, T., Sanjo, H., Takeuchi, O., Sugiyama, M., Okabe, M., Takeda, K., and Akira, S. 2003. Role of adaptor TRIF in the MyD88-independent toll-like receptor signaling pathway. Science 301: 640–643.

Yamamoto, M., Sato, S., Hemmi, H., Sanjo, H., Uematsu, S., Kaisho, T., Hoshino, K., Takeuchi, O., Kobayashi, M., Fujita, T., Takeda, K., and Akira, S. 2002a. Essential role for TIRAP in activation of the signalling cascade shared by TLR2 and TLR4. Nature 420: 324–329.

Yamamoto, M., Sato, S., Mori, K., Hoshino, K., Takeuchi, O., Takeda, K., and Akira, S. 2002b. Cutting edge: a novel Toll/IL-1 receptor domain-containing adapter that preferentially activates the IFN-beta promoter in the Toll-like receptor signaling. J. Immunol. 169: 6668–6672.

Yang, D., Chen, Q., Hoover, D.M., Staley, P., Tucker, K.D., Lubkowski, J., and Oppenheim, J.J. 2003. Many chemokines including CCL20/MIP-3alpha display antimicrobial activity. J. Leukoc. Biol. 74: 448–455.

Yang, D., Biragyn, A., Kwak, L.W., and Oppenheim, J.J. 2002. Mammalian defensins in immunity: more than just microbicidal. Trends Immunol. 23: 291–296.

Yang, D., Chen, Q., Chertov, O., and Oppenheim, J.J. 2000. Human neutrophil defensins selectively chemoattract naive T and immature dendritic cells. J. Leukoc. Biol. 68: 9–14.

Yang, D., Chertov, O., Bykovskaia, S.N., Chen, Q., Buffo, M.J., Shogan, J., Anderson, M., Schroder, J.M., Wang, J.M., Howard, O.M., and Oppenheim, J.J. 1999. Beta-defensins: linking innate and adaptive immunity through dendritic and T cell CCR6. Science 286: 525–528.

Yin, Z. and Craft, J. 2000. gamma delta T cells in autoimmunity. Springer Semin Immunopathol 22: 311–320.

Zasloff, M. 2002. Antimicrobial peptides of multicellular organisms. Nature 415: 389–395.

Zeng, W., Ghosh, S., Lau, Y.F., Brown, L.E., and Jackson, D.C. 2002. Highly immunogenic and totally synthetic lipopeptides as self-adjuvanting immunocontraceptive vaccines. J. Immunol. 169: 4905–4912.

Zhang, G. and Ghosh, S. 2002. Negative regulation of toll-like receptor-mediated signaling by Tollip. J. Biol. Chem. 277: 7059–7065.

Zhang, L., Yu, W., He, T., Yu, J., Caffrey, R.E., Dalmasso, E.A., Fu, S., Pham, T., Mei, J., Ho, J.J., Zhang, W., Lopez, P., and Ho, D.D. 2002. Contribution of human alpha-defensin 1, 2, and 3 to the anti-HIV-1 activity of CD8 antiviral factor. Science 298: 995–1000.

Zhou, F. and Huang, L. 1993. Monophosphoryl lipid A enhances specific CTL induction by a soluble protein antigen entrapped in liposomes. Vaccine 11: 1139–1144.

Chapter 4

Mucosal Immunity and Vaccine Design

Cecil Czerkinsky, Ali M. Harandi and Jan Holmgren

Abstract

The mucosal immune system consists of an integrated network of lymphoid cells which works in concert with innate host factors to promote host defense. Mucosal immunization can be used both to protect mucosal surfaces against colonization and invasion by microbial pathogens and to provide a means to prevent local and systemic inflammatory immune responses to non-degraded food and airborne antigens or allergens. The latter property has recently been utilized in attempts to suppress auto- and allo-reactive responses associated with organ-specific autoimmune diseases and to prevent graft rejection.

However, in practice, induction of productive immunity as well as induction of peripheral immune suppression by the mucosal route of administration require large amounts of antigens and even so have relatively short-lasting effects. To circumvent these limitations and to bypass the powerful natural mechanical and physicochemical barrier function of mucosal epithelia, major efforts have been devoted to the development of delivery systems and adjuvants/immunomodulators to formulate efficient mucosal vaccines.

Among the most studied vector/delivery systems and adjuvants for mucosal immunization, cholera toxin (CT) and the closely related *E. coli* heat-labile enterotoxin (LT) have proven to be very useful tools to study mucosal immune responses induced by various routes. Because of the inherent toxicity of CT and LT which precludes their use in humans, detoxified derivatives of these toxins with retained adjuvant activity have been generated. The clinically most advanced of these derivatives is the completely non-toxic, recombinantly produced cholera toxin B-subunit (CTB). CTB is a protective component of a widely registered oral vaccine against cholera. CTB has also in preclinical studies proved to be a very promising vector for either giving rise to anti-infective immunity or for inducing peripheral anti-inflammatory tolerance to chemically or genetically linked foreign antigens administered mucosally. Promising advances have recently been made in the design of another class of efficient mucosal adjuvants based on CpG-motif containing bacterial DNA or synthetic oligo-deoxynucleotides, as well as various imidazoquinoline compounds binding to different Toll-like receptors on mucosal antigen-presenting cells.

INTRODUCTION

Mucosal immunization has recently attracted much interest both as a means to induce protective immunity against many infections and, conversely as a possible approach towards specific immunological treatment of diseases caused by tissue-damaging immune responses against certain autoantigens, allergens or antigens derived from persistent microbial pathogens (Czerkinsky *et al.*, 1999; Wu and Weiner, 2003).

There are important reasons for choosing a mucosal route of vaccination instead of the more conventional route of parenteral injection. First, the majority of infectious agents and allergens (airborne and food-derived) use the mucosal epithelium as their portal of entry and their absorption into host tissues can best be prevented by inducing an antibody response at these very same sites. In these situations, topical application of a vaccine has often proven to be superior for inducing local, so-called 'secretory', antibody production. This is the case for instance with gastrointestinal infections caused by *Helicobacter pylori*, *Vibrio cholerae*, enterotoxigenic *Escherichia coli* (ETEC), *Shigella* spp., *Clostridium difficile*, rotaviruses and caliciviruses; respiratory infections caused by *Mycoplasma pneumoniae*, influenza virus and respiratory syncytial virus; and genital infections caused by human papillomavirus, HIV, *Chlamydia*, *Neisseria gonorrhoeae* and herpex simplex virus, to mention just a few examples of contagious diseases of major public health importance.

Second, mucosal vaccines, especially oral vaccines and to a lesser extent nasal vaccines, should also be easier to administer than parenteral vaccines and safer than injectable vaccines, thus potentially improving compliance in many settings.

Alternatively, although less well appreciated than vaccination against infections, mucosal vaccination could also be used to induce immunological suppression, in order to interfere with the development of harmful immune responses. This phenomenon, called mucosal tolerance and often referred to as 'oral tolerance' (because it was initially documented as a consequence of antigen ingestion), is characterized by the fact that an individual who has ingested or inhaled an antigen may become refractory to developing an immune response when exposed to the same antigen, when reintroduced by a systemic route. This phenomenon is an important physiological mechanism to avoid development of T cell-driven inflammatory reactions and other allergic reactions to ingested food proteins and other antigens such as airborne allergens, should these antigens reach the body interior in an undegraded form. Since mucosal tolerance, at variance with many other forms of immunotherapy, is specific for the antigen initially ingested or inhaled, it has become an attractive strategy for prevention and potentially also for halting illnesses caused by untoward immune responses against allergens and autoantigens (Wu and Weiner, 2003).

Mucosal tolerance and induction of mucosal immunity are however not mutually exclusive. Mucosal tolerance (or ignorance) is the default response to ingested food proteins or autoantigens and is difficult to induce with strongly immunogenic antigens, and the converse is true for inducing mucosal immune responses. However, sometimes the same mucosal immunization may concomitantly give rise both to a local significant IgA antibody response and to diminished immune responsiveness in the periphery. Although the mechanisms underlying the induction of this dual form of immunity are still not fully elucidated, certain cytokines, such as transforming growth factor (TGF) β and interleukin 4 (IL-4), are known to be involved both in the production of secretory IgA antibodies at the mucosal surface and in the induction of mucosal tolerance.

However, despite the many attractive features of mucosal immunization it has often proven difficult in practice to stimulate strong mucosal IgA immune responses and the results to date have, with a few notable exceptions, been rather disappointing. Indeed, only half a dozen of the vaccines that are currently approved for human use are administered mucosally: the oral polio vaccine, two types of oral vaccines against cholera (composed of either killed whole-cell cholera vibrios plus CTB or of a live-attenuated cholera vaccine strain), an oral live-attenuated typhoid vaccine, an oral adenovirus vaccine (restricted to military personnel), a nasal cold-adapted influenza virus vaccine (Flumist®) and an oral BCG strain used in Brazil for vaccination against tuberculosis. Two additional mucosal vaccines, an oral live-attenuated vaccine against rotavirus diarrhea and a nasal enterotoxin-adjuvanted inactivated influenza vaccine, were withdrawn after a short time on the market because of potential serious adverse reactions (intussusception and facial paresis, respectively), thus illustrating the complexity of mucosal vaccine development.

Likewise, in the area of mucosal tolerance, although promising results were obtained in patients with multiple sclerosis, rheumatoid arthritis, and in recently diagnosed type I diabetic patients (Faria and Weiner, 1999), larger randomized placebo-controlled multicenter trials failed to yield significant therapeutic benefits. In contrast, and also less appreciated, this approach has given much promise in patients with allergic disorders. Thus, clinical trials of mucosal (mostly oral-sublingual) tolerance therapy have given positive results in patients with type I respiratory allergies (Morris, 1999; Morris et al., 2003; Passalacqua et al., 2003; Mortemousque et al., 2003). These latter observations may seem surprising since T helper 2-driven responses (which play a major role in type I allergy) are usually more difficult to suppress than Th1 responses (assumed to drive most autoimmune disorders). A possible explanation is that the autoantigens selected for clinical trials of autoimmunotherapy may not have been the most pertinent ones while the situation in type I allergy is somewhat different (most respiratory allergens have been identified). Even in the latter situation, the efficacy of mucosal/sublingual immunotherapy in type I allergic patients has been limited (generally 30% improvement in clinical scores) and there is ample space for improving the efficacy of such an approach.

To overcome the obstacles to the development of a broader range of mucosal vaccines and mucosal immunotherapies, there is a need to find more efficient means of delivering the appropriate antigens to the mucosal immune system, and/or to develop effective, safe mucosal adjuvants or immunomodulating agents which, depending on the indication and the adjuvant formulations used, could provide protective immunity against infectious agents or induce suppression of pathological immunity, respectively.

ADJUVANTS FOR MUCOSAL VACCINATION

Among the numerous candidate delivery systems and adjuvants proposed for mucosal immunization, we will describe the advances made with the two most promising classes of mucosal antigen-delivery and adjuvant systems available to date. The first group comprises cholera toxin (CT) and the structutally related heat-labile enterotoxin (LT) produced by certain strains of *Escherichia coli*, and different detoxified derivatives of CT and LT, including their completely non-toxic B subunit components (CTB or LTB). The other class of recently described mucosal adjuvants is represented by bacterial DNA or synthetic oligo-deoxynucleotide analogues containing so-called CpG-motifs and novel imidazoquinoline amines, which can bind to different Toll-like receptors and thereby stimulate both innate and adaptive immune responses.

Dendritic cells and macrophages have a central role in the adjuvanticity of CT-like molecules, bacterial DNA, and imidazoquinoline compounds. Agents that modulate the function of these cells within the mucosal microenvironment will thus be of considerable interest for the development of vaccines against mucosal infection.

MUCOSAL VACCINATION WITH CHOLERA TOXIN B SUBUNIT IN HUMANS

CT is the enterotoxin causing severe diarrhea in cholera disease. It consists of a pentamer of B subunits (CTB) associated with a single toxic A subunit (CTA). CTB binds specifically to GM1 ganglioside receptors expressed on most nucleated cells and especially on mucosal epithelial cells, and facilitates the entry of CTA. CTA ADP-ribosylates the Gs protein of adenylate cyclase leading to increased cAMP production in the target cell (de Haan and Hirst, 2000).

CT is an exceptionally potent mucosal immunogen and one of the strongest immune adjuvants known to this day. The toxicity of CT has however precluded its use in human vaccines. Instead, the non-toxic CTB has been extensively used as a mucosal immunogen in humans without any side-effects. Indeed, recombinantly produced CTB is an important component of the oral cholera vaccine (Dukoral®, SBL Vaccin, Sweden), which also contains inactivated cholera vibrios (Holmgren and Svennerholm, 1998; WHO, 2001). This vaccine has proven to be safe and immunogenic in both adults and children. Thus, when given in two or three oral doses, the cholera vaccine has been found to stimulate the same levels of intestinal IgA antitoxin and antibacterial antibodies as seen in convalescents from cholera disease. It also induces long-lasting (more than 5 years) immunologic memory in the intestinal mucosa. A high protective efficacy of the vaccine has been documented, reaching 85% for the first 6 months after vaccination, and remaining at above 60% for at least 2 years in vaccinated adults and children above 5 years of age. In children below age 5, who are particularly vulnerable to severe cholera disease, the short-term efficacy of the vaccine is very high (100% for the first 6 months when tested in a field trial in Bangladesh), but wanes more rapidly than in older children.

Based on its excellent records in terms of safety and immunogenicity in humans when given by the oral route, CTB has also been tested in humans as a probe to evaluate alternative routes of mucosal administration. Indeed, much of our current knowledge of the anatomical dissemination of mucosal immune responses after different routes of immunization has emerged from studies in human volunteers given CTB by the oral, intratonsillar, nasal, rectal, and vaginal routes. Altogether, these studies have indicated that the so-called 'common mucosal immune system' (McDermott and Bienenstock, 1979) exhibits a certain degree of anatomical compartmentalization. Indeed, such studies have clearly shown that the strongest response usually takes place at the site of vaccine exposure and the next best responses at adjacent mucosae or at specifically interconnected inductive-expression mucosal sites such as the gut–mammary gland–salivary glands axis (Czerkinsky and Holmgren, 1995). However, a notable exception is the fact that nasal immunization not only evokes an immune response in the nasal and in the lower respiratory tract mucosa but also in the genital tract mucosa (Rudin *et al.*, 1998; Johansson *et al.*, 2001). Interestingly, in contrast with the intestinal immune response to oral vaccination with CTB, which was maximal already 2 weeks after immunization, both the local specific IgA and IgG antibody response in nasal secretions after intranasal vaccination increased for a period of 6–12 months after vaccination (Rudin *et al.*, 1998). Mucosal vaccination studies with CTB have further shown that for the induction of an immune response in the genital tract, both nasal and vaginal vaccination are effective in stimulating local genital antibody formation in women. However, the response to the vaginal immunization is also more prominent in the cervix and is highly dependent on when in the menstruation cycle the vaccine is given (Johansson *et al.*, 2001). In contrast, nasal vaccination with CTB evoked only modest cervical responses but was superior to vaginal immunization for inducing a specific IgA response in vaginal secretions. Vaginal and nasal vaccinations both resulted in significant IgA and IgG anticholera toxin B subunit responses in serum. A combination of nasal and vaginal vaccination might thus be the best vaccination strategy for inducing protective antibody responses in both cervical and vaginal secretions, provided that the vaginal vaccination is given at optimal times during the menstruation cycle.

CTB has also been used as a model vaccine in a study showing that topical rectal immunization in humans is highly effective in inducing a strong local-rectal immune response (Jertborn et al., 2001). All volunteers responded to the rectal immunization with increases in CTB-specific IgA antibody titer in rectal secretions and displayed serum IgG antibody responses.

Thus, collectively the results of these and several other studies indicate that oral, nasal, vaginal or rectal immunization in humans with CTB, and probably also with other vaccine-relevant immunogens linked to CTB, could work to elicit local mucosal IgA and IgG immune responses and thus to bring about effective immunity at the respective mucosal portal of entry for specific pathogens.

BACTERIAL TOXINS AND DERIVATIVES AS MUCOSAL ADJUVANTS

Besides being strong mucosal immunogens, both CT and LT are powerful mucosal adjuvants. They strongly potentiate the immunogenicity of most other antigens, whether these are linked to or simply coadministered. These effects, which alone or in combination might explain their strong adjuvant action after mucosal immunization, include: (1) increased permeability of the epithelium leading to enhanced uptake of coadministered antigen; (2) promotion of isotype differentiation in B cells leading to increased IgA formation; (3) complex stimulatory as well as inhibitory effects on mucosal T cell subsets; (4) modulation of antigen presentation by various APCs; and, most probably linked to the latter effect; and (5) abrogation of mucosal tolerance to coadministered antigens (Holmgren et al., 1993; Lycke, 1997).

Among these many effects, those leading to enhanced antigen presentation by various APCs are probably of the greatest importance for the adjuvant activity. CT markedly increases antigen presentation by dendritic cells (DCs), macrophages and B cells and has also been claimed, at least in vitro, to render intestinal epithelial cells effective APCs. Consistent with this activity, CT up-regulates the expression of MHC/HLA-DR molecules, CD80/B7.1 and CD86/B7.2 costimulatory molecules as well as chemokine receptors such as CCR7 and CXCR4 on both murine and human DCs and other APCs, including B cells (Gagliardi et al., 2002). Importantly, CT also induces the secretion of IL-1β from DCs (Eriksson et al., 2003). thus supporting similar observations made earlier for macrophages. IL-1 not only induces the maturation of DCs, but is also by itself an efficient mucosal adjuvant when coadministered with protein antigens (Staats and Ennis, 1999) and might thus contribute a significant part of CT adjuvanticity.

It has also been claimed that CT preferentially induces Th2 type immune responses characterized by CD4[+] T cells producing IL-4, IL-5, IL-6 and IL-10 and by the production of IgA, IgG1 and IgE antibodies. LT, on the other hand, has been reported to induce a mixed Th1- and Th2-type immune response. However, other studies have shown that also CT can induce mixed Th1- and Th2-types of immune responses, in contrast to CTB, which appears to induce a more restricted Th2 type of immune response (Eriksson et al., 2003). Thus, DCs which had been pre-treated in vitro with a protein antigen (ovalbumin, OVA) linked to or admixed with CT and then injected into mice in an antigen-specific manner induced both Th1 and CTL responses in addition to a Th2 response. In contrast, DCs pulsed *in vitro* with OVA linked to CTB only gave rise to a Th2 type of immune response. Interestingly, and consistent with these observations, infusion of DCs pulsed with a conjugate consisting of a CTL epitope linked to CT induced CTL responses and rejection of a tumor expressing this same epitope in recipient mice (Eriksson *et al.*, 2004).

DEVELOPMENT OF NON-TOXIC ENTEROTOXIN DERIVATIVES AS MUCOSAL ADJUVANTS

To avoid toxicity, isolated CTB and LTB have been explored for their ability to augment immune responses to coadministered antigens. However, their capacity to serve as mucosal adjuvants has proven to be much less impressive than corresponding holotoxins. Indeed, both CTB and LTB are poor adjuvants when given to animals together with non-coupled antigens by the oral route, although they display a more significant adjuvant activity when administered nasally. Mice vaccinated intranasally with influenza virus HA vaccine together with LTB had higher levels of antiviral IgA and IgG both in sera and in nasal or lung secretions compared with mice given the subunit vaccine alone, and were also protected against an intranasal viral challenge (Haan *et al.*, 2001). Adjuvanticity of CTB or LTB is much improved when coupled to antigens, due to the increased uptake of coupled antigen across the mucosal barrier and its more efficient targetting of DCs, macrophages and B cells (George-Chandy *et al.*, 2001; Eriksson *et al.*, 2003).

Recently, site-directed mutagenesis has permitted the generation of LT and CT mutants with reduced toxicity, but which retain significant adjuvanticity when given to animals by the nasal mucosal route or, even though they then perform less well, by the oral route (Pizza *et al.*, 2001). Two such mutants, LTK63 and LTK72, are currently evaluated as adjuvants for intranasally administered influenza vaccine (Chong *et al.*, 1998; A. Podda *et al.*, unpublished).

Another approach that is being explored to circumvent the harmful drawbacks of CT or LT adjuvants is to link the enzymatically active A subunit domain of the toxin to a cell-binding moiety other than the natural B subunit, such as the cell-binding domain of *Staphylococcus aureus* protein A (CTA1-DD) (Agren *et al.*, 1999). CTA1-DD, like most other toxin derivates, functions when applied nasally but not when given orally. This limitation has recently been overcome by the incorporation of CTA1-DD fused to a short peptide into immune stimulating complexes (ISCOMS). Oral vaccination with the ISCOM-CTA1–DD complex-induced systemic and mucosal responses with both Th1 and Th2 characteristics (Mowat *et al.*, 2001).

To achieve detoxification of CT, yet another type of mutants was recently developed in which peptides are added to the CTA1 amino end. The added peptides seem to reduce both enterotoxicity and ADP-ribosylating activity, probably by steric hindrance of the CTA1 active site (Sanchez *et al.*, 2002). In general, in these (like in all other detoxified) constructs, adjuvanticity is decreased with the loss of enterotoxicity/ADP-ribosylation activity. However, a mutant (eCT6), with 10 to 20-fold lower enterotoxicity, displayed a level of adjuvanticity comparable to that of the wild type CT. Another mutant with a longer peptide linked to CTA1 (eCT23) and no detectable toxic activity, although being also much less potent in adjuvant activity than either CT or eCT6, was nevertheless superior to CTB both as a mucosal immunogen per se and as an adjuvant for a coadministered antigen.

TOLL-LIKE RECEPTOR LIGANDS AS MUCOSAL ADJUVANTS
The innate immune system recognizes conserved motifs in pathogens termed PAMPs through Toll-like receptors (TLRs) (Medzhitov and Janeway, 2000). Ligation of TLRs by PAMPs triggers a signaling pathway involving activation of MAP kinases, subsequent nuclear translocation of active NF-kappa B leading to expression of proinflammatory genes (Aderem and Ulevitch, 2000). Based on this, it seems an attractive strategy for vaccine and immunotherapy purposes to trick the immune system to react to TLR ligands in the same way as it naturally responds to a real infectious pathogen, e.g. by using the TLR9 ligand CpG DNA, or recently discovered novel TLR7/8 ligands. As described below, recent work, both by us and by others, has shown that these ligands, when administered at mucosal surfaces, can strongly stimulate innate and adaptive immunity in mucosal tissues.

Toll-like receptor 9 ligands (immunostimulatory CpG DNA) as mucosal adjuvants
The concept of immunostimulatory DNA was born nearly 2 decades ago when Tokunaga *et al.* described that DNA purified from BCG inhibited the growth of various syngeneic animal tumors, augmented NK cell activity and induced IFN-α/β and -γ from mouse spleen cells and human peripheral blood lymphocytes (Tokunaga *et al.*, 1984). Since then, a series of studies conducted by several laboratories has revealed that unmethylated cytidine-phosphate-guanosine (CpG) with appropriate flanking regions (CpG motifs) are responsible for the stimulatory effects of bacterial DNA on vertebrate immune systems (Krieg, 2002). The fact that CpG motifs are underrepresented and methylated in vertebrate DNA suggests that the CpG motifs may serve as a 'danger signal' to the immune system. Interactions between unmethylated CpG motifs in bacterial DNA or synthetic oligodeoxynucleotides (ODN) stimulate dendritic cells and macrophages through the Toll/IL-1-receptor signaling pathway to produce Th1 cytokines such as IFN-γ, IL-1β and IL-12. Further, such interactions upregulate costimulatory molecules on APCs, and promote B cell proliferation and differentiation in antibody-forming cells (Wagner, 2002).

Parental delivery of immunostimulatory CpG DNA, in the absence of antigen, has been demonstrated to induce non-specific Th1-like innate immune responses which were associated with partial protection against challenge with *Plasmodium yoelii*, *Listeria monocytogenes*, and *Leishmania major*. This conceptual framework was extended to mucosal innate immunity by our recent findings that a single vaginal administration of immunostimulatory CpG ODN, in the absence of any antigen, elicits rapid production of Th1-associated cytokines IFN-γ, IL-12, and IL-18 and CC chemokines RANTES, MIP-1α, and MIP-1β in the murine female genital tract and/or in the draining genital lymph nodes (Harandi *et al.*, 2003). Further, such treatment led to lymph node enlargement associated with marked increases in numbers of B cells, NK cells, NKT cells, and T cells in the genital lymph nodes in the absence of any appreciable changes in either size or cell contents of the spleen, reflecting the local/regional nature of the response. Importantly, a single vaginal dose of CpG ODN, in the absence of any exogenous viral antigen, elicited protective immunity against genital herpes infection and disease and the observed protection further led to the development of specific memory responses conferring complete protection against reinfection.

In this context, it is also noteworthy that infection of CD4$^+$ T cells by HIV-1 can be antagonized by RANTES, MIP-1α, and MIP-1β, the natural ligands of the HIV coreceptor CCR5 (Cocci *et al.*, 1995), i.e. by CC chemokines that we found were strongly increased in the female genital tract mucosa after topical treatment with CpG ODN. In this respect, nasal immunization with inactivated human immunodeficiency virus plus CpG oligodeoxynucleotides was shown to induce genital immune responses and protection against intravaginal challenge (Dumais *et al.*, 2002). These findings warrant further exploration of immunostimulatory CpG DNA for mucosal-vaginal administration as a novel strategy to elicit innate protective immunity against other sexually transmitted infections such as HIV and HPV infections.

Recently, orally administered immunostimulatory CpG DNA without any bacterial antigen codelivery has been shown to elicit innate immunity in the murine gastrointestinal tract mucosa. Thus, intragastric administration of CpG ODN to mice was found to induce strong local production of CC chemokines RANTES, MIP-1α and MIP-1β and CXC chemokine IP-10 in the stomach and/or intestine. Further, intragastric delivery of CpG ODN, but not non-CpG control ODN, in the absence of any exogenous bacterial antigen suppressed bacterial colonization in the stomach of mice with an already established *Helicobacter pylori* infection (S. Raghavan *et al.*, unpublished).

In addition to its impact on innate mucosal immune response, several immunostimulatory features of CpG DNA, including the generation of a Th1-like cytokine milieu, an antiapoptotic effect on B cells and DCs, and upregulation of costimulatory molecules expression on APCs, suggest that CpG DNA could also be efficient as a vaccine adjuvant. The vast majority of studies using CpG DNA as adjuvant have been carried out with a systemic route of administration. However, an early study had shown that mucosal immunization with CpG DNA coadministered with influenza virus vaccine evoked both mucosal and systemic virus-specific immune responses (Moldoveanu *et al.*, 1998). Intranasal codelivery of CpG DNA with specific antigens has proven to be effective for inducing protective immunity in remote mucosal tissues such as the murine female genital tract (Dumais *et al.*, 2002; Gallichan *et al.*, 2001). Further, the efficacy of CpG DNA as a mucosal adjuvant for vaccination has been documented in primate and non-primate systems with other pathogen-related antigens (Holmgren *et al.*, 2003).

TLR7/8 ligands imidazoquinolines as mucosal adjuvants

The imidazoquinoline compounds, of which imiquimod, formulated as Aldara™, is the best characterized to date, act by activating macrophages and dendritic cells via binding to cell surface receptors, such as Toll receptor 7 and/or TLR 8, thereby inducing production of proinflammatory cytokines, mainly interferon (IFN)-alpha, tumour necrosis factor (TNF)-alpha, GM-CSF, G-CSF, IL-1, IL-6, and IL-12. This locally biased Th1 cytokine milieu favors cell-mediated immune responses with the generation of cytotoxic effectors, and this has been exploited clinically in the treatment of viral infections (human papillomavirus, herpes simplex virus, molluscum contagiosum) and skin cancer (Miller *et al.*, 1999; Harrison *et al.*, 2001; Dockrell *et al.*, 2001; Hemmi *et al.*, 2002; Stanley, 2002). Imiquimod has been shown to be effective in clearing genital warts, and this is related to its ability to generate proinflammatory cytokines and a Th1 response. Thus, topical administration of TLR7/TLR8 ligand imiquimod or resiquimod represents a new approach for the treatment of viral diseases at the site of mucocutaneous entry. These compounds also have adjuvant properties which have been documented in animal models and in a recent clinical trial and could thus significantly enhance conventional mucosal vaccine strategies.

MUCOSAL IMMUNOTHERAPY BASED ON CHOLERA TOXIN B SUBUNIT

As mentioned previously, mucosal tolerance is a mechanism whereby the immune system refrains from responding to the plethora of harmless antigens from food, commensal microorganisms and airborne antigens that regularly encounter mucosal surfaces. This permits mammals to coexist with their normal flora and to absorb large amounts of foreign proteins without responding with potentially harmful systemic immune responses. Although described in scientific journals as far back as in the turn of the twentieth century and utilized empirically (as antidote) even in the Antiquity, the immunological basis of this phenomenon is not fully understood. At least three different mechanisms which may coexist have been described: (1) ignorance of the antigen by the immune system; (2) anergy or deletion of antigen-specific T cells; and/or (3) the generation of regulatory T cells that down-modulate the inflammatory response (Faria and Weiner, 1999). Thus, various mucosally delivered 'vaccines' that mimic the natural induction of oral tolerance could potentially be useful as prophylactic or therapeutic treatments for various allergic and other inflammatory diseases. However, just as for the induction of mucosal immune responses, mucosal tolerance requires large (alimentary) quantities of tolerogens. Furthermore, even when administered repeatedly and using massive doses, these tolerogens are not very effective in suppressing an established state of systemic immunity. It is therefore not too surprising that the clinical testing of this concept in patients with autoimmune diseases has largely failed to show significant effect over that of placebo in large multicenter trials. It appears clear that, just as adjuvants are required for effective induction of mucosal immunity, there is a need for delivery systems and/or appropriate adjuvants to efficiently promote mucosal tolerance for immunotherapeutic applications.

Studies that we initiated 10 years ago have shown that physical coupling of selected antigens to CTB led to unexpected effects; when given by various mucosal routes (nasal, oral, rectal), CTB induced a strong mucosal IgA immune response to itself and in some cases also to the conjugated antigen, but instead of abrogating systemic tolerance like CT or LT, enhanced it profoundly (Sun et al., 1994).

Since then, CTB has emerged as the most promising combined mucosal antigen delivery and adjuvant system for inducing peripheral T cell tolerance. The use of antigen coupled to CTB has been found to minimize by several hundred-fold the amount of antigen/tolerogen and to drastically reduce the number of doses that would otherwise be required by reported protocols of orally induced tolerization. Further, and most important, at divergence from the use of free antigen, CTB-linked antigens have been shown to work also in an already sensitized individual (Czerkinsky et al., 1999). Below we will summarize the results of studies using this approach as a means to prevent or treat pathological immune responses associated with experimental autoimmune diseases, type I allergies, and allograft rejection.

TREATMENT OF AUTOIMMUNE DISEASES

Mucosal administration of relevant autoantigens linked to CTB could inhibit the development of clinical disease in animal models of experimentally inducible autoimmune diseases, such as allergic encephalomyelitis (Sun et al., 1996; Sun et al., 2000b), autoimmune diabetes (Bergerot et al., 1997; Arakawa et al., 1998) and collagen-induced arthritis (Tarkowski et al., 1999). In the latter model, nasal administration of a collagen type II–CTB conjugate could inhibit disease progression, even when treatment was initiated after onset of clinically overt disease. Similarly, oral treatment of female NOD mice with a CTB–insulin conjugate could suppress autoimmune type I diabetes even when given at a time when all mice had developed insulitis (Bergerot *et al.*, 1997). Taken together, these observations indicate that CTB-driven mucosal tolerance can affect not only the afferent but also the efferent phase of systemic T-cell-mediated inflammatory responses.

A particularly interesting recent development in the field of oral tolerance induction with CTB-antigen conjugates relates to work indicating that oral treatment with a disease-specific human heat-shock protein 60 (HSP60) derived peptide linked to CTB can suppress uveitis and other inflammatory manifestations in patients with Beçhet's disease (BD) (Stanford *et al.*, unpublished). BD patients have T cells reacting with a specific peptide (p336–351) within HSP60. Systemic or mucosal immunization with this peptide can induce uveitis in rats, and recent work has shown that such experimentally induced uveitis could efficiently be prevented by oral tolerization with the specific peptide linked to CTB (Phillips *et al.*, 2003). This has led us to test this strategy for treatment of BD in humans in a phase I-II clinical trial (M.R. Stanford *et al.*, unpublished). Oral administration of a CTB–BD peptide conjugate, three times weekly, had no adverse effects and enabled gradual withdrawal of immunosuppressive drugs in five out of eight unselected patients with BD, without any relapse of uveitis. Indeed, relapse of uveitis was prevented after complete withdrawal of existing immunosuppressive treatment in four of five patients, in whom such a treatment had maintained the patient in clinical remission prior to initiating the tolerizing regime. Most strikingly, remission has been maintained up to 1 year following withdrawal of the peptide–CTB treatment, without a need for any systemic immunosuppressive drug. Associated with the control of uveitis in the BD patients was a lack of peptide-specific CD4$^+$ T cell proliferation. This study is the first instance where mucosal tolerization with a CTB-specific antigen conjugate has been tested in humans. The promising results of this study clearly need to be confirmed by a placebo controlled phase III trial. However, if the efficacy of the peptide–CTB oral tolerance treatment observed here were to be confirmed, this novel treatment strategy may be applicable generally to autoimmune diseases in which oral tolerization with the specific antigen alone has not been effective.

PREVENTION OF GRAFT REJECTION
By coupling thymocytes to cholera B subunit and feeding this conjugate to mice, it has been possible to significantly prolong the survival of transplanted hearts in allogeneic mouse recipients (Sun *et al.*, 2000a). Similarly, feeding CTB-derivatized keratinocytes has been shown to prevent corneal allograft rejection in mice (Ma *et al.*, 1998).

PREVENTION OF TYPE I ALLERGIES
The possibility of preventing type I allergic reactions by mucosal administration of a prototype allergen (ovalbumin, OVA) linked to CTB or LTB has also recently been examined in a mouse model of ovalbumin (OVA)-induced allergic reactions. Thus, mice nasally administered with OVA conjugated to *E. coli* LTB prior to allergic sensitization showed suppressed skin DTH responses to OVA and also suppressed serum IgE antibody responses to the inhaled allergen (Tamura *et al.*, 1997). Further, these mice showed markedly decreased anaphylactic responses to intravenously administered OVA. Similar findings were made with orally administered OVA linked to CTB (Rask *et al.*, 2000). Together with results from measurement of different cytokines, the latter observations

indicate that under certain conditions, mucosal administration of soluble protein together with CTB or LTB can suppress both systemic Th1- and Th2-driven responses. The fact that the same type of regimen is also known to favour S-IgA responses in mucosal tissues makes this concept even more attractive since IgA is know to be non-phlogistic and could theoretically outcompete IgE for binding to a given allergen. However, it should also be pointed out that suppression of Th2-driven responses such as IgE antibody responses appears considerably more difficult to achieve than corresponding Th1 responses (e.g. DTH) in an animal already systemically sensitized to the allergen; in the latter situation, mucosal treatment with CTB-conjugated allergen required prolonged administration of the conjugate and was effective only with certain allergens.

MODE OF ACTION OF CTB IN INDUCTION OF ORAL TOLERANCE
Depending on the nature of the conjugated antigen, the route of administration (oral, nasal) of the conjugate, and the animal species used, treatment with CTB–antigen conjugates variably affected the capacity of T cells to produce Th1 or Th2 cytokines. The most striking observation in all models of autoimmune diseases tested so far was the finding that treatment with CTB–antigen suppressed leukocyte infiltration into the target organ. This suggests that the mechanisms governing induction of tolerance by feeding or inhaling CTB-linked antigens may involve modifications of the migratory behaviour of inflammatory cells.

The specific mechanisms involved in the strong enhancement of oral tolerance by CTB–antigen conjugates are complex and may include: (1) increased uptake of tolerizing antigen across the mucosal surface; (2) increased high affinity delivery of both specific antigen and CTB to the relevant mucosal APCs; and (3) a direct immunomodulatory effect of bound CTB on these APCs. Effective treatment with different CTB–antigen conjugates or fusion proteins are associated with the development of actively tolerogenic APCs as well as of TGF-β-secreting suppressive-regulatory T cells in mucosal tissues and draining lymph nodes (Sun *et al.*, 2000b; Anjuere *et al.*, unpublished).

Furthermore, tolerization also results in a local down-regulation in the target tissue of certain chemokines, such as MCP-1 and RANTES, known to selectively promote both the attraction and differentiation of inflammatory-pathogenic Th1 cells (Sun *et al.*, 2000b). CTB has also been shown to be anti-inflammatory *per se*. Oral feeding of CTB both prevents and cures Th1-driven experimental colitis induced by an hapten in mice, through an unidentified mechanism involving a reduced production of IL-12 within the large bowel (Boirivant *et al.*, 2001).

MUCOSAL VACCINES FOR SIMULTANEOUS INDUCTION OF ANTI-INFECTIOUS AND ANTI-PATHOLOGICAL IMMUNITY
Vaccinologists have usually believed that a reciprocal relationship exists between induction of immunity and tolerance. The observation that secretory IgA antibodies may develop concomitantly with systemic immunological tolerance contradicts this notion and has led to the belief that vaccines against mucosal pathogens should primarily stimulate immunity without inducing tolerance. It is clear that such goal must be met if one were to develop a mucosal vaccine against an invasive microbial pathogen such as HIV or *Salmonella*.

However, from a theroretical standpoint, the possibility to manipulate the mucosal immune system towards both immunity and tolerance appears especially attractive to design strategies aimed at protecting the host from colonization or invasion by mucosal pathogens. It also might allow to interfere with the development of potentially harmful systemic immunological reactions against the same pathogens or their products.

The notion that immunological tolerance may provide the host with a protective mechanism against an infectious disease has been elegantly illustrated by recent studies in transgenic mice. Whereas mice with a susceptible (BALB/c) background develop an early Th2-driven IL-4 response and ultimately succumb to an infection with *Leishmania major*, mice rendered tolerant by transgenic expression in the thymus of LACK, a protective surface antigen of *Leishmania*, fail to produce this early response and resolve their infection. Importantly, tolerization of post-thymic, mature parasite-specific T cells could also be accomplished in the periphery after nasal administration of as little as 10 µg of *L. major* LACK antigen conjugated to CTB (McSorley *et al.*, 1998). Such treatment markedly delayed the onset of lesion development in infected mice and reduced parasite burden in the skin and draining lymph nodes of infected mice.

Similar findings have been made in mice that had already been infested with the parasitic trematode, *Schistosoma mansoni* and treated with a CTB–parasite conjugate vaccine (Sun *et al.*, 1999; Lebens *et al.*, 2001). Thus, nasal treatment of mice with *S. mansoni* glutathione S-transferase (GST) or defined GST peptides conjugated to CTB suppressed granuloma formation and decreased parasite burden and egg deposition in the liver of infested animals. Protection with this nasal CTB–GST vaccine was associated with decreased hepatic production of IFN-γ, IL-5 and IL-3 but apparently intact IL-4 production. Most importantly, such treatment could significantly prolong the survival of parasitized animals, even when initiated as late as 6 weeks after initial infection, that is at a time when liver granulomatous reactions are most pronounced (Sun *et al.*, 2001).

While this type of approach has only been attempted in two parasitic diseases, there are obvious diseases caused by microbial pathogens (who use mucosal membranes as their portals for entry) that could theoretically benefit from the induction of S-IgA immune responses and a concomitant downregulation of T-cell-driven immunopathology. Examples of such diseases include gastroduodenal ulcers caused by *Helicobacter pylori*, genital ulcers caused by papillomaviruses, bronchopneumonitis induced by parainfluenzae viruses and respiratory syncytial virus, or chronic pelvic inflammatory diasease, trachoma and urethritis caused by *Chlamydia pneumoniae*.

CONCLUSIONS

The last decade has brought much progress in the development of especially CTB but also LTB as mucosal vaccine immunogens protecting against cholera and/or ETEC diarrhea as well as serving as model immunogens in humans for studying immune responses in different mucosal tissues after oral, nasal, vaginal or rectal immunizations. Together with findings showing that CTB or LTB can also serve as efficient mucosal carriers for inducing mucosal immune responses to various antigens or peptides chemically linked to or genetically fused to CTB/LTB it seems likely that mucosal vaccines against various microbial pathogens may be developed based on CTB or LTB, or analogues as vectors. Significant progress has also been made in developing detoxified CT and LT molecules that display adjuvant activity with little or no toxicity. Based on the rapid pace of investigation in the field, it seems likely that the future holds much promise for the detoxified CT and LT derivatives in the realm of mucosal adjuvants for human use.

The discovery of PAMPs as potential ligands for TLRs has made a strong impact also in the field of mucosal immunomodulators and adjuvants. Among the

PAMPs, bacterial immunostimulatory CpG DNA, a TLR9 ligand, shows especially promising immunomodulating activity at mucosal surfaces. Recently, also non-PAMP imidazoquinoline compounds, which are TLR7/8 ligands, have been identified as powerful immunostimulators/adjuvants on genital tract immune responses. Based on this it seems likely that future investigation of both PAMP and non-PAMP TLR ligands will continue to be a fruitful area of research for development of novel mucosal immunomodulators and adjuvants.

Finally, the prospects for using CTB (or LTB) for inducing so-called oral tolerance to various chemically linked or genetically fused organ-specific antigens or selected allergens for immunotherapeutic purposes has taken a big step forward with the proof of concept obtained in a first clinical trial in patients with Beçhet's disease. If the promising results of this study are confirmed, this novel strategy may find broad medical indications, ranging from allergic disorders to autoimmune diseases in which oral tolerization with specific antigens given alone has proven to be ineffective.

References

Aderem, A., and Ulevitch, R. (2000). Toll-like receptors in the induction of the innate immune response. Nature 406: 782–787.

Agren, L.C., Ekman, L., Lowenadler, B., Nedrud, J.G., and Lycke, N. 1999. Adjuvanticity of the cholera toxin A1-based gene fusion protein, CTA1-DD, is critically dependent on the ADP-ribosyltransferase and Ig-binding activity. J. Immunol. 162: 2432–2440.

Arakawa, T., Yu, J., Chong, D.K., Hough, J., Engen, P.C., and Langridge, W.H. 1998. A plant-based cholera toxin B subunit-insulin fusion protein protects against the development of autoimmune diabetes. Nature Biotechnol. 16: 934–938.

Bergerot, I., Ploix, C., Petersen, J. et al. 1997. A cholera toxoid-insulin conjugate as an oral vaccine against spontaneous autoimmune diabetes. Proc. Natl. Acad. Sci. USA 94: 4610–4614.

Boirivant, M., Fuss, U., Ferroni, L., De Pascale, M., and Strober, W. 2001. Oral administration of recombinant cholera toxin subunit B inhibits IL-12-mediated murine experimental (trinitrobenzene sulfonic acid) colitis. J. Immunol. 166: 3522–3532.

Chong, C., Friberg, M., and Clements, J.D. 1998. LT (R192G), a non-toxic mutant of the heat-labile enterotoxin of Escherichia coli, elicits enhanced humoral and cellular immune responses associated with protection against lethal oral challenge with Salmonella spp. Vaccine 16: 732–740.

Cocchi, F., DeVico, A.L., Garzino-Demo, A, Arya, S.K., Gallo, R.C., and Lusso, P., 1995. Identification of RANTES, MIP-1 alpha, and MIP-1 beta as the major HIV-suppressive factors produced by CD8[+] T cells. Science 270: 1811–1815.

Czerkinsky, C., and Holmgren, J., 1995. The mucosal immune system and prospects for anti-infectious and anti-inflammatory vaccines. Immunologist 3: 97–103.

Czerkinsky, C., Anjuere, F., McGhee, J.R., et al. 1999. Mucosal immunity and tolerance: relevance to vaccine development. Immunol. Rev. 170: 197–222.

de Haan, L., and Hirst, T.R. 2000. Cholera toxin and related enterotoxins: a cell biological and immunological perspective. J. Nature Toxins 9: 281–297.

Dumais, N., Patrick, A., Moss, R.B., Davis, H.L., and Rosenthal, .KL. 2002. Mucosal immunization with inactivated human immunodeficiency virus plus CpG oligodeoxynucleotides induces genital immune responses and protection against intravaginal challenge. J. Infect. Dis. 186: 1098–1105.

Dockrell, D., and Kinghorn, G. 2001. Imiquimod and resiquimod as novel immunomodulators. J. Antimicrob. Chemother. 48: 751–755.

Eriksson, K., Fredriksson, M., Nordström, I., and Holmgren, J. 2003. Cholera toxin and its B subunit promote dendritic cell vaccination with different influence on Th1/Th2 development. Infect. Immun. 71: 1740–1747.

Eriksson, K., Sun, J.B., Nordstrom, I., Fredriksson, M., Lindblad, M., Li, B.L., and Holmgren, J. 2004. Coupling of antigen to cholera toxin for dendritic cell vaccination promotes the induction of MHC class I-restricted cytotoxic T cells and the rejection of a cognate antigen-expressing model tumor. Eur. J. Immunol. 34: 1272–1281.

Faria, A.M and Weiner, H.L. 1999. Oral tolerance: mechanisms and therapeutic applications. Adv. Immunol. 73: 153–264.

Gagliardi, M., Sallusto, F., Marinaro, M., Vendetti, S., Riccomi, A., and De Magistris, M. 2002. Effects of the adjuvant cholera toxin on dendritic cells: stimulatory and inhibitory signals that result in the amplification of immune responses. Int. J. Med. Microbiol. 291: 571–575.

Gallichan, W., Woolstencroftn R., Guarasci, T., McCluskie, M., Davis, H., and Rosenthal, K. 2001. Intranasal immunization with CpG oligodeoxynucleotides as an adjuvant dramatically increases IgA and protection against herpes simplex virus-2 in the genital tract. J. Immunol. 166: 3451–3457.

George-Chandy, A., Eriksson, K., Lebens, M., Nordstrom, I., Schon, E., and Holmgren, J. 2001. Cholera toxin B subunit as a carrier Mol.ecule promotes antigen presentation and increases CD40 and CD86 expression on antigen- presenting cells. Infect. Immun. 69: 5716–5725.

Haan, L., Verweij, W., Holtrop, M., *et al.* 2001. Nasal or intramuscular immunization of mice with influenza subunit antigen and the B subunit of *Escherichia coli* heat-labile toxin induces IgA- or IgG-mediated protective mucosal immunity. Vaccine 19: 2898–2907.

Harandi, A.M., Eriksson, K., and Holmgren, J. 2003. A protective role of locally administered immunostimulatory CpG oligodeoxynucleotide in a mouse model of genital herpes infection. J. Virol. 77: 953–962.

Harrison, C.J., Miller, R.L. and Bernstein, D.I. 2001. Reduction of recurrent HSV disease using imiquimod alone or combined with a glycoprotein vaccine. Vaccine 19: 1820–1826.

Hemmi, H., Kaisho, T., Takeuchi O., *et al.* 2002. Small anti-viral compounds activate immune cells via the TLR7 MyD88-dependent signalling pathway. Nature Immunol. 3: 196–200.

Holmgren, J., Lycke, N., and Czerkinsky, C. 1993. Cholera toxin and cholera B subunit as oral-mucosal adjuvant and antigen vector system. Vaccine 11: 1179–1184.

Holmgren, J., and Svennerholm, A-M. 1998. Vaccines against diarrheal diseases. In: Handbook of Experimental Pharmacology, Vol. 133: Vaccines, Perlmann, P. and Wigzell, H. eds, Springer-Verlag, Berlin, pp. 291–328.

Holmgren, J., Harandi, AM., and Czerkinsky, C. 2003. Mucosal adjuvants and anti-infection and anti-immunopathology vaccines based on cholera toxin, cholera toxin B subunit and CpG DNA. Expert Rev. Vaccines. 2: 205–17.

Jertborn, M., Nordström, I., Kilander, A., Czerkinsky, C., and Holmgren, J. 2001. Local and systemic immune responses to rectal administration of recombinant cholera toxin B subunit in humans. Infect. Immun. 69: 4125–4128.

Johansson, E-L., Wassén, L., Holmgren, J., Jertborn, M., and Rudin, A. 2001. Nasal and vaginal vaccinations have differential effects on antibody responses in vaginal and cervical secretions in humans. Infect. Immun. 69: 7481–7486.

Krieg, A., and Davis, H. 2001. Enhancing vaccine with immune stimulatory CpG DNA. Curr. Opin. Mol. Ther. 3: 15–24.

Krieg, A.M. 2002. CpG motifs in bacterial DNA and their immune effects. Annu. Rev. Immunol. 20: 709–760.

Lebens, M., Sun, J.-B, Mielcarek N., *et al.* 2001. A mucosally administered recombinant fusion protein vaccine against schistosomiasis protecting against immunopathology and infection. Vaccine 3435: 1–7.

Lin, B-L., Sun, J.-B., and Holmgren, J. 2001. Adoptive transfer of mucosal T cells or dendritic cells from animals fed with cholera toxin B subunit alloantigen conjugate induces allogeneic T cell tolerance. Adv. Exp. Med. Biol. 495: 271–275.

Lycke, N. The mechanism of cholera toxin adjuvanticity. 1997. Res. Immunol. 148: 504–520.

Ma, D., Mellon, J., and Niederkorn, J.Y. 1998. Conditions affecting enhanced corneal allograft survival by oral immunization. Invest. Ophthalmol. Vis. Sci. 39: 1835–1846.

McCluskie, M.J., Weeratna, R.D., Krieg, A.M., and Davis, H.L. 2000. CpG DNA is an effective oral adjuvant to protein antigens in mice. Vaccine 19: 950–957.

McDermott, M.R., and Bienenstock, J. 1979. Evidence for a common mucosal Immunologic system. I. Migration of B immunoblasts into intestinal, respiratory, and genital tissues. J. Immunol. 122: 1892–1898.

McSorley, S.J., Rask, C., Pichot, R., Julia, V., Czerkinsky, C. and Glaichenhaus, N. 1998. Selective tolerization of Th1-like cells after nasal administration of a cholera toxoid-LACK conjugate. Eur. J. Immunol. 28: 44–430.

Medzhitov, R., and Janeway, C., Jr. 2000. The toll receptor family and microbial recognition. Trends Microbiol. 8: 452–456.

Miller, R., Imbertson, L., Reiter, M., and Gerster, J. 1999. Treatment of primary herpes simplex virus infection in guinea pigs by imiquimod. Antiviral Res. 44: 31–42.

Moldoveanu, Z., Love-Homan, L., Huang, W.Q., and Krieg, A.M. 1998. CpG DNA, a novel immune enhancer for systemic and mucosal immunization with influenza virus. Vaccine 16: 1216–1224.

Morris, DL. 1999. WHO position paper on oral (sublingual) immunotherapy. Ann. Allergy Asthma Immunol. 83: 423–4.

Morris, D.L., Kroker, G.F., Sabnis, V.K., and Morris, M.S. 2003. Local immunotherapy in allergy. Chem. Immunol. Allergy 82: 1–10.

Mortemousque, B., Bertel, F., De Casamayor, J., Verin, P., and Colin, J. 2003. House-dust mite sublingual-swallow immunotherapy in perennial conjunctivitis: a double-blind, placebo-controlled study. Clin. Exp. Allergy 33: 464–9.

Mowat, A.M., Donachie, A.M., Jagewall, S., *et al.* 2001. CTA1-DD-immune stimulating complexes: a novel, rationally designed combined mucosal vaccine adjuvant effective with nanogram doses of antigen. J. Immunol. 167: 3398–3405.

Passalacqua, G., Fumagalli, F., Guerra, L. and Canonica, G.W. 2003. Safety of allergen-specific sublingual immunotherapy and nasal immunotherapy. Chem. Immunol. Allergy 82: 109–18.

Pizza, M., Giuliani, M., Fontana, M., *et al.* 2001. Mucosal vaccines: non toxic derivatives of LT and CT as mucosal adjuvants. Vaccine 19: 2534–2541.

Phipps, P.A., Stanford, MR., Sun, J.B. *et al.* 2003. Prevention of mucosally induced uveitis with a HSP60-derived peptide linked to cholera toxin B subunit. Eur. J. Immunol. 33: 224–232.

Rask, C., Holmgren, J., Fredriksson, M., *et al.* 2000. Prolonged oral treatment with low doses of allergen conjugated to cholera toxin B subunit suppresses immonoglobulin E antibody responses in sensitized mice. Clin. Exp. Allergy 30: 1024–1032.

Rudin, A., Johansson, E.-L., Bergquist, C., Holmgren, J. 1998. Differential kinetics and distribution of antibodies in serum and nasal and vaginal secretions after nasal and oral vaccination in humans. Infect. Immun. 66: 3390–3396.

Sanchez, J., Wallerstrom, G., Fredriksson, M., Angstrom, J., and Holmgren, J. 2002. Detoxification of cholera toxin without removal of its immunoadjuvanticity by the addition of (STa-related) peptides to the catalytic subunit. A potential new strategy to generate immunostimulants for vaccination. J. Biol. Chem. 277: 33369–33377.

Staats, H.F., and Ennis, F.A., Jr. 1999. IL-1 is an effective adjuvant for mucosal and systemic immune responses when coadministered with protein immunogens. J. Immunol. 162: 6141–6147.

Stanley, M.A. 2002. Imiquimod and the imidazoguinolones: mechanism of action and therapeutic potential. Clin. Exp. Dermatol. 27: 571–577.

Sun, J.-B., Holmgren, J., and Czerkinsky, C. 1994. Cholera toxin B subunit: An efficient transmucosal carrier-delivery system for induction of peripheral Immunological tolerance. Proc. Natl. Acad. Sci. USA 91: 10795–10799.

Sun, JB., Rask, C., Olsson, T., Holmgren, J., and Czerkinsky, C. 1996. Treatment of experimental autoimmune encephalomyelitis by feeding myelin basic protein conjugated to cholera toxin B subunit. Proc. Natl. Acad. Sci. USA 93: 7196–7201.

Sun, J.-B., Mielcarek, N., Lakew, M., *et al.* 1999. Intranasal administration of a *Schistosoma mansoni* glutathione S-transferase-cholera toxoid conjugate vaccine evokes antiparasitic and antipathological immunity in mice. J. Immunol. 163: 1045–1052.

Sun, J.-B., Li, B.-L., Czerkinsky, C., and Holmgren, J. 2000a. Enhanced immunological tolerance against allograft rejection by oral administration of allogeneic antigen linked to cholera toxin B subunit. J. Clin. Immunol. 97: 130–139.

Sun, J.-B., Xiao B.-G., Lindblad, M. *et al.* 2000b. Oral administration of cholera toxin B subunit conjugated to myelin basic protein protects against experimental autoimmune encephalomyelitis by inducing transforming growth factor-β-secreting cells and suppressing chemokine expression. Int. Immunol. 12: 1449–1457.

Sun, J.-B., Stadecker, M.J., Mielcarek, N., *et al.* 2001. Nasal administration of *Schistosoma mansoni* egg antigen-cholera B subunit conjugate suppresses hepatic granuloma formation and reduces mortality in S. mansoni-infected mice. Scand. J. Immunol. 54: 440–447.

Tamura, S., Hatori, E., Tsuruhara, T., Aizawa, C., and Kurata, T. 1997. Suppression of delayed-type hypersensitivity and IgE antibody responses to ovalbumin by intranasal administration of *Escherichia coli* heat-labile enterotoxin B subunit-conjugated ovalbumin. Vaccine 15: 225–229.

Tarkowski, A., Sun, J.-B., Holmdahl, R., Holmgren, J., and Czerkinsky, C. 1999. Treatment of experimental autoimmune arthritis by nasal administration of a type II collagen-cholera toxoid conjugate vaccine. Arthritis. Rheum. 42: 1628–1634.

Tokunaga, T., Yamamoto, H., Shimada, S., *et al.* 1984. Antitumor acitivity of deoxyribonucleic acid fraction from *Mycobacterium bovis* BCG. I. Isolation, physicochemical characterization, and antitumor activity. J. Natl. Cancer Inst. 72: 955–962.

Wagner, H. 2002. Interactions between bacterial CpG-DNA and TLR9 bridge innate and adaptive immunity. Curr. Opin. Immunol. 5: 62–69.

WHO position paper: Cholera vaccines. 2001. In: Weekly Epidemiological Record. World Health Organization, Geneva, 76: 117–124.

Wu, H.Y., and Weiner, H.L. 2003. Oral tolerance. Immunol. Res. 28: 265–84.

Chapter 5

Immunization Using the Skin: New Approaches

Gregory M. Glenn, David C. Flyer, Mohammad Al-Khalili and Larry R. Ellingsworth

Abstract

The skin has a large component of immune cells, and is well equipped to detect invasion by pathogens and orchestrate vaccine responses. Notably, the gold standard, yet crude skin immunization technique is responsible for eradication of smallpox worldwide. Vaccine delivery into the skin must overcome the natural barriers to delivery and result in effective, functional immune responses. There are currently a great deal of preclinical data suggesting that this may happen for human vaccines. Clinical testing of this concept has confirmed the preclinical observations that adjuvants can be delivered to safely induce strong immune responses. In this chapter, we discuss various approaches to optimizing vaccine delivery to the skin.

INTRODUCTION

Today, most licenced vaccines are injected into the muscle. The origins of this less than optimal but proven technique are complex but lie somewhere between empiric practice, leading to convention, and a lack of understanding of the immune system. This practice, which began in the 1800s, is now being challenged by the overwhelming perception that the skin and mucosa might be superior targets for deposition of vaccine antigens, largely due to the immune defenses that are effectively used to combat the daily immune challenges at these sites.

The outermost layer of the living skin has a large component of immune cells committed to host defense against pathogens. The skin is closely juxtaposed to the microbial world and is well equipped to detect invasion by pathogens and orchestrate effective immune responses. There is some suggestion that a homeostasis exists that maintains immune health through constant challenge with skin and gut pathogens. Beyond this basal activity, the skin immune system is sensitive to the danger signals presented by microbes that trigger effective immune responses. Vaccinologists seek to replicate effective immune response to infections by presenting all or some portions of a microbe in a form that leads to protective immune responses without creating the symptoms of disease. The recent advances in characterization of the skin immune system, and the demonstration that new delivery technologies and adjuvants can take advantage of the rich populations of dendritic cells in the skin to stimulate immune responses, together suggest that skin immunization techniques will dominate new and established immunization protocols.

The gold standard skin immunization technique for smallpox involves intradermal inoculation with a bifurcated needle. A small volume of 0.0025 mL of vaccine adheres by capillary action between the tines of the needle and the skin is stroked 15 times so that a trace of blood appears at the vaccination site. This seemingly crude technique, which results in 100% vaccine uptake, is, in part, responsible for eradication of smallpox worldwide (Henderson *et al.*, 2004), and is suggestive of the promise of future skin immunization techniques.

Recent work in our laboratories and those of others has focused on vaccine delivery into the skin using a patch or similar means for vaccine delivery. The skin, as a non-invasive route for vaccine delivery, has great potential for safe use of potent immune stimulating compounds that can target the dense population of immune cells found in the skin. The use of such compounds to stimulate the skin immune system leads to strong and effective immune responses, and this immune responsiveness, in combination with an apparent high safety margin, has fostered a great deal of interest in targeting the skin with vaccines. The basic insights gained through initial studies have led to several efforts to formulate and test human use vaccines. Commercialization of skin delivery has a unique set of hurdles, however, it seems almost certain that skin delivery techniques will play an important future role.

BACKGROUND

Mammalian skin is composed of three primary layers (Figure 5.1). The stratum corneum (SC), the outermost layer of the skin, is composed of 10–20 layers of quiescent, cornified epidermal skin cells called keratinocytes that are continuously shed. During the formation of the SC, the keratinocytes secrete lipids that form a type of lipid mortar that encases the

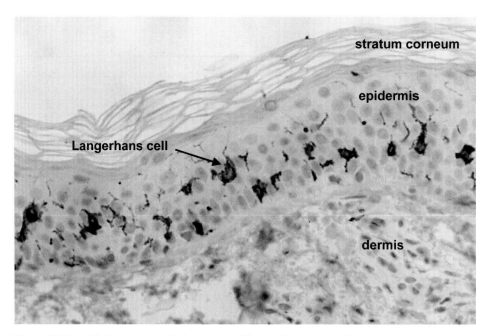

Figure 5.1 The skin is composed of three principal layers: the dermis, epidermis, and stratum corneum. Existing vaccine delivery involves perforation through the skin, bypassing the immune-rich layers of the skin. New technologies targeting the skin take advantage of the skin immune system elements, such as epidermal Langerhans cells, shown above. Adapted from Glenn GM, Taylor DN, Li X. Transcutaneous immunization: a human vaccine delivery strategy using a patch. Nature Med. 2000; 6: 1403–1406, with permission.

dead and dying keratinocytes. The human SC is 10–20 μm thick in a 'bricks and mortar' format, and represents an effective but fragile barrier to microbes, fluids and foreign material. The epidermis underlies the SC and is composed of epidermal keratinocytes and other skin elements in a continuous growing layer of epithelium. The epidermis is also a dynamic immune environment, with active traffic of immune cells in and out of the epidermis. The primary antigen-presenting cell (APC) found in the epidermis is the Langerhans cell (LC), a bone-marrow-derived dendritic cell that migrates from the bone marrow into the skin and plays the dual role of immune surveillance and antigen presentation (Jakob and Udey, 1999). Confocal microscopy in human skin demonstrated that LCs cover 25% of the total skin surface area, although they account for approximately only 1–3% of the epidermal cells (Yu et al., 1994). Their density, accessibility and antigen presentation function create an ideal target for vaccine delivery. The final layer of the skin, the dermis, supports the epidermis with connective tissue, contains the blood vessels (generally the target for transdermal drug delivery) and lymphatics, and provides a foundation for the epidermal appendages such as hair and sweat glands. The dermis contains dendritic cells (DCs) and Langerhans cells in transit, but the density of APCs in the dermis does not match that of the epidermis (Udey, 1997). Hair follicles, which extend into the dermis, have their own unique microenvironment of immune cells (Christoph et al., 2000). The normal practice of vaccine delivery by needle perforates the skin to deliver antigens to other tissues, bypassing the highly attractive skin immune system. In transcutaneous immunization, antigen and immune activating adjuvants are applied to the skin. The activated LCs take up antigen and migrate to the draining lymph node, where they orchestrate potent systemic immune responses.

OPTIMIZATION OF DELIVERY

The stratum corneum is an effective barrier to penetration of fluids, large molecules, particles and microbes. Disruption of the SC leads to greater immune responses, which are the most relevant surrogates for measuring antigen delivery. There are a variety of techniques to overcome this barrier function, including chemical and physical penetration techniques. Long-held maxims of skin penetration have stated that even with use of skin penetration techniques, delivery of drugs and bioactive molecules greater than 500 Da was not possible. However, it has become clear that these maxims were often based on transdermal delivery of drugs to the blood vessels in the dermis or due to the failure to deliver larger moieties such as insulin through the combined barrier created by the SC, epidermis, and dermis. However, vaccine antigens and adjuvants targeting the skin, defined here as transcutaneous immunization (TCI), merely require delivery to the epidermis.

The superficial nature of anatomical targets for antigen delivery suggests that few restrictions for antigen size apply to TCI. In human skin, which is the most relevant setting for testing vaccine delivery concepts, we have shown that with crude patches and minimal SC disruption, very large recombinant antigens on the order of 1,500,000 Da can be delivered to elicit strong systemic immune responses (Güereña-Burgueño et al., 2002). This study followed initial observations that the heat-labile enterotoxin of E. coli (LT) (86,000 Da) was effectively delivered through human skin by simply applying LT in wet gauze to the skin without any other manipulation (Glenn et al., 2000). Most currently licensed vaccine antigens fall within this size range, (e.g. tetanus toxoid ~ 160,000 Da). Extensive animal data has shown that whole viruses (Hammond et al., 2000), recombinants (Yu et al., 2002), and even whole bacterial cells (L.R. Ellingsworth, unpublished observations) can be effectively delivered to the skin immune system. These observations suggest that the delivery of a variety of antigens and adjuvants is feasible, but that each product will require optimization and formulation to make a commercially viable product.

Disruption of the SC is important for efficient delivery and lends itself to relatively simple techniques. Occlusion, wetting of the skin, and other methods lead to hydration of the SC. Hydration of the SC results in swelling of the keratinocytes and pooling of fluid in the intercellular spaces, leading to dramatic microscopic changes in the SC structure (Roberts and Walker, 1993) that have no lasting effect once the skin is allowed to dry. Hydrated SC clearly allows antigens to pass through the skin (Glenn *et al.*, 2000). The transit pathways utilized by antigens (as well as transdermal drugs) to traverse the SC are not well characterized. Transdermal drug delivery of polar small molecule drugs is thought to occur through aqueous intercellular channels formed between the keratinocytes in hydrated skin, and it is possible that similar pathways are engaged for antigen delivery by TCI (Roberts and Walker, 1993).

Physical and chemical penetration enhancement techniques that disrupt the integrity of the SC have also been described (Glenn and Alving, 1999b; Chen *et al.*, 2001a; Mikszta *et al.*, 2002; Glenn *et al.*, 2003a; Guebre-Xabier *et al.*, 2004). We have tested concepts with clinical relevance to patch delivery in model systems and subsequently applied them to human skin where penetration enhancement appears to represent an improvement over simple hydration of the skin. For product development, we have focused on the use of simple, inexpensive materials with clinical utility in other settings, and simple methods of use/application that lead to consistent, heightened immune responses. Device-based techniques also disrupt the SC and use various means for delivery of antigens and adjuvants into the epidermis. With the exception of gas-powered gun delivery, these techniques have not to date been proven to work in the clinic and only limited animal immunization data exists.

Modeling skin delivery of vaccines is not straightforward, as with many transdermal drugs. Hairless guinea pigs can be used to examine the effect of mild abrasives or devices to disrupt the stratum corneum, as they have an epidermis and SC that is similar in thickness to humans and have been widely used for studying penetration enhancement techniques. Biopsy of skin treated to disrupt the SC suggested that this method might aid in efficiency of antigen delivery and allow optimization and testing of agents to disrupt the SC (Glenn *et al.*, 2003a). However, the hairless guinea pig is not suitable for topical immunization studies due to the high lipid content of its skin, and thus is not useful for comparison with other pretreatment techniques such as the use of microneedles (Mikszta *et al.*, 2002). It has been suggested that hair follicles play an important role in topical administration, but this hypothesis would not explain the enhancement seen with SC disruption (discussed below). The likelihood that follicles are not significant antigen transit pathways is supported by the observation that out-bred CD1 mice with normal hair follicle development, and hairless SKH mice (same genetic background) with sparse, vestigial follicles, respond equally well to topical immunization and disruption of the SC (Glenn *et al.*, 2003a).

Although the SC is the most significant barrier to topical immunization, it is a fragile barrier that can be easily disrupted, possibly allowing antigens to more readily diffuse into the superficial epidermis. Despite the differences in the thickness of human and mouse SC and epidermis, murine studies have been remarkably predictive for human immune responses and, in conjunction with guinea pig models using histology to guide SC disruption techniques, clinically acceptable and simple SC disruption techniques have been optimized (Glenn *et al.*, 2000; Scharton-Kersten *et al.*, 2000; Güereña-Burgueño *et al.*, 2002; Yu *et al.*, 2002; Glenn *et al.*, 2003a). Disruption of the SC using mild abrasive materials is a technique used clinically for enhancing conductivity of electrical fields through the skin to record EKGs. The same materials used in conjunction with hydrating solution improve antigen delivery, creating a single simple pretreatment swab for use prior to patch placement. Studies in our laboratory have explored this concept and demonstrated its feasibility and effect on the delivery of both an antigen and adjuvant. In preclinical studies, the optimized application of a simple, wet patch compares well with the efficiency of adjuvanted, injected antigen. The effect of pretreatment in mouse models can be seen using split virus influenza vaccine (A/Panama) combined with LT applied to intact skin that has been pretreated to disrupt the SC. As illustrated in Figure 5.2, shaved but untreated mouse skin was wetted with saline, and pretreated with emery paper (EKG prep, 10 gentle strokes on wet skin) or stripped with D-Squame tape (10 applications) or 3M™ tape (10 applications). Two weeks after three topical applications, the serum antibody response to the influenza antigens was increased 100- to 300-fold when compared with hydration alone. The pretreatment techniques for SC disruption, skillfully done, are well tolerated but can be accompanied by mild, local and self-limiting rashes, and are likely to have an

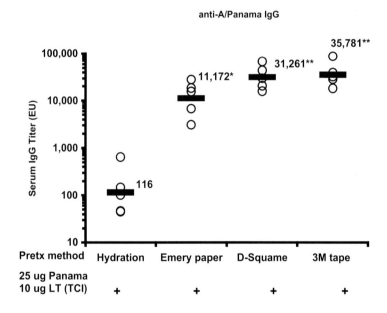

Figure 5.2 Improved topical delivery of influenza split-virus vaccine by disruption of the stratum corneum. C57Bl/6 mice were shaved on the dorsal caudal surface two days prior to topical immunization. Exposed skin was hydrated by gently rubbing (20 strokes) with a saline saturated gauze sponge. The SC was disrupted by mild abrasion with emery paper (10 strokes) or tape stripping with D-Squame (10×) or 3M™ tape (10×). A solution consisting of 25 μg A/Panama and 10 μg LT was applied to the pretreated skin for 1 hr and then washed off with warm water. Groups were immunized three times (day 0, 14 and 28) and serum collected two weeks after the third immunization on day 42. Serum antibody titers to A/Panama were determined by ELISA, and titers were reported as ELISA Units (EU). The geometric mean titer for each group is indicated. Serum elicited by hydration pretreatment was compared to antibody titers elicited by skin pretreatment with emery paper or by tape stripping. *$P = 0.012$; **$P \leq 0.006$. From Glenn GM, Kenney RT, Ellingsworth LR, *et al*. Transcutaneous immunization and immunostimulant strategies: capitalizing on the immunocompetence of the skin. Expert Rev.Vaccines 2003; 2: 253–267, with permission.

improved safety profile compared with the acceptable level of reactions that occur with parenteral immunization. When pretreatment is used, the delivery of antigen is sufficient to elicit immune responses similar to that seen with the same dose delivered by the parenteral route. As shown in Figure 5.3, mice given trivalent split virus vaccine by TCI respond equally to vaccine delivered by the i.m. route. Note also, the importance of the addition of adjuvant to achieve robust responses on the skin.

Although transdermal drug delivery developers use guinea pig or other mammalian skin equivalent models to track or quantitate the amount of drug delivered after a topical application, this may be difficult to emulate with skin immunization due to the fact that standard transdermal delivery quantitation models required drug transit through the skin into a reservoir. By contrast, transcutaneous techniques deliver antigen into the skin, likely as extremely small amounts of material, but sufficient to elicit robust immune responses. In general, vaccine antigens delivered by any route must encounter antigen-presenting cells to prime the immune response. Thus, quantitation or estimation of an antibody response might be the most relevant measurement of antigen delivery. Biodistribution of DNA vaccine delivered by gene gun into the skin lends itself to PCR analysis which is a sensitive, amplified signal for detecting delivery in pigs' skin, a relevant model for gun delivery of DNA (Pilling *et al.*, 2002). At day 2, the plasmid was detected only at the treatment site and the inguinal nodes; by day 57 it was detected only at the treatment site, and by day 141, it appeared to have cleared. These data suggest that skin delivery results in antigen localized only in the skin or draining lymph nodes (DLN). This is consistent with our findings that labeled adjuvant and antigen can only be detected in the DLN after topical application and not in distal nodes (Glenn *et al.*, 2003a; Guebre-Xabier *et al.*,

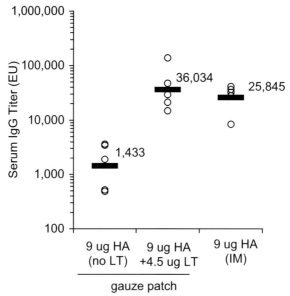

Figure 5.3 C57 BL6 mice were immunized using commercially obtained trivalent split virus influenza vaccine (Flushield) at day 0, 14 and 28. Intramuscular injection was done in the lateral thigh. Patch groups were immunized as previously described using the trivalent vaccine with or without LT applied to a gauze patch. Data shown using sera collected 2 weeks after the third immunization. Sera assayed against a single representative strain, New Caledonia, as previously described.

2003). However, more recent data suggest that some DCs loaded with adjuvant may also migrate to the mucosa in mice (Belyakov et al., in press; Enioutina et al., 2000). Nasal immunization leads to more broadly distributed plasmid (Oh et al., 2001), but the relevance of this model for human biodistribution of skin vaccination is doubtful (Zurbriggen et al., 2003).

Some early attempts to track antigen after TCI with radiolabeled cholera toxin (CT) suggested that the majority of CT remained in the skin (Glenn et al., 1999). More recently, tracking studies with fluorescently tagged antigen and adjuvant suggested that antigen delivered by simple wetting of the skin with antigen (no pretreatment) in solution in a gauze patch is somewhat less efficient at loading antigen APCs in the skin compared with direct injection. In mice injected with labeled ovalbumin (OVA) by the intradermal route (i.d.) or exposed to six times the dose in a simple topical application, the total number of labeled cells in the TCI application approximated the number seen after i.d. injection, which is in essence 'complete delivery' of antigen. With the addition of adjuvant, the number of antigen-laden APCs increases significantly both with admixture of antigen and adjuvant on the skin and with application of adjuvant in a patch over the i.d. injection. Thus, the adjuvant makes up some of the difference in efficiency due to the limitations of passive delivery where no physical or chemical disruption of the stratum corneum is used. It is also of interest that human tracking studies using radiolabeled antigen delivered by intradermal injection have shown that ~5% of the injected dose reaches the DLN (Uren et al., 2003). This suggests that despite the premise that injection represents efficient delivery of antigen, in fact, only a small portion is taken into the immune environment even after intradermal injection, which is thought to be the most efficient method for targeting antigen-presenting cells and has been posited to represent 'complete delivery' of antigen. Taken together, these studies suggest that the efficiency of antigen loading of APCs for TCI without optimization, and i.d. injection, 'complete antigen delivery', are not too dissimilar. As the addition of adjuvant by the safe and acceptable means of SC disruption leads to several log increases in the immune response compared with antigen alone, one could surmise that immune responses to injected antigens might be lower compared with TCI. An optimized system using pharmaceutically formulated patches, optimized for efficient delivery, may achieve the goal of providing a more efficient use of antigen and thereby lower the antigen dose in a particular vaccine compared with needle-based delivery. Clearly, a goal of the development program will be to optimize delivery in certain products and overall use of smaller amounts of antigen than by needle-based routes.

ADJUVANTS AND THE SKIN

The delivery of antigens and adjuvants to the skin for the purpose of TCI is consistently dependent on the presence of an adjuvant in the formulation for induction of robust immune responses (Glenn et al., 1998a; Glenn and Alving, 1999a; Baca-Estrada et al., 2000; Scharton-Kersten et al., 2000; Chen et al., 2001a; Güereña-Burgueño et al., 2002). In general, adjuvants greatly augment the immune responses to coadministered antigens and there are a wide variety of adjuvants that may be used (Kenney and Edelman, 2003). The bacterial ADP-ribosylating exotoxins (bAREs) are potent adjuvants in the context of the skin and include CT, LT, and their mutants and subunits. bAREs have had extensive use as adjuvants via intranasal and oral routes, and are causative agents in self-limiting diarrheal diseases, the latter suggesting that their topical use would not be accompanied by long-term side-effects (Dickinson and Clements, 1995; Snider, 1995; Freytag and Clements, 1999; Michetti *et al.*, 1999; Glück *et al.*, 2000; O'Hagan, 2000; Scharton-Kersten *et al.*, 2000; Weltzin *et al.*, 2000; Kenney and Edelman, 2003;).

The adjuvanticity of the bAREs on the skin appears to correlate with the level of ribosyl-transferase activity as it does in oral and most nasal immunization studies (Scharton-Kersten *et al.*, 2000). Purified cholera toxin B-subunit (pCTB) and mutant toxins that retain ribosyl-transferase activity act as adjuvants on the skin, in contrast to recombinant CTB that is devoid of ribosyl-transferase activity and is subsequently far less potent as an adjuvant (Scharton-Kersten *et al.*, 2000). Other adjuvants, including bacterial DNA, cytokines, LPS, and LPS analogues, have been shown to have activity in the context of the skin, but their comparative potency on the skin needs to be further evaluated (Scharton-Kersten *et al.*, 2000).

TCI is similar to intranasal or oral immunization, as the simple admixture of LT with a coadministered antigen such as tetanus toxoid (TTx) or influenza hemagglutinin results in markedly higher antibody levels compared with the administration of antigens alone, which can themselves elicit immune responses (Glenn *et al.*, 1998a; Güereña-Burgueño *et al.*, 2002; Scharton-Kersten *et al.*, 2000). Similarly, use of bAREs by TCI induces cell-mediated immunity to the coadministered antigens such as CD4+ or CD8+ T cells with a balanced T helper profile (Hammond *et al.*, 2001b; Neidleman *et al.*, 2000; Porgador *et al.*, 1997; Seo *et al.*, 2000).

THE SAFETY OF LT AS A TOPICAL ADJUVANT

For specific product development, we have focused on the adjuvant LT, one of the family of bARE adjuvants that includes CT, *Pseudomonas* exotoxin A, and diphtheria toxin. Each member has distinctive features, i.e. cell surface binding targets, size, and qualitative immune effects. LT is the causative agent in enterotoxigenic *E. coli* (ETEC) travelers' diarrhea. As an adjuvant, LT has a unique safety database since millions of persons are exposed yearly to this self-limiting disease with no short-term or long-term adverse events. In developing countries with an endemic ETEC, the majority of the population develop anti-LT antibodies through repeated exposure to ETEC, and adults in developed countries frequently have high levels of serum anti-LT IgG, suggesting travel-related exposure to ETEC. The immune responses to LT after challenge studies are similar in magnitude to responses elicited by transcutaneous immunization (D.N. Taylor, unpublished observations) and thus suggest that this level of exposure and response to LT occurs without significant effects beyond the self-limited diarrheal disease. Additionally, there exists a unique and extensive publication record on the safety/toxicology of LT, providing helpful guidance for reviewers and regulatory authorities.

LT and its mutants have been subjected to extensive formal toxicology studies (Peppoloni *et al.*, 2003; Zurbriggen *et al.*, 2003). This includes ferrets, rats, miniature pigs, NZW rabbits, and baboons, and using routes including nasal, oral, and intravenous (i.v.). The most invasive route, i.v. injection, required 630 human doses to reach an LD_{50}, whereas the oral route using equivalent doses did not induce mortality or clinical changes (Zurbriggen *et al.*, 2003). Ocular exposure in NZW mice and nasal use of LT in baboons resulted in no local or distal changes in a detailed CNS histopathologic study (Zurbriggen *et al.*, 2003). Toxicology studies in guinea pigs using LT with a recombinant antigen, CS6, previously demonstrated the preclinical safety of LT as adjuvant on the skin (Yu *et al.*, 2002). Six carefully controlled GLP toxicology studies have confirmed these findings

(S.A. Frech, unpublished observations). Claims that CT may induce chronic diseases based on contrived mouse models (using spinal cord proteins as immunogens given in conjunction with i.v. infusion of pertussis toxin (Riminton *et al.*, 2004)) have been made. Previous similar claims have been made for oil-in-water adjuvants (autoimmune disease, cancer), and Hib vaccination (diabetes). These specific claims have been discounted with extensive, carefully conducted human studies showing that these models have no predictive value for safety in human vaccination studies (Page *et al.*, 1993; Graves *et al.*, 1999; Offit and Hackett, 2003).

Although the native toxins are highly sensitive to the low pH found in the stomach, the use of mutant toxins as adjuvants are molecular approaches to address the potential concerns associated with oral vaccination using native toxins delivered to the small intestine, which can cause diarrhea upon ingestion in fasting subjects in whom the gastric acid has been neutralized (Levine *et al.*, 1983a; Michetti *et al.*, 1999). The relevance of these concerns for topical use of adjuvants such as LT is doubtful. Given the common use of potentially toxic drugs in transdermal patches, such as nicotine, and the potential for misuse of other pharmaceuticals, e.g. acetaminophen, when used as directed, patches are likely to have no significant side-effects. The ability to safely use potent adjuvants on the skin that might not be used otherwise is precisely the strength of skin-targeting technologies.

In phase I human trials, the use of LT on the skin appears to be safe and well tolerated (Glenn *et al.*, 2000; Güereña-Burgueño *et al.*, 2002; Glenn *et al.*, 2003a). Local, mild rashes on the skin have been described in conjunction with topical use of LT (Güereña-Burgueño *et al.*, 2002). The use of gene guns to deliver DNA to the skin results in mild, self-limiting local rashes in 100% of the subjects but these do not appear to be a serious concern. Studies with smallpox and BCG result in local scarring, the eschar of smallpox vaccination suggesting a clinical 'take' of the vaccine, but this clearly is not acceptable as a routine reaction for skin delivery of new vaccines. The oral use of LT appears to have enough side-effects (including diarrhea) to discourage its use as an oral adjuvant (Kotloff *et al.*, 2001), and the possible relationship between the increased incidence of Bell's palsy in subjects and the administration of an intranasal flu vaccine with LT, and controversy suggesting LT may migrate along the olfactory bulb (Zurbriggen *et al.*, 2003) suggests that the skin may be the most acceptable route by which LT may be used as an adjuvant. Others have pursued the use of mutant LT adjuvants for intranasal products and are in phase I trials (Peppoloni *et al.*, 2003). Our group has completed large, double-blind placebo control trials, and repeat dosing trials which have confirmed the finding of the six well-controlled GLP toxicology studies showing that LT may be safely used on the skin. These findings are in concert with the scientific data on the mechanism of adjuvanticity, the epidemiology of enteric diseases as toxin-based, self-limiting events with no long-term sequalae, and suggest that LT is an ideal adjuvant for use on the skin.

IMMUNE RESPONSES TO TCI – ADJUVANT AND ANTIGEN IN A PATCH

The early observation that CT could be used as an adjuvant for topical immunization with toxoid antigens (Glenn *et al.*, 1998a) led to numerous studies showing that a wide variety of adjuvants and antigens can be used to induce systemic and mucosal immunity (Glenn *et al.*, 1999; El-Ghorr *et al.*, 2000; Glenn *et al.*, 2000; Gockel *et al.*, 2000; Hammond *et al.*, 2000; Scharton-Kersten *et al.*, 2000; Beignon *et al.*, 2002; Godefroy *et al.*, 2003). The mechanisms by which adjuvants exert their effects at the level of the skin are becoming increasingly clear and the enhancing effects are well documented. LT and its derivatives appear to be unmatched in their potency and can be safely used in the context of the skin (Freytag and Clements, 1999; Güereña-Burgueño *et al.*, 2002). Given the availability of LT in commercial GMP supply, LT has been the focus of our development programs. However, it is clear that most adjuvants have a similar biological effect, and given sufficient commercial and biological rationale, could conceivably be developed in a product targeting the skin.

TCI represents a departure from other routes of immunization, yet results in 'classic' immune responses similar to those induced by other routes of immunization. The use of adjuvant on the skin results in both primary and secondary serum antibody responses to coadministered antigens when boosting is conducted using adjuvants (Glenn *et al.*, 1999). Repeated immunization with the same adjuvant but different antigens may readily be achieved despite the preexisting high-titer antibodies to the adjuvant (Glenn *et al.*, 1999; O'Hagan, 2000). Additionally, TCI appears to induce boostable, long-lasting, stable immune responses (Glenn and Kenney, 2004). The magnitude of the adjuvanticity correlates with the ribosyl-transferase activity and this is evident using a variety of adjuvants. Mice immunized with the model antigen TTx along with the adjuvants CT, rCTB, pCTB (which contains trace holotoxin activity), LT, or LTR192G, LTK63, LTR72 (Dickinson and Clements, 1995; Kotloff *et al.*, 2001; Tierney *et al.*, 2003) show similar boostable antibody responses to TTx, with the exception of rCTB, which lacks the ribosyl-transferase activity associated with the A subunit (Scharton-Kersten *et al.*, 2000). Tetanus-specific T-cell proliferative responses in spleen and lymph nodes suggest that boosting is related to the T-cell responses (Hammond *et al.*, 2001b). Priming by the intramuscular (i.m.) route with TTx and alum, which induces T-cell memory, can be followed by a booster immunization on the skin to induce secondary responses (Hammond *et al.*, 2001b). These and many other studies demonstrate that TCI induces T-cell responses and boostable antibody responses, and confirm that immunization via the skin can be expected to induce immune responses with characteristics similar to other routes of immunization.

It was clear in early studies that the use of an adjuvant is critical to the induction of high levels of antibodies to a coadministered antigen (Glenn *et al.*, 1998a) and results in functional immune responses. This has been confirmed in several other settings, such as gene-gun immunization (Chen *et al.*, 2001a; Matriano *et al.*, 2002). In an early TCI study, TTx delivered with increasing doses of LT as adjuvant produced robust levels of anti-TTx antibodies that are clearly dependent on the presence of adjuvant (Scharton-Kersten *et al.*, 2000). The same animals were fully protected by systemic tetanus toxin challenge, and only animals receiving adjuvant with the antigen were fully protected (Scharton-Kersten *et al.*, 2000; Tierney *et al.*, 2003). In a live RSV (Godefroy *et al.*, 2003) and *Chlamydia* challenge (Berry *et al.*, 2004), the adjuvant was shown to play a crucial role in protective responses (Godefroy *et al.*, 2003), and others have shown that antidiphtheria toxin antibodies generated by TCI in the presence of adjuvant neutralize the highly potent diphtheria toxin (Hammond *et al.*, 2001a). Conversely, skin immunization with recombinant protection antigen (RPA) was protective in a live *Bacillus anthracis* challenge both with and without adjuvant, despite log higher titers in the presence of adjuvant (Matyas *et al.*, 2004), suggesting in this model that even modest levels of antibodies are protective. These data have confirmed the assertion that skin-delivered antigen and adjuvants result in robust, functional, protective immune responses.

The critical role of the adjuvant for human immunogenicity was shown using a recombinant *E. coli*/ETEC antigen, CS6. This large antigen (>1.5 million daltons) was delivered with and without LT using a simple patch. As shown in Figure 5.4, only subjects receiving both antigen and adjuvant produced anti-CS6 antibodies (Figure 5.4C and D). This very clear and seminal study (discussed in detail below) confirmed the universal preclinical observation that adjuvants play an important role in inducing robust immune responses to antigens delivered to the skin.

MUCOSAL RESPONSES TO SKIN IMMUNIZATION

In early studies it was observed that topical immunization with LT and CT as adjuvants induced both IgG and IgA antibodies in mucosal secretions of mice (Enioutina *et al.*, 2000; Glenn *et al.*, 1998b). The mucosa and skin share similar elements, including LCs and secretory organs, the presence of IgA such as that found in the sweat glands (Gebhart *et al.*, 1987; Okada *et al.*, 1988) and microorganisms coated with immunoglobulins, including IgA and the secretory component of IgA (Hard, 1969; Metze *et al.*, 1991). The topical application of bAREs, such as LT, CT, and coadministered antigens, induces mucosal antibodies (Glenn *et al.*, 1998b; El-Ghorr *et al.*, 2000; Scharton-Kersten *et al.*, 2000), and mucosal cellular responses (Gockel *et al.*, 2000). Mice immunized transcutaneously with CT produce anti-CT neutralizing IgG and IgA antibodies in the stool and pulmonary secretions (Glenn *et al.*, 1998b; Glenn *et al.*, 1999). IgG antibodies to the coadministered antigen are routinely detected in the mucosa (El-Ghorr *et al.*, 2000; Scharton-Kersten *et*

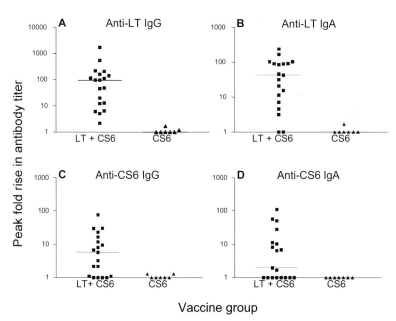

Vaccine group

Figure 5.4 Human serum IgG and IgA responses to coadministered CS6 and LT. Normal adult volunteers were enrolled in a dose-escalating study of 250, 500, 1000 or 2000 μg CS6 alone or with 500 μg LT dosed at 0, 1, and 3 months. The peak fold-rise in antibody for each individual is shown (reported as fold rise over baseline), combining the dose groups as the responses were not significantly different, and the geometric mean for each group is shown as a bar. From Guereña-Burgueño F, Hall ER, Taylor DN, *et al*. Safety and immunogenicity of a prototype enterotoxigenic *Escherichia coli* vaccine administered transcutaneously. Infect. Immun. 2002; 70: 1874–1880, with permission.

al., 2000), and IgA to recombinant *E. coli* antigens (CS6), as well as chlamydia, tetanus and herpes antigens, have been detected in mice immunized topically with CT and TTx or inactivated herpes virus (El-Ghorr *et al.*, 2000; Gockel *et al.*, 2000; Yu *et al.*, 2002 Berry *et al.*, 2004). These data suggest that antibody-secreting cells have homed to the mucosa. Goeckel *et al.* have shown that anti-TTx ASCs can be detected in the vaginal mucosa of mice immunized topically using CT and TTx (Gockel *et al.*, 2000). Migration of dendritic cells to the gut may also explain these findings, as shown in experiments with injected dendritic cells (Enioutina *et al.*, 2000). More recent studies have shown that transcutaneous immunization with a helper peptide derived for HIV IIIB and the immunodominant CTL epitope from the V_3 loop of the HIV IIIB strain of HIV-induced CTLs in the Peyer's patches (Belyakov *et al.*, 2004). The CTL response correlated with protection against intrarectal challenge with gp 160 expressing vaccinia virus. Interestingly, whereas the majority of DCs clearly migrated to the draining lymph nodes, some DCs containing fluorescently labeled LT appeared in the Peyer's patches and that DCs isolated after immunization could present antigen, suggesting that a population of DCs can present antigen directly to the mucosal immune system.

Antibodies detected in TCI studies may represent transudates into the mucosa, yet recent data have shown that anti-LT antibodies detected in the stool and lung wash contain the secretory component of IgA, indicating that local mucosal antibody production occurs (Yu *et al.*, 2002). In a study using plasmid DNA immunization delivered by TCI, induction of both serum IgG and fecal IgA against the M protein encoded in the plasmid conferred protection upon live influenza virus challenge (Watabe *et al.*, 2001). Anti-LT IgG and IgA antibodies were detected in humans immunized topically with LT, consistent with the repeated observations in mice (Glenn *et al.*, 2000). The presence of mucosal antibodies in response to TCI raises interesting mechanistic questions, and this finding suggests that induction of mucosal and systemic responses by TCI may enhance vaccine efficacy in certain settings.

IMMUNOSTIMULANT PATCH

The potent immune stimulation observed by the use of adjuvants on the skin and the highly regional trafficking of the activated LCs to the DLN in response to LT suggested that the delivery of adjuvants to the skin might be used to enhance immune responses to *injected* vaccines. We hypothesized that adjuvant-activated epidermal LCs could exert bystander immunostimulatory effects on immune cells loaded with antigen by injection if they targeted the same DLN, leading to enhanced immune responses to the injected vaccines. This allows separate, potentially safer delivery of adjuvants, and a general approach for enhancing vaccine delivery in multiple applications.

The practicality of separating the delivery of adjuvant and antigen might not be readily apparent. However, in practice, the addition of an immunostimulant (IS™) patch to an immunization appears to be quite straightforward, substituting the Band-Aid™ placed after immunization with an adjuvant-laden patch. Adjuvants can play an important role with poorly immunogenic vaccine antigens, in dose sparing (both amount of antigen and number of immunizations), or possibly in settings of immune compromise such as the senescent immune system (Singh and O'Hagan, 1999; Gasparini *et al.*, 2001). Topical delivery of adjuvants to the skin to augment immune responses to vaccines delivered concurrently by injection has the potential added benefit of safety.

The effects at the LC level undergird a large body of data showing that adding an IS™ patch after immunization greatly enhances antibody, T-cell, and effector responses in immunization protocols. The model antigen tetanus toxoid was injected in combination with an IS™ patch, and the anti-TT antibody response was greatly augmented after a single dose when an IS™ patch was added (Glenn *et al.*, 2003b). Patches used include a crude gauze patch compared with proprietary IOMAI formulations that are manufacturable and that have suitable shelf stability and improved delivery efficiency. Formulated patches may in fact be more efficient delivery platforms for antigens and adjuvants. The IS™ patch has also been used with split virus antigen from influenza. The immune response to trivalent split virus vaccine injected by the i.m. or i.d. route is augmented by addition of an IS™ patch (Guebre-Xabier *et al.*, 2003). In these studies, enhanced antigen-specific IgG, HAI titers, mucosal antibodies, T-cell responses, and lung antibody-secreting cells were seen (Guebre-Xabier *et al.*, 2003). These studies have been followed by a wide variety of protocols including biological warfare agent vaccines, recombinant antigens, whole cells, peptides, cancer immunotherapy and infectious disease challenge models demonstrating the IS effect.

The LT immunostimulant (LT-IS™) patch may be useful in influenza vaccination of the elderly, which normally falls well short of fully protecting the recipients due to the low response rates to the vaccine (de Bruijn *et al.*, 1999). To explore this application, aged and young mice were immunized with trivalent influenza vaccine with or without the LT-IS™ patch. While the age-related immune deficit was seen, the LT-IS™ patch was able to repair this deficit, improving the antibody response to a level equal to or greater than the response in young mice (Figure 5.5) (Guebre-Xabier *et al.*, 2004).

The present data show that an LT-IS™ patch elicits qualitative and quantitative enhancement of antigen-specific responses. This strategy may be used in several contexts, such as enhancing immune responses to influenza and pneumococcal vaccines in elderly vaccinees, in established cancer immunotherapy regimens that lack sufficient immune stimulation, or in dose sparing where vaccine antigen supply is critical (pandemic influenza). As the response rates to influenza vaccination are unsatisfactory in the elderly and are much lower compared with healthy adults (de Bruijn *et al.*, 1999), the use of an LT-IS™ patch may both enhance the influenza-specific immune response and improve the tolerability of adjuvant use. The clinical applicability of an IS strategy has been confirmed in the context of influenza immunization of the elderly (S.A. Frech, unpublished observations). The LT-IS™ patch is a practical strategy, allowing safe use of adjuvants with existing vaccines or new vaccines that are more effectively delivered by injection, and thus provides an additional important tool for immunization strategies.

HUMAN STUDIES

The safety and immunogenicity of TCI and related approaches was shown by early-stage clinical investigations. The challenges in the early studies were to show delivery of LT in the context of human skin and to demonstrate the role of LT as an adjuvant, extending our preclinical observations. These points are now firmly established (Glenn *et al.*, 2000) and have been confirmed in subsequent studies (Güereña-Burgueño *et al.*, 2002). The next level of development will require further extension of safety observations, demonstration of the clinical utility of TCI with various antigens, optimization of their delivery by studying skin pretreatment and patch types, and assessment of the immune responses induced.

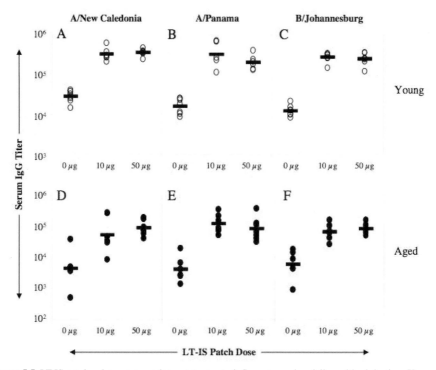

Figure 5.5 LT-IS patch enhances secondary responses to influenza vaccine delivered by injection. Young (~2 months) and aged (18 months) C57BL/6 mice were immunized i.d. on day 0, 14 and 28 with 5 μg with trivalent split influenza virus vaccine. Patches containing 25 μl of PBS (0 μg LT), 10 μg or 50 μg LT were applied on the skin over the injection site immediately after parenteral injection for 18 h. All mice were immunized on study day 0 and serum was collected 2 weeks post-immunization (day 14). Serum IgG titers to A/New Caledonia (A, D), A/Panama (B, E) and B/Johannesburg (C, F) were determined by an ELISA method. Individual titers are displayed with open circles (young mice) or closed circles (aged mice). The geometric mean of each group is indicated with horizontal bars. Prebleed samples had titers < 80 EU for young and < 230 EU for aged mice. From Guebre-Xabier M, Hammond SA, Ellingsworth LR, *et al.* 2004. Immunostimulant patch enhances immunity to influenza vaccine in aged mice, J. Virol. 78: 7610–7618, with permission.

Capitalizing on its ability to act as both an antigen and an adjuvant, the initial clinical study used a liquid application of LT alone in a simple patch on untreated skin in a dose escalation format to assess the safety and immune response (Glenn *et al.*, 2000). Volunteers received an LT solution in a gauze pad under an adhesive patch, and were immunized at 0, 1, and 9 months. No serious vaccine-related adverse reactions were observed, and histological sections of biopsies taken at the dosing sites were normal, consistent with the absence of DTH clinically. Subjects in the high dose group produced a greater than four-fold rise in serum antibodies against LT, along with IgG or IgA antibodies against LT in either the urine or stool. Antibodies against LT were durable and persisted long after the second immunization, with a clear booster response after the second and third dose. This was the first demonstration that a passively delivered vaccine antigen could elicit a systemic immune response in humans.

The importance of the role of an adjuvant in the induction of immune responses to a coadministered antigen was initially tested in the context of *E. coli*-related traveler's diarrhea using the colonization factor CS6, a multi-subunit intestinal epithelial cell-binding protein (Wolf *et al.*, 1997). Volunteers were given CS6 in a dose escalating fashion at 0, 1, and 3 months (Güereña-Burgueño *et al.*, 2002). Seventy-four percent of volunteers in the combined groups had mild DTH skin reactions with the second or third dose, possibly to the colonization factor CS6 or LPS in the CS6 buffer. No other adverse events correlated with vaccine administration. As shown in Figure 5.4, only volunteers receiving LT as adjuvant produced serum anti-CS6 IgG and IgA. The anti-CS6 response compared favorably to responses seen after challenge infection using the live B7A ETEC strain, which results in full protection on rechallenge (Levine *et al.*, 1983b; Wolf *et al.*, 1999). Antibody secreting cells (ASCs) to CS6 were also detected in the peripheral blood. The lack of response to CS6 without LT and clear responses in the presence of LT confirmed the universal finding in animal studies that the adjuvant plays a critical role in TCI. This study also confirmed that large antigens such as CS6 (>1,000,000 Da) can be readily delivered to the human skin immune system (Yu *et al.*, 2002).

As noted above, preclinical studies suggested the dose of LT could be reduced with retention of immunogenicity by disruption of the SC. The effect of mild disruption of the SC on the delivery of LT was explored with commercially available medical products, including abrasive pads used to enhance EKG signal conductivity, or adhesive tape used to evaluate skin hydration. These strategies are in clinical practice to enhance the flux of drugs for topical application or electrical conductivity to improve the quality of electrocardiograms. To evaluate the penetration enhancement of various skin pretreatment methods in humans, we conducted a phase I study in healthy adults. Subjects were pretreated prior to vaccination with one of the following techniques: (a) hydration alone with a glycerol/isopropyl alcohol (IPA) solution (groups 1 and 5); (b) tape-stripping followed by glycerol/IPA hydrating solution (group 2); (c) glycerol/IPA hydrating solution followed by 10 strokes of pumice-impregnated IPA pad (group 3); or (d) glycerol/IPA hydrating solution followed by ten strokes of emery paper (group 4). Following pretreatment, all groups were then vaccinated twice, 21 days apart, with a patch composed of gauze containing 50 μg LT (groups 1–4) or 400 μg LT (group 5), covered by Tegaderm™. No significant adverse events were observed after either LT vaccination, apart from a mild, self-limited maculopapular rash that occasionally developed with or without associated pruritus at the site of vaccination.

Results from this study suggest that pretreatment with either emery paper or tape stripping delivered LT more efficiently than with glycerol/IPA hydration alone (Figure 5.6), as responses, defined as a two-fold rise in LT IgG, were greatest in these groups. Following each vaccination, LT IgG geometric mean titers (GMT) showed greater response following pretreatment with glycerol/IPA hydration and emery paper (group 4) and tape-stripping (group 2) when compared with glycerol/IPA hydration alone (group 1). The improvements in LT IgG GMT seen in the treatment groups (emery and tape-stripping), with respect to hydration alone, suggest improved LT delivery with SC disruption using emery pretreatment. Subjects pretreated with tape stripping (group 2) or emery (group 4) and vaccinated with 50 μg showed no significant difference in GMT for LT IgG when compared with those receiving hydration alone and 400 μg LT (group 5). These data indicate that an eight-fold reduction in LT from 400 μg to 50 μg is possible when emery pretreatment, or its equivalent, is used. This study established the general tolerability of various penetration enhancement techniques, as well as the potential dose sparing such pretreatment can yield. Current trials using IS™ patch applications use 45 μg doses and have demonstrated similar immunogenicity with as little as 15 μg of LT based on these and other studies. In general, 45 μg LT dosed twice by TCI yields geometric mean IgG titers

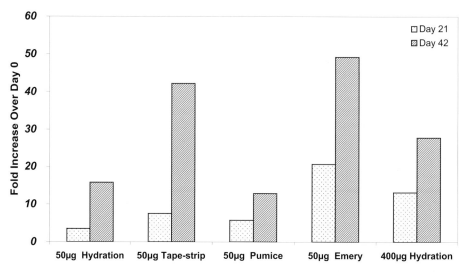

Figure 5.6 Human LT IgG response after one and two doses in NLT105. Eight subjects per group were pretreated with the indicated methods as described, then vaccinated with 50 μg or 400 μg LT on day 0 and day 21. LT IgG ELISA was run on sera from day 0, 21, and 42, reported as fold increase of relative ELISA units. From Glenn GM, Kenney RT, Ellingsworth LR, *et al.* Transcutaneous immunization and immunostimulant strategies: capitalizing on the immunocompetence of the skin. Expert Rev. Vaccines 2003; 2: 253–267, with permission.

of 5000–10,000 and results in seroconversion in over 90% of the subjects (G.M. Glenn, unpublished observations).

OTHER SKIN DELIVERY TECHNOLOGIES

The epidermal powder immunization (EPI) technology developed by PowderJect is designed to deliver vaccine antigens into the epidermal layer of the skin. EPI delivers vaccine antigens in the form of microscopic particles composed of a vaccine antigen and a carrier particle. Theoretically, any vaccine that is stable as a dried powder or in a particulate form can be delivered using EPI, and PowderJect has successfully induced significant immune responses with a number of plasmids that contain genes of interest (Fynan *et al.*, 1993; Schirmbeck *et al.*, 1995; Yoshida *et al.*, 2000; Chen *et al.*, 2000;) as well as recombinant proteins (Chen *et al.*, 2001b; Chen *et al.*, 2002; Osorio *et al.*, 2003) and inactivated viruses (Chen *et al.*, 2001b; Chen *et al.*, 2003). Depending upon the type of vaccine antigen, PowderJect has used a number of different particle formulations. For particle-mediated DNA immunization, plasmid DNA(s) are precipitated onto 1–3 μm gold beads. Protein antigens can either be precipitated onto similar gold particles or formulated as a dense powder with sugar excipients to produce 20–70 μm particles.

Numerous reports have shown that EPI is capable of inducing potent humoral (systemic as well as mucosal) and cellular (CD4[+] and CD8[+] T cell mediated) immune responses in a variety of animal models (Dean *et al.*, 2003). Active immunization has been achieved with both DNA and protein-coated gold particles as well as protein-formulated sugar particles, and the addition of adjuvants such as QS-21 (Chen *et al.*, 2003), CpG DNA (Chen *et al.*, 2001b; Osorio *et al.*, 2003), CT and LT (Arrington *et al.*, 2002; Osorio *et al.*, 2003) to these formulated antigen vaccines significantly enhances these immune responses.

Given the success and widespread use of gene guns in preclinical models, particularly those using rhesus monkeys, the path to clinical trials has been slow; the most recent clinical report was published in 1999. Two phase I clinical trials testing the safety and immunogenicity of a particle-mediated hepatitis B DNA vaccine have been completed. The most recent trial was an open-label, phase I safety and immunogenicity trial in healthy adults using gold particles coated with plasmid DNA (Roy *et al.*, 2000). Volunteers received three administrations of DNA encoding the surface antigen of hepatitis B virus (HBV) at 1, 2, or 4 μg. The DNA vaccine was found to be safe and well tolerated and all volunteers developed protective antibody responses following the third vaccination. Vaccinations were given at either two anatomical sites (1 or 2 μg DNA) or four anatomical sites (4 μg of DNA). Increase in serconversion appears to correlate with increasing DNA dose following the second vaccination. Protective immunity was defined as serum antibody levels greater than 10 mIU/mL of HbsAg-specific antibody (1987). Although 100% of the volunteers developed protective antibody responses, the antibody titers were 4–10-fold lower than those reported for the currently licenced recombinant hepatitis B protein vaccine (Van Damme *et al.*, 1989; West, 1989). Furthermore, a single dose of the recombinant subunit vaccine induces a significantly higher number of individuals with detectable anti-HbsAG antibody than a single dose of the DNA vaccine (50–60% vs 16%). Although DNA immunization induced lower levels of antibody overall, patients were specifically primed and a subsequent vaccination with recombinant HbsAg-induced elevated antibody responses.

In addition to antibody responses, DNA immunization induced significant cellular immune responses in both the CD4$^+$ and CD8$^+$ cellular compartment. Following the third immunization, ELISPOT assays utilizing recombinant HbsAg protein indicated the presence of IFN-γ secreting cells in all 12 volunteers while IL-5 secreting cells could only be detected in 3 of 12 volunteers. These three individuals had relatively equal numbers of IL-5 and IFN-γ cytokine secreting cells indicating a balanced TH1/TH2 response while the remaining 9 individuals exhibiting little or no IL-5 response, indicating the preferential induction of a TH1 response. These TH cell responses were detected following the first immunization in the majority of volunteers, suggesting the vaccine regimen used was more conducive to the induction of cellular immune responses than humoral responses.

The HLA-A2 class I restricted HbsAg335–343 peptide was used to evaluate the induction of HbsAg-specific CD8$^+$ T cell responses in the eight HLA-A2 volunteers within the study. Here, ELISPOT analysis demonstrated the presence of peptide-specific, CD8$^+$ IFN-γ-secreting cells in the PBMC of all eight volunteers, again indicating the efficacy of EPI in the induction of cellular immune responses.

EPI using DNA adsorbed gold particles allows for the introduction of the HbsAg gene directly into cells. The targeting of Langerhans cells results in efficient antigen presentation of the encoded protein and subsequent antibody and cellular immune responses. While the antibody levels generated are protective for HbsAg, they are significantly lower than that observed with the standard injected recombinant protein vaccine. Perhaps optimization of the vaccine dose and delivery regimen or the incorporation of an immunological adjuvant will result in the generation of comparable antibody titers.

ELECTROPORATION

Electroporation (EP) involves the application of a high voltage electric current across a biologic membrane leading to a reversible electric breakdown of that membrane. Originally the phenomenon was observed on the cellular level in cultured cells, leading to various developments in genetic research, especially those focused on introduction of

DNA molecules into tumor cells (Wells *et al.*, 2000; Heller and Coppola, 2002). Although the SC differs markedly from normal cell membranes (being composed of multilamellar, intercellular lipid bilayers with few phospholipids and no living cells) it is considered to be electrically insulating and behaves as the dielectric layer of a capacitor when a pulse electric field is applied. However, when the strength of the applied electric field exceeds that needed for the electric breakdown of the SC dielectric material, pores (in the nanometer range) are believed to form, allowing the movement of molecules smaller than the pore size across the SC and into the more diffusive living epidermis (Prausnitz *et al.*, 1993). Typically, skin EP involves the application of a pulse electric field in the range of 50 to 1000 V for micro- or millisecond period, and it has been shown to enhance the permeation of a broad range of compounds including small therapeutic compounds (Vanbever *et al.*, 1994), oligonucleotides (Zewert *et al.*, 1995), protein molecules (Zewert *et al.*, 1999) and drug-loaded microparticles (Prausnitz *et al.*, 1996).

Conceptually, the accessibility of the skin and the presence of potent APCs make it a good target for electroporation-enhanced skin vaccination, especially in the field of DNA vaccination, although to date little preclinical and no clinical data exists for this application. Generally, direct injection of naked DNA or bombardment of somatic cells with particles coated with plasmid DNA results in low levels of transgene expression (Drabick *et al.*, 2001). However, it was shown that using electroporating pulse enhances cellular uptake and, subsequently, the gene expression of intradermally injected DNA in both mice and human skin xenografts on nude mice (Zhang *et al.*, 2002). Moreover, in a freshly excised hairless rat model, it was shown that EP not only enhanced the permeation of the FITC-labeled oligonucleotides across intact SC, but also resulted in higher cellular uptake within a few minutes after pulse application (Regnier and Preat, 1998). Application of EP in conjunction with intradermally injected DNA resulted in the transfection of several skin cell types, in addition to the appearance of transfected cells in the lymphatic drainage feeding the application site, as well as immune responses. Analysis of subclasses of antibodies (IgG1 and IgG2a) produced after immunization using DNA encoding the hepatitis B surface antigen resulted in a mixed qualitative antibody response (both Th1 and Th2) compared with a Th2 dominant response using the recombinant protein (Drabick *et al.*, 2001). Electroporation may not be limited to DNA vaccination. Misra *et al.* (1999) used EP to enhance the delivery of myristylated peptide and diphtheria toxoid administered into the skin. It was shown that EP-administered myristylated peptide elicited higher responses than the i.d. injected peptide, but lower than intraperitonial (i.p.) immunization. On the other hand, EP-assisted transcutaneous administration of diphtheria toxoid elicited less response than that administered i.d.

The safety of the application of high-voltage pulses on skin was assessed *in vivo* using pig skin, based on histological scores, alteration of skin function such as transepidermal water loss, and by scaling the degree of erythema, edema and the presence of petechia and pulse sensation or pain. Data showed that short pulses at high voltages were well tolerated, and that erythema and irritation were mild and short-lived (Vanbever and Preat, 1999). In summary, EP has potential as a technology applicable to vaccination using the skin but is in early stage development, and it remains to be seen whether EP can offer significant advantages over other delivery technologies.

SONOPHORESIS

Sonophoresis is a new, emerging technology that uses ultrasound waves to perturb the SC and facilitate the permeation of chemicals of various sizes through the skin. Low frequency ultrasounds in the range of 0.02–0.1 MHz were used successfully to enhance the permeation of small molecules (Tang *et al.*, 2001). Mitragotri *et al.* (Mitragotri *et al.*, 1995) reported the possibility of using low frequency sonophoresis to deliver molecules in the range of 6 to 50 kDa across the skin both *in vitro* and *in vivo*. However, the efficacy of sonophoresis at the reported intensities to deliver large molecules is still controversial.

The technique may have potential in the field of TCI to deliver small epitopes. Weimann and Wu (Weimann and Wu, 2002) showed that using high intensity (2–50 W/cm^2) low frequency ultrasounds resulted in higher permeation than that reported in Mitragotri's study (<2 W/cm^2) for the same compounds and also resulted in the formation of micropores in the SC. Although several have reported low frequency sonophoresis at intensities >2.5 W/cm^2, the safety of the techniques needs to be addressed further.

OTHER TECHNOLOGIES

SC disruption via other physical penetration enhancement techniques includes use of arrays of microneedles, laser removal of the SC, and electroporation. Microneedles, which might not perforate the skin, were described in the 1970s, but their potential application has only recently gained traction. Microneedle skin pretreatment followed by topical application of plasmid resulted in enhanced delivery of DNA, as indicated by improved immune responses in mice (Mikszta *et al.*, 2002). Another microneedle technology, macroflux microprojections, was tested for penetration into hairless guinea pig skin and found to penetrate at an average depth of 100 μm with no projections deeper than 300 μm, using an applicator device (Matriano *et al.*, 2002). In antigen delivery evaluations, 1 to 80 μg of OVA were delivered via 1- or 2-cm^2 microneedle patches by varying the coating solution concentration. The delivery rates measured suggested that up to 20 μg of antigen could be delivered in 5 seconds. In a prime and boost immunization study, OVA-coated needles induced higher antibody titers when OVA was administered with the microprojection array compared with i.d. administration at lower doses, but was greater than that observed after the same dose given by the subcutaneous or i.m. route. The use of the adjuvant, glucosaminyl muramyl dipeptide, further augmented the OVA-specific antibody responses. Similarly, EP using a heated probe to 'vaporize' the SC has been shown to enhance immune responses to adenoviral-based vaccines (Bramson *et al.*, 2003).

CONCLUSION

The skin provides both an attractive immune environment for vaccine antigen delivery and a safe and confined anatomical space for the use of potent adjuvants. It has been our presumption that Langerhans cells, as a class of dendritic cells, should stimulate potent immune responses when presented with antigens and adjuvants, and this continues to be validated. Progress on SC disruption and simple pretreatment of the skin has led to well-developed, simple use protocols not dissimilar from current protocols used to cleanse the skin prior to injection. In addition, antigen and adjuvant formulation optimization has progressed, leading to phase II testing of the patch technologies in formulated, manufacturable patches. While delivery optimization and product testing is inevitably challenging, the major biological observations underlying TCI and the IS™ patch, and gas-powered gun delivery, have been clearly established in that large protein antigens have been delivered clinically, resulting in immune responses with good safety profiles. While the focus of this review may seem to be weighted towards patch technology, the review reflects the proportionality of scientific publications and stage of clinical development. At the time of publication, over 16 clinical trials with LT patches, including several phase II trials have been conducted and over 40 publications using transcutaneous immunization are in the literature, representing the bias of the authors that the most critical lessons on skin delivery technologies will be learned in the clinic. Over the next five years, the challenge will be to conduct a development program that leads to safe and effective vaccination in the context of specific applications.

Acknowledgement

The authors wish to thank Wanda Hardy for her help in the preparation of this manuscript.

References

Arrington, J., Braun, R.P., Dong, L., Fuller, D.H., Macklin, M.D., Umlauf, S.W., Wagner, S.J., Wu, M.S., Payne, L.G., and Haynes, J.R. 2002. Plasmid vectors encoding cholera toxin or the heat-labile enterotoxin from *Escherichia coli* are strong adjuvants for DNA vaccines. J. Virol. 76: 4536–4546.

Baca-Estrada, M.E., Foldvari, M., Ewen, C., Badea, I., and Babiuk, L.A. 2000. Effects of IL-12 on immune responses induced by transcutaneous immunization with antigens formulated in a novel lipid-based biphasic delivery system. Vaccine 18: 1847–1854.

Beignon, A.S., Briand, J.P., Rappuoli, R., Muller, S., and Partidos, C.D. 2002. The LTR72 mutant of heat-labile enterotoxin of *Escherichia coli* enhances the ability of peptide antigens to elicit CD4(+) T cells and secrete gamma Interferon after coapplication onto bare skin. Infect. Immun. 70: 3012–3019.

Belyakov, I.M., Hammond, S.A., Ahlers, J.D., Glenn, G.M., and Berzofsky, J.A. 2004. Transcutaneous immunization induces mucosal and protective immunity by migration of primed skin dendritic cells. J. Clin. Invest. 113: 998–1007.

Berry, L.J., Hickey, D.K., Skelding, K.A., Bao, S., Rendina, A.M., Hansbro, P.M., Gockel, C.M., and Beagley, K.W. 2004. Transcutaneous immunization with combined cholera toxin and CpG adjuvant protects against *Chlamydia muridarum* genital tract infection. Infect. Immun. 72: 1019–1028.

Bramson, J., Dayball, K., Evelegh, C., Wan, Y.H., Page, D., and Smith, A. 2003. Enabling topical immunization via microporation: a novel method for pain-free and needle-free delivery of adenovirus-based vaccines. Gene Ther. 10: 251–260.

Chen, D., Endres, R., Maa, Y.F., Kensil, C.R., Whitaker-Dowling, P., Trichel, A., Youngner, J.S., and Payne, L.G. 2003. Epidermal powder immunization of mice and monkeys with an influenza vaccine. Vaccine 21: 2830–2836.

Chen, D., Endres, R.L., Erickson, C.A., Weis, K.F., McGregor, M.W., Kawaoka, Y., and Payne, L.G. 2000. Epidermal immunization by a needle-free powder delivery technology: immunogenicity of influenza vaccine and protection in mice. Nature Med. 6: 1187–1190.

Chen, D., Erickson, C.A., Endres, R.L., Periwal, S.B., Chu, Q., Shu, C., Maa, Y.F., and Payne, L.G. 2001a. Adjuvantation of epidermal powder immunization. Vaccine 19: 2908–2917.

Chen, D., Weis, K.F., Chu, Q., Erickson, C., Endres, R., Lively, C.R., Osorio, J., and Payne, L.G. 2001b. Epidermal powder immunization induces both cytotoxic T-lymphocyte and antibody responses to protein antigens of influenza and hepatitis B viruses. J. Virol. 75: 11630–11640.

Chen, D., Zuleger, C., Chu, Q., Maa, Y.F., Osorio, J., and Payne, L.G. 2002. Epidermal powder immunization with a recombinant HIV gp120 targets Langerhans cells and induces enhanced immune responses. AIDS Res. Hum. Retroviruses 18: 715–722.

Christoph, T., Muller-Rover, S., Audring, H., Tobin, D.J., Hermes, B., Cotsarelis, G., Ruckert, R., and Paus, R. 2000. The human hair follicle immune system: cellular composition and immune privilege. Br. J. Dermatol. 142: 862–873.

de Bruijn, I.A., Remarque, E.J., Jol-van der Zijde, C.M., van Tol, M.J., Westendorp, R.G., and Knook, D.L. 1999. Quality and quantity of the humoral immune response in healthy elderly and young subjects after annually repeated influenza vaccination. J. Infect. Dis. 179: 31–36.

Dean, H.J., Fuller, D., and Osorio, J.E. 2003. Powder and particle-mediated approaches for delivery of DNA and protein vaccines into the epidermis. Comp. Immunol. Microbiol. Infect. Dis. 26: 373–388.

Dickinson, B.L., and Clements, J.D. 1995. Dissociation of *Escherichia coli* heat-labile enterotoxin adjuvanticity from ADP-ribosyltransferase activity. Infect. Immun. 63: 1617–1623.

Drabick, J.J., Glasspool-Malone, J., King, A., and Malone, R.W. 2001. Cutaneous transfection and immune responses to intradermal nucleic acid vaccination are significantly enhanced by in vivo electropermeabilization. Mol. Ther. 3: 249–255.

El-Ghorr, A.A., Williams, R.M., Heap, C., and Norval, M. 2000. Transcutaneous immunisation with herpes simplex virus stimulates immunity in mice. FEMS Immunol. Med. Microbiol. 29: 255–261.

Enioutina, E.Y., Visic, D., and Daynes, R.A. 2000. The induction of systemic and mucosal immune responses to antigen-adjuvant compositions administered into the skin: alterations in the migratory properties of dendritic cells appears to be important for stimulating mucosal immunity. Vaccine 18: 2753–2767.

Freytag, L.C., and Clements, J.D. 1999. Bacterial toxins as mucosal adjuvants. Curr. Top. Microbiol. Immunol. 236: 215–236.

Fynan, E.F., Webster, R.G., Fuller, D.H., Haynes, J.R., Santoro, J.C., and Robinson, H.L. 1993. DNA vaccines: protective immunizations by parenteral, mucosal, and gene- gun inoculations. Proc. Natl. Acad. Sci. USA 90: 11478–11482.

Gasparini, R., Pozzi, T., Montomoli, E., Fragapane, E., Senatore, F., Minutello, M., and Podda, A. 2001. Increased immunogenicity of the MF59-adjuvanted influenza vaccine compared to a conventional subunit vaccine in elderly subjects. Eur. J. Epidemiol. 17: 135–140.

Gebhart, W., Metze, D., and Jurecka, W. 1987. IgA in human skin appendages. In: Immunodermatology, R. Caputo, ed. (CIC Edizioni Internationali), p. 185.

Glenn, G.M., and Alving, C.R. 1999a. Adjuvant for transcutaneous immunization. U.S. Patent No. 5,980,898.

Glenn, G.M., and Alving, C.R. 1999b. Use of penetration enhancers and barrier disruption agents to enhance the transcutaneous immune response induced by ADP-ribosylating exotoxin. European Patent No. 1061951.

Glenn, G.M., and Kenney, R.T. 2004. Transcutaneous immunization. In: New Generation Vaccines, M. M. Levine, J. B. Kaper, R. Rappuoli, M. Liu, and M. Good, eds. New York, Marcel Dekker, Inc., pp. 401–402.

Glenn, G.M., Kenney, R.T., Ellingsworth, L.R., Frech, S.A., Hammond, S.A., and Zoeteweij, J.P. 2003a. Transcutaneous immunization and immunostimulant strategies: capitalizing on the immunocompetence of the skin. Expert Rev. Vaccines 2: 253–267.

Glenn, G.M., Kenney, R.T., Hammond, S.A., and Ellingsworth, L.R. 2003b. Transcutaneous immunization and immunostimulant strategies. In: Immunology and Allergy Clinics of North America: Vaccines in the 21st Century, S. E. Barth, ed. Philadelphia, PA, W.B. Saunders Company, pp. 787–813.

Glenn, G.M., Rao, M., Matyas, G.R., and Alving, C.R. 1998a. Skin immunization made possible by cholera toxin. Nature 391: 851.

Glenn, G.M., Scharton-Kersten, T., Vassell, R., Mallett, C.P., Hale, T.L., and Alving, C.R. 1998b. Transcutaneous immunization with cholera toxin protects mice against lethal mucosal toxin challenge. J. Immunol. 161: 3211–3214.

Glenn, G.M., Scharton-Kersten, T., Vassell, R., Matyas, G.R., and Alving, C.R. 1999. Transcutaneous immunization with bacterial ADP-ribosylating exotoxins as antigens and adjuvants. Infect. Immun. 67: 1100–1106.

Glenn, G.M., Taylor, D.N., Li, X., Frankel, S., Montemarano, A., and Alving, C.R. 2000. Transcutaneous immunization: A human vaccine delivery strategy using a patch. Nature Med. 6: 1403–1406.

Glück, R., Mischler, R., Durrer, P., Furer, E., Lang, A.B., Herzog, C., and Cryz, S.J., Jr. 2000. Safety and immunogenicity of intranasally administered inactivated trivalent virosome-formulated influenza vaccine containing *Escherichia coli* heat-labile toxin as a mucosal adjuvant. J. Infect. Dis. 181: 1129–1132.

Gockel, C.M., Bao, S., and Beagley, K.W. 2000. Transcutaneous immunization induces mucosal and systemic immunity: A potent method for targeting immunity to the female reproductive tract. Mol. Immunol. 37: 537–544.

Godefroy, S., Goestch, L., Plotnicky-Gilquin, H., Nguyen, T.N., Schmitt, D., Staquet, M.J., and Corvaia, N. 2003. Immunization onto shaved skin with a bacterial enterotoxin adjuvant protects mice against respiratory syncytial virus (RSV). Vaccine 21: 1665–1671.

Graves, P.M., Barriga, K.J., Norris, J.M., Hoffman, M.R., Yu, L., Eisenbarth, G.S., and Rewers, M. 1999. Lack of association between early childhood immunizations and beta-cell autoimmunity. Diabetes Care 22: 1694–1697.

Guebre-Xabier, M., Hammond, .A., Ellingsworth, L.R., and Glenn, G.M. 2004. Immunostimulant patch enhances immune responses to infuenza vaccine in aged mice. J. Virol. 78: 7610–7618.

Guebre-Xabier, M., Hammond, S.A., Epperson, D.E., Yu, J., Ellingsworth, L., and Glenn, G.M. 2003. Immunostimulant patch containing heat labile enterotoxin from *E. coli* enhances immune responses to injected influenza vaccine through activation of skin dendritic cells. J. Virol. 77: 5218–5225.

Güereña-Burgueño, F., Hall, E.R., Taylor, D.N., Cassels, F.J., Scott, D.A., Wolf, M.K., Roberts, Z J., Nesterova, G.V., Alving, C.R., and Glenn, G.M. 2002. Safety and immunogenicity of a prototype enterotoxigenic *Escherichia coli* vaccine administered transcutaneously. Infect. Immun. 70: 1874–1880.

Hammond, S.A., Guebre-Xabier, M., Yu, J., and Glenn, G.M. 2001a. Transcutaneous immunization: an emerging route of immunization and potent immunostimulation strategy. Crit. Rev. Ther. Drug Carrier Sys. 18: 503–526.

Hammond, S.A., Tsonis, C., Sellins, K., Rushlow, K., Scharton-Kersten, T., Colditz, I., and Glenn, G.M. 2000. Transcutaneous immunization of domestic animals: opportunities and challenges. Adv. Drug Delivery Rev. 43: 45–55.

Hammond, S.A., Walwender, D., Alving, C.R., and Glenn, G.M. 2001b. Transcutaneous immunization: T-cell responses and boosting of existing immunity. Vaccine 19: 2701–2707.

Hard, G.C. 1969. Electron microscopic examination of *Corynebacterium ovis*. J. Bacteriol. 97: 1480–1485.

Heller, L.C., and Coppola, D. 2002. Electrically mediated delivery of vector plasmid DNA elicits an antitumor effect. Gene Ther. 9: 1321–1325.

Henderson, D.A., Borio, L.L., and Lane, J.M. 2004. Smallpox and vaccinia. In: Vaccines, S.A. Plotkin, and W.A. Orenstein, eds. Philadelphia, Saunders, pp. 123–153.

Jakob, T., and Udey, M C. 1999. Epidermal Langerhans cells: from neurons to nature's adjuvants. Adv. Dermatol. 14: 209–258.

Kenney, R.T., and Edelman, R. 2003. Survey of human-use adjuvants. Expert Rev. Vaccines 2: 167–188.

Kotloff, K.L., Sztein, M.B., Wasserman, S.S., Losonsky, G.A., DiLorenzo, S.C., and Walker, R.I. 2001. Safety and immunogenicity of oral inactivated whole-cell *Helicobacter pylori* vaccine with adjuvant among volunteers with or without subclinical infection. Infect. Immun. 69: 3581–3590.

Levine, M.M., Kaper, J.B., Black, R.E., and Clements, M.L. 1983a. New knowledge on pathogenesis of bacterial enteric infections as applied to vaccine development. Microbiol. Rev. 47: 510–550.

Levine, M.M., Ristaino, P., Sack, R.B., Kaper, J.B., Orskov, F., and Orskov, I. 1983b. Colonization factor antigens I and II and type 1 somatic pili in enterotoxigenic *Escherichia coli*: relation to enterotoxin type. Infect. Immun. 39: 889–897.

Matriano, J.A., Cormier, M., Johnson, J., Young, W.A., Buttery, M., Nyam, K., and Daddona, P.E. 2002. Macroflux microprojection array patch technology: a new and efficient approach for intracutaneous immunization. Pharm. Res. 19: 63–70.

Matyas, G.R., Friedlander, A.M., Glenn, G.M., Little, S., Yu, J., and Alving, C.R. 2004. Needle-free skin patch vaccination method for anthrax. Infect. Immun. 72: 1181–1183.

Metze, D., Kersten, A., Jurecka, W., and Gebhart, W. 1991. Immunoglobulins coat microorganisms of skin surface: a comparative immunohistochemical and ultrastructural study of cutaneous and oral microbial symbionts. J. Invest. Dermatol. 96: 439–445.

Michetti, P., Kreiss, C., Kotloff, K.L., Porta, N., Blanco, J.L., Bachmann, D., Herranz, M., Saldinger, P.F., Corthesy-Theulaz, I., Losonsky, G., *et al.* 1999. Oral immunization with urease and *Escherichia coli* heat-labile enterotoxin is safe and immunogenic in *Helicobacter pylori*-infected adults. Gastroenterology 116: 804–812.

Mikszta, J.A., Alarcon, J.B., Brittingham, J.M., Sutter, D.E., Pettis, R.J., and Harvey, N.G. 2002. Improved genetic immunization via micromechanical disruption of skin- barrier function and targeted epidermal delivery. Nature Med. 8: 415–419.

Misra, A., Ganga, S., and Upadhyay, P. 1999. Needle-free, non-adjuvanted skin immunization by electroporation-enhanced transdermal delivery of diphtheria toxoid and a candidate peptide vaccine against hepatitis B virus. Vaccine 18: 517–523.

Mitragotri, S., Blankschtein, D., and Langer, R. 1995. Ultrasound-mediated transdermal protein delivery. Science 269: 850–853.

Neidleman, J.A., Ott, G., and O'Hagan, D. 2000. Mutant heat-labile enterotoxins as adjuvants for CTL induction. In: Vaccine Adjuvants: Preparation Methods and Research Protocols, D. O'Hagan, ed. Totowa, NJ, Humana Press, pp. 327–336.

O'Hagan, D.T., ed. 2000. Methods in Molecular Medicine, Vol. 42. Totowa, NJ, Humana Press, Inc.

Offit, P.A., and Hackett, C.J. 2003. Addressing parents' concerns: do vaccines cause allergic or autoimmune diseases? Pediatrics 111: 653–659.

Oh, Y.K., Kim, J.P., Hwang, T.S., Ko, J.J., Kim, J.M., Yang, J.S., and Kim, C.K. 2001. Nasal absorption and biodistribution of plasmid DNA: an alternative route of DNA vaccine delivery. Vaccine 19: 4519–4525.

Okada, T., Konishi, H., Ito, M., Nagura, H., and Asai, J. 1988. Identification of secretory immunoglobulin A in human sweat and sweat glands. J. Invest Dermatol 90: 648–651.

Osorio, J.E., Zuleger, C.L., Burger, M., Chu, Q., Payne, L.G., and Chen, D. 2003. Immune responses to hepatitis B surface antigen following epidermal powder immunization. Immunol. Cell. Biol 81: 52–58.

Page, W.F., Norman, J.E., and Benenson, A.S. 1993. Long-term follow-up of army recruits immunized with Freund's incomplete adjuvanted vaccine.Vaccine Res. 2: 141–149.

Peppoloni, S., Ruggiero, P., Contorni, M., Morandi, M., Pizza, M., Rappuoli, R., Podda, A., and Del Giudice, G. 2003. Mutants of the *Escherichia coli* heat-labile enterotoxin as safe and strong adjuvants for intranasal delivery of vaccines. Expert Rev. Vaccines 2: 285–293.

Pilling, A.M., Harman, R.M., Jones, S.A., McCormack, N.A., Lavender, D., and Haworth, R. 2002. The assessment of local tolerance, acute toxicity, and DNA biodistribution following particle-mediated delivery of a DNA vaccine to minipigs. Toxicol. Pathol. 30: 298–305.

Porgador, A., Staats, H.F., Faiola, B., Gilboa, E., and Palker, T.J. 1997. Intranasal immunization with CTL epitope peptides from HIV-1 or ovalbumin and the mucosal adjuvant cholera toxin induces peptide-specific CTLs and protection against tumor development in vivo. J. Immunol. 158: 834–841.

Prausnitz, M.R., Bose, V.G., Langer, R., and Weaver, J.C. 1993. Electroporation of mammalian skin: a mechanism to enhance transdermal drug delivery. Proc. Natl. Acad. Sci. USA 90: 10504–10508.

Prausnitz, M.R., Gimm, J.A., Guy, R.H., Langer, R., Weaver, J.C., and Cullander, C. 1996. Imaging regions of transport across human stratum corneum during high-voltage and low-voltage exposures. J. Pharm Sci. 85: 1363–1370.

Recommendations of the Immunization Practices Advisory Committee Update on Hepatitis B Prevention. 1987. MMWR 36: 353.

Regnier, V., and Preat, V. 1998. Localization of a FITC-labeled phosphorothioate oligodeoxynucleotide in the skin after topical delivery by iontophoresis and electroporation. Pharm. Res. 15: 1596–1602.

Riminton, D.S., Kandasamy, R., Dravec, D., Basten, A., and Baxter, A.G. 2004. Dermal enhancement: bacterial products on intact skin induce and augment organ-specific autoimmune disease. J. Immunol. 172: 302–309.

Roberts, M.S., and Walker, M. 1993. Water, The Most Natural Penetration Enhancer, Vol. 59. New York, Marcel Dekker.

Roy, M.J., Wu, M.S., Barr, L. ., Fuller, J.T., Tussey, L.G., Speller, S., Culp, J., Burkholder, J.K., Swain, W.F., Dixon, R.M., *et al.* 2000. Induction of antigen-specific CD8$^+$ T cells, T helper cells, and protective levels of antibody in humans by particle-mediated administration of a hepatitis B virus DNA vaccine. Vaccine 19: 764–778.

Scharton-Kersten, T., Yu, J., Vassell, R., O'Hagan, D., Alving, C R., and Glenn, G.M. 2000. Transcutaneous immunization with bacterial ADP-ribosylating exotoxins, subunits, and unrelated adjuvants. Infect. Immun. 68: 5306–5313.

Schirmbeck, R., Bohm, W., Ando, K., Chisari, F.V., and Reimann, J. 1995. Nucleic acid vaccination primes hepatitis B virus surface antigen-specific cytotoxic T lymphocytes in nonresponder mice. J. Virol. 69: 5929–5934.

Seo, N., Tokura, Y., Nishijima, T., Hashizume, H., Furukawa, F., and Takigawa, M. 2000. Percutaneous peptide immunization via corneum barrier-disrupted murine skin for experimental tumor immunoprophylaxis. Proc. Natl. Acad. Sci. USA 97: 371–376.

Singh, M., and O'Hagan, D. 1999. Advances in vaccine adjuvants. Nature Biotechnol. 17: 1075–1081.

Snider, D.P. 1995. The mucosal adjuvant activities of ADP-ribosylating bacterial enterotoxins. Crit. Rev. Immunol. 15: 317–348.

Tang, H., Mitragotri, S., Blankschtein, D., and Langer, R. 2001. Theoretical description of transdermal transport of hydrophilic permeants: application to low-frequency sonophoresis. J. Pharm. Sci. 90: 545–568.

Tierney, R., Beignon, A.S., Rappuoli, R., Muller, S., Sesardic, D., and Partidos, C.D. 2003. Transcutaneous immunization with tetanus toxoid and mutants of *Escherichia coli* heat-labile enterotoxin as adjuvants elicits strong protective antibody responses. J. Infect. Dis. 188: 753–758.

Udey, M.C. 1997. Cadherins and Langerhans cell immunobiology. Clin. Exp. Immunol. 107 Suppl. 1: 6–8.

Uren, R.F., Howman-Giles, R., and Thompson, J.F. 2003. Patterns of lymphatic drainage from the skin in patients with melanoma. J. Nucl. Med. 44: 570–582.

Van Damme, P., Vranckx, R., Safary, A., Andre, F.E., and Meheus, A. 1989. Protective efficacy of a recombinant deoxyribonucleic acid hepatitis B vaccine in institutionalized mentally handicapped clients. Am. J. Med. 87: 26S–29S.

Vanbever, R., Lecouturier, N., and Preat, V. 1994. Transdermal delivery of metoprolol by electroporation. Pharm. Res. 11: 1657–1662.

Vanbever, R., and Preat, V.V. 1999. In vivo efficacy and safety of skin electroporation. Adv. Drug Delivery Rev. 35: 77–88.

Watabe, S., Xin, K., Ihata, A., Liu, L., Honsho, A., Aoki, I., Hamajima, K., Wahren, B., and Okuda, K. 2001. Protection against influenza virus challenge by topical application of influenza DNA vaccine. Vaccine 19: 4434–4444.

Weimann, L.J., and Wu, J. 2002. Transdermal delivery of poly-l-lysine by sonomacroporation. Ultrasound Med. Biol 28: 1173–1180.

Wells, J.M., Li, L.H., Sen, A., Jahreis, G.P., and Hui, S.W. 2000. Electroporation-enhanced gene delivery in mammary tumors. Gene Ther. 7: 541–547.

Weltzin, R., Guy, B., Thomas, W.D., Jr., Giannasca, P.J., and Monath, T.P. 2000. Parenteral adjuvant activities of *Escherichia coli* heat-labile toxin and its B subunit for immunization of mice against gastric *Helicobacter pylori* infection. Infect. Immun. 68: 2775–2782.

West, D.J. 1989. Clinical experience with hepatitis B vaccines. Am. J. Infect. Control 17: 172–180.

Wolf, M., Hall, E., Taylor, D., Coster, T., Trespalacios, F., Cassels, F., deLorimier, A., and McQueen, C. 1999. Use of the human challenge model to characterize the immune response to the colonization factors of enterotoxigenic *Escherichia coli* (ETEC). The 35th US–Japan Cholera and Other Bacterial Enteric Infections Joint Panel Meeting, Baltimore, MD.

Wolf, M.K., de Haan, L.A., Cassels, F.J., Willshaw, G.A., Warren, R., Boedeker, E.C., and Gaastra, W. 1997. The CS6 colonization factor of human enterotoxigenic *Escherichia coli* contains two heterologous major subunits. FEMS Microbiol. Lett. 148: 35–42.

Yoshida, A., Nagata, T., Uchijima, M., Higashi, T., and Koide, Y. 2000. Advantage of gene gun-mediated over intramuscular inoculation of plasmid DNA vaccine in reproducible induction of specific immune responses. Vaccine 18: 1725–1729.

Yu, J., Cassels, F., Scharton-Kersten, T., Hammond, S.A., Hartman, A., Angov, E., Corthesy, B., Alving, C., and Glenn, G. 2002. Transcutaneous immunization using colonization factor and heat labile enterotoxin induces correlates of protective immunity for enterotoxigenic *Escherichia coli*. Infect. Immun. 70: 1056–1068.

Yu, R.C., Abrams, D.C., Alaibac, M., and Chu, A.C. 1994. Morphological and quantitative analyses of normal epidermal Langerhans cells using confocal scanning laser microscopy. Br. J. Dermatol. 131: 843–848.

Zewert, T.E., Pliquett, U.F., Langer, R., and Weaver, J.C. 1995. Transdermal transport of DNA antisense oligonucleotides by electroporation. Biochem. Biophys. Res. Commun. 212: 286–292.

Zewert, T.E., Pliquett, U.F., Vanbever, R., Langer, R., and Weaver, J.C. 1999. Creation of transdermal pathways for macromolecule transport by skin electroporation and a low toxicity, pathway-enlarging molecule. Bioelectrochem. Bioenerg. 49: 11–20.

Zhang, L., Nolan, E., Kreitschitz, S., and Rabussay, D.P. 2002. Enhanced delivery of naked DNA to the skin by non-invasive in vivo electroporation. Biochim. Biophys. Acta 1572: 1–9.

Zurbriggen, R., Metcalfe, I.C., Glück, R., Viret, J.-F., and Moser, C. 2003. Nonclinical safety evaluation of *Escherichia coli* heat-labile toxin mucosal adjuvant as a component of a nasal influenza vaccine. Expert Rev. Vaccines 2: 295–304.

Chapter 6

Cellular Vaccines: Current Status

Alessandra Nardin and Jean-Pierre Abastado

Abstract

Cellular vaccines represent a novel generation of vaccines specifically designed for immunotherapy of cancer and chronic infectious diseases. Similarly to classical vaccines, they comprise both antigenic and adjuvant activities. However, these two components are engineered to provide the immunogenicity required to overcome a potential immunodeficit associated with the disease, so that a sustained, protective immune response can be elicited. Dendritic cells which were differentiated, activated, and loaded *ex vivo* with tumor-derived antigens have been shown to represent a safe vaccine, inducing immune and clinical responses following injection in some cancer patients. Given the numerous methods used to prepare dendritic cells, the definition of common criteria for assessing their potency is one of the main technological challenges. Vaccination with killed autologous or allogeneic tumor cells constitutes another approach for eliciting immunity to relevant tumor rejection antigens, many of which are still unknown. Although this may seem a less technologically demanding strategy as it does not require the preparation of viable, active cells, it remains critical to provide an effective adjuvant together with the antigen. We review here the current methods for preparing cell-based vaccines and discuss the new technological avenues that are being explored in this field.

INTRODUCTION: WHY CELLULAR VACCINES?

The possibility of harnessing the immune system against cancer was recognized over a century ago when W. Coley injected bacterial toxins into patients with sarcoma and observed some spectacular, although anecdotal, remissions. Ever since, vaccinating people against their cancer has been the holy grail of tumor immunologists, and between 10% and 20% of clinical responses have been observed in the most successful studies. Initially, cancer vaccines were prepared from the patient's own tumor, which was processed to eliminate its tumorigenic potential and increase its immunogenicity. Only recently, these approaches began to be based on both a solid knowledge of tumor antigens and a clear understanding of immunological mechanisms involved.

Cellular vaccines are therapeutic preparations of living or irradiated cells designed to stimulate specific immune responses. Such a definition covers dendritic cells (DCs) and related products (which function as adjuvants), as well as various types of tumor cell preparations (used as antigen source). The composition of cellular vaccines is clearly more complex than that of standard vaccines made of attenuated or killed viruses and bacteria or recombinant proteins. We review here the current status of these technologies and try to identify the main challenges for future developments.

Dendritic cells

Active immunotherapy of cancer and infectious diseases by administration of *ex vivo* generated DCs is currently the most actively developed application of cellular vaccines. As of November 2004, DCs are being tested in at least 29 clinical trials (source: NIH database, www.clinicaltrials.gov), some of which are phase III studies. Considering that DCs, first described by P. Langerhans in 1868, were rediscovered only in 1973 (Steinman and Cohn, 1973), and that the first methods of *in vitro* DC generation were developed in the 1990s (Caux *et al.*, 1992; Romani *et al.*, 1994; Sallusto and Lanzavecchia, 1994), it is clear that rapid progress has been made in scaling-up and optimizing DC production for clinical applications.

DCs are bone marrow-derived professional antigen-presenting cells (APCs). In both human and mouse, several subsets with distinct properties have been described, widely distributed around the body, in lymphoid and non-lymphoid tissues (Shortman and Liu, 2002). DCs are strategically located at sites of potential pathogen entry (skin, mucosae). They constitutively take up antigens and migrate to draining lymphoid organs, where, upon infection and inflammation, they prime helper and cytotoxic T cells (Banchereau and Steinman, 1998). In steady-state conditions, DCs probably contribute to the shaping of the T cell repertoire by deletion or inactivation of self-reactive T cells and play an important role in the maintenance of peripheral tolerance to self-antigens (Steinman *et al.*, 2003). It was originally thought that distinct DC subsets (e.g. myeloid versus lymphoid, $CD8^+$ versus $CD8^-$) were responsible for immunostimulation and tolerance respectively (Suss and Shortman, 1996; Fazekas de St Groth, 1998). The situation is likely to be more complex. Most DC subsets are capable of both functions, probably depending on their state of activation and on environmental signals. This plasticity has profound consequences on the protocols used to generate cellular vaccines, to ensure that the vaccines are inducing an immune response rather than specifically suppressing it.

The aim of vaccination is to induce an effective and long-lasting protective, antigen-specific immune response. Conventional vaccines are prophylactic. In such a setting, the immune system is generally intact. With viral antigens, cellular and humoral protective responses can often be generated by the mere inoculation of the antigen in combination with a standard adjuvant. Chronic viral infections and cancers represent a more challenging situation in which active immunotherapy aims to modify and/or redirect the existing immune response. Animal models and human studies indicate that, in these settings, antigen formulation with classical adjuvants may not be sufficient for the induction of relevant cellular immunity, namely cytotoxic lymphocyte responses. Many elements probably contribute to this deficiency, including the nature of tumor-associated antigens, most of which are part of the self-repertoire (Kourilsky and Fazilleau, 2001). The development of cancer is a multievent process in which tumor cells escape both from normal growth control mechanisms and from immune recognition. Therefore, tumor cells seem to be predominantly poorly immunogenic (for a review of tumor immunoediting, see Dunn *et al.*, 2002). Furthermore, tumor growth is often associated with a suppressive microenvironment. For example, APCs in cancer patients can be functionally defective (Gabrilovich *et al.*, 1997). However, normal professional APCs can be generated *ex vivo* from cancer patients starting from precursors. In addition, increased frequencies of $CD4^+CD25^+$ cells able to mediate inhibition of autologous T cell proliferation have been found among lymphocytes of patients bearing different types of cancer, including advanced ovarian carcinoma (Woo *et al.*, 2001), non-small cell lung cancer (Woo *et al.*,

2002), colorectal, pancreas and breast cancers (Liyanage *et al.*, 2002; Somasundaram *et al.*, 2002). Immunosuppressive phenomena and defective immune responses may be initially local, but eventually become systemic. A majority of cancer patients are aged, which also contributes to the observed immunodeficit.

DCs represent the most promising cellular vaccine because they are effective natural adjuvants. DCs are capable of initiating and modulating immune responses by priming and polarizing naive T cells. Some cancer patients have a pre-existing antitumor response. However, since the tumor is able to escape immune-surveillance, this natural response is likely to be inappropriate. For example, it may come too late, be too limited, or be directed towards antigens which are no longer expressed or presented by tumor cells (Campoli *et al.*, 2002). Alternatively, T cells in cancer patients may present defects in migration or effector function (Schule *et al.*, 2002). DCs may overcome some of these deficiencies by providing strong costimulation, secreting Th1 polarizing cytokines and T cell growth factors, and generating cognate help for cytotoxic lymphocytes in order to provide durable memory responses that will prevent relapses. A key difference of vaccination with DCs over classical adjuvants is the clonal diversification of cytotoxic T lymphocytes generated, whereas in classical vaccination these T cell populations are mostly monoclonal (Coulie *et al.*, 2002). In addition, it is proposed that antigen presentation segregated in different APCs may allow to overcome immunodominance *in vivo*, and therefore leads to polyclonal lymphocyte responses (Palmowski *et al.*, 2002a).

Although the vast majority of ongoing clinical trials with DC vaccines are conducted in cancer, some studies target HIV. A clinical trial has also focused on EBV peptide-pulsed DCs as a therapy for EBV-positive nasopharyngeal carcinoma (Lin *et al.*, 2002). The conceptual and technological application of cellular vaccines to chronic infectious diseases is the same as for cancer. However, additional hurdles are associated with the manipulation of infected biological materials from patients.

Tumor cells

Immunization with whole tumor cells, autologous or allogeneic, represents another instance of cellular cancer vaccines. In this approach, the cancer cell carries the target antigens, and it needs to be combined with an adjuvant. As such, it does not differ from conventional vaccination strategies, and thus only a brief overview will be presented on such technological developments. For review see Schadendorf *et al.* (2000).

TECHNOLOGY

Cellular vaccines constitute a novel type of therapy. In this field, advances in basic immunology and clinical development are leading to a better understanding of the immune system that permits its rational exploitation for treating cancer and other chronic diseases. Various constraints (e.g. regulatory guidelines) linked to clinical development need to be taken into consideration early during the preclinical research. Such a long-term perspective is difficult to apply in an academic environment, and likely represents one of the fundamental differences in the strategy of industrial versus research groups developing cellular vaccines. Good manufacturing practices (GMP) need to be integrated in the process of DC differentiation, loading, and maturation. Finally, securing access to intellectual property constitutes another category of constraints faced by most biotechnology companies developing new drugs.

Dendritic cell production and selection criteria

Differentiation

In principle, both autologous and allogeneic, HLA-matched, APCs could be used to induce an immune response. Vaccination with allogeneic APCs (Peiper et al., 1997; Fujii et al., 2001) is attractive from an industrial point of view due to the high degree of product standardization that can be achieved. It poses however scientific and safety concerns. For example, the need to irradiate allogeneic cells prior to administration raises several questions with regards to their functional competence (ability to migrate, to secrete cytokines) in vivo. A CD34[+] acute myeloid leukemia cell line that can differentiate into DCs upon culture in presence of GM-CSF and IL-4 has been developed (Masterson et al., 2002). Allogeneic DCs obtained from siblings have also been tested in clinical studies in the HIV field (Peshwa et al., 1998).

In the autologous setting, DCs can either be directly isolated from blood (where they represent less than 1% of circulating leukocytes) or differentiated from circulating precursors. Specifically, there are three main methods for obtaining DCs for immunization:

1 by direct isolation from blood apheresis (with enrichment, for example on a metrizamide gradient or immunoselection) (Small et al., 2000; Fong et al.; 2001a; Lopez et al., 2003);
2 from proliferating CD34[+] progenitors enriched from blood apheresis and cultured ex vivo with cytokines and growth factors (e.g. GM-CSF and TNF-α ± Flt3 ligand) (Romani et al., 1994; Banchereau et al., 2001);
3 from non-proliferating blood monocyte precursors isolated from blood and cultured ex vivo with cytokines and growth factors (e.g. GM-CSF and IL-4 or IL-13).

Generation of DCs from human bone marrow mononuclear cells has also been described (Bai et al., 2002).

Few clinical studies have been performed to directly compare the characteristics and biological activities of APCs obtained via these different methods. Overall, in vitro studies indicate that biological properties of CD34-derived DCs resemble those of monocyte-derived DCs (Herbst et al., 1997; Ferlazzo et al., 2000; Chen et al., 2001; Bykovskaia et al., 2002). One report suggested that DCs differentiated from CD34[+] progenitors are more effective than monocyte-derived DCs for the activation of low-frequency peptide-specific cytotoxic lymphocytes (Mortarini et al., 1997). During culture, CD34[+] progenitors differentiate toward both the Langerhans cell and the interstitial DC lineages (Caux et al., 1996; Banchereau et al., 2001). Although it may be an advantage to provide the activity of both subsets, it will also be more difficult to characterize and standardize the final product.

Regardless of the method chosen for DC generation, treatment of the patients with G-CSF (Banchereau et al., 2001), GM-CSF (Triozzi et al., 2000), or Flt3 ligand (Fong et al., 2001b) are common procedures used to enhance the number of precursor cells prior to apheresis (a technique referred to as 'patient mobilization'). For example, Fong and collegues reported that Flt3 ligand mobilization allows up to a 60-fold increase in DCs: from an average of 5×10^6 to 271×10^6 cells per apheresis (Fong et al., 2001b). The purity of DC preparations after direct isolation from blood is often lower than 50% (Small et al., 2000; Fong et al., 2001a).

In vivo mobilization and *in vitro* expansion of CD34$^+$ progenitors are thus effective methods to increase final DC yield. However, DC differentiation from blood CD14$^+$ monocytes remains the simplest (and today most widely used) method for obtaining large APC numbers. The possibility to prepare all vaccine doses starting from a single apheresis has the advantage of leading to a better standardized manufacturing.

The first protocol for generation of DCs from CD14$^+$ monocytes was described in 1994 (Sallusto and Lanzavecchia, 1994). According to this now classical procedure, peripheral blood leukocytes are obtained by Ficoll/Hypaque separation or by apheresis, and then monocytes are isolated by adherence to plastic and cultured for 7 days in the presence of GM-CSF and IL-4. Alternative monocyte purification methods include immunoselection of CD14$^+$ cells with magnetic beads (Stift *et al.*, 2003a), depletion of T and B cells (Suen *et al.*, 2001), or monocyte elutriation (Bernard *et al.*, 1998).

Depending on the cytokine combination during culture, monocytes can be driven to differentiate not only towards a lineage of interstitial DCs (GM-CSF+IL-4 or GM-CSF+IL-13; Morse *et al.*, 1999b; Goxe *et al.*, 2000), but also towards a Langerhans cell-like phenotype. Langerin-expressing cells have been obtained in the presence of GM-CSF, IL-4 and TGF-α (Geissmann *et al.*, 1998) or GM-CSF and IL-15 (Mohamadzadeh *et al.*, 2001). In addition, potent APCs can also be obtained by culturing monocytes in the presence of GM-CSF and IFN-α (Paquette *et al.*, 1998; Santini *et al.*, 2000). Some recent methods describe the preparation of APCs from monocytes within 2–3 days of culture instead of the traditional 7 days (Dauer *et al.*, 2003; Di Pucchio *et al.*, 2003). Although potentially interesting, further characterization of APCs thus obtained is still awaited.

One of the critical steps for generation of DCs from CD14$^+$ monocytes is the initial isolation of precursors. Monocyte adhesion to plastic is subject to variability, and extensive manipulation can lead to contamination. In order to simplify the process and improve clinical compatibility, we have developed a single-use kit for the differentiation of monocyte-derived DCs (cell processor). This is a closed system in which cells from unfractionated apheresis are seeded in gas-permeable bags in serum-free medium. DC differentiation occurs within 7 days in the presence of GM-CSF and IL-13. DCs are then purified by elutriation (Goxe *et al.*, 2000). A schematic representation of the process is shown in Figure 6.1. From the analysis of 37 different preparations, a mean production yield is 9.2 (± 4.6) $\times 10^8$ DCs per apheresis (with an efficiency of differentiation from monocytes of $52 \pm 15\%$), with a mean viability of 98% and a mean purity of 95%. As T cells are devoid of IL-13 receptor, IL-13-driven DC differentiation can be performed in bulk leukocytes. This procedure leads not only to higher yields ($48 \pm 9\%$ differentiation yield from bulk culture compared with $28 \pm 5\%$ from monocyte-enriched preparations), but also to stronger stimulatory activity (our unpublished observation). Interestingly, an independent report indicates that bulk culture may also improve differentiation of DCs generated in the presence of GM-CSF and IL-4. In addition, it is suggested that non-adherent PBMC may participate in enhancing DC maturation (Hinkel *et al.*, 2000, personal observation).

To eliminate the variability in cell culture, Aastrom developed a completely closed and automated process. Its core technology is based on the Aastrom Replicell™ System, an integrated system of instrumentation and single-use disposable kits for the commercial-scale production of human cells. Aastrom has developed DC-I (DCs for fusion and transfection), DCV-I (complex antigen-loaded DCs) and DCV-II (peptide-loaded DCs) production systems. These APCs have yet to be extensively tested in clinical trials.

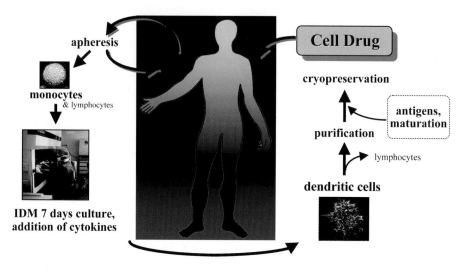

Autologous Cell Drug™ Therapy

Figure 6.1 Schematic representation of IDM technology for DC differentiation. Peripheral blood mononuclear cells are collected by apheresis, washed, and seeded in serum-free medium in non-adherent, gas-permeable, bags. GM-CSF and IL-13 are added to drive the differentiation of monocytes into immature DCs. After 7 days of culture, DCs are purified by elutriation, loaded with antigen and activated. Vaccine doses are then cryopreserved for re-infusion into the patient after batch release assays. This closed culture system allows the preparation of, on average, 900 million antigen-loaded DCs.

Lastly, we wish to emphasize that DC differentiation depends not only on the type of precursors, but also on the combination of cytokines added to the culture, the type of plasticware (Guyre *et al.*, 2002), the culture medium used (for example, presence or absence of serum) (Duperrier *et al.*, 2000; Loudovaris *et al.*, 2001), or the cytokine source and concentration (leading to APCs with different phenotypic and functional properties). Standardized assays for comparison of functional properties of all these APCs are needed, as discussed later.

Maturation

Maturation is the process by which DCs increase their costimulation properties, reduce antigen uptake, augment the processing and presentation of MHC class I and class II-restricted epitopes, secrete immunomodulatory cytokines, and acquire responsiveness to chemokine gradients which induce migration to draining lymphoid organs (Mellman and Steinman, 2001). DC maturation is triggered by microbial or inflammatory signals, and it is thought to be the hallmark distinguishing between stimulatory and steady-state 'tolerogenic' DCs. It is therefore critical, in the production of DC-based vaccines, to provide *ex vivo* the relevant signals inducing DC final differentiation and activation. Such signals in cancer patients may either be not appropriate, or down-regulated by the tumor (Kiertscher *et al.*, 2000). Indeed, it has been reported that administration of immature DCs results in the induction of either anergic T cells (Jonuleit *et al.*, 2001), or IL-10-secreting antigen-specific CD8[+] cells with regulatory properties (Dhodapkar *et al.*, 2001).

The choice of the maturation agent for DC-based vaccines is driven by criteria of activity, GMP-grade availability, and compliance with regulatory requirements. When evaluating potential maturation agents, three standard features are usually measured on the APCs: up-regulation of surface markers (e.g. costimulatory and antigen-presentation molecules, DC-specific activation markers such as CD83), cytokine secretion (in particular IL-12, a critical Th1-polarizing cytokine), and increased migration in chemotactic assays. Functional assays can also be performed: in this case, mature and immature DCs are evaluated for their ability to prime naïve T cells. It is important to underline that not all maturation agents have equivalent activities. For example, while some Toll-like receptor (TLR) agonists such as lipopolysaccharide (LPS) and double-stranded RNA (Cella *et al.*, 1999) induce phenotypic maturation as well as secretion of bioactive IL-12, this latter cytokine is not produced in response to stimuli such as TNF-α or monocyte-conditioned medium (mimicked by a cocktail containing TNF-α, IL-6, IL-1β, prostaglandin E_2). CD40L is also rather inefficient in inducing IL-12 secretion, unless used in combination with a microbial stimulus or IFN-γ (Hilkens *et al.*, 1997). IFN-γ, but also IL-1β (Luft *et al.*, 2002a) or type I IFN (Luft *et al.*, 2002c), positively modulate IL-12 secretion. On the other hand, IL-12 is inhibited by vitamin D_3 (Penna and Adorini, 2000) or by agents that increase cyclic AMP such as prostaglandin E_2 or cholera toxin (Kalinski *et al.*, 1998; Gagliardi *et al.*, 2000). To make things more complex, these latter agents have been recently shown to provide an essential complementary signal for inducing responsiveness to CCR7 ligands in monocyte-derived DCs (Luft *et al.*, 2002b; Scandella *et al.*, 2002). This led to the hypothesis that cytokine-secreting, 'inflammatory' DCs, and 'migratory' DCs represent two segregated phenotypes of monocyte-derived DCs, and that the developmental programs for DC localization and DC maturation are controlled independently. Therefore, the method of maturation may have to be chosen also based on (a) the route of injection (i.e. i.d. or s.c. versus intranodal) and (b) the method of DC generation (Luft *et al.*, 2002b).

Bacterial extracts or cells (e.g. *M. bovis* bacillus Calmette–Guerin, BCG) are highly efficient maturation agents for DCs (Boccaccio *et al.*, 2002). A vast array of bacterial or viral-derived natural and synthetic TLR ligands have been identified, which have potential application as DC maturation factors: they include for example *Klebsiella pneumoniae* outer membrane protein A (Jeannin *et al.*, 2000), OM-197-MP-AC (Byl *et al.*, 2003), monophosphoryl lipid A (MPL) (Ismaili *et al.*, 2002), JBT3002 (Eue *et al.*, 1998), and polyriboinosinic polyribocytidylic acid (polyI:C) (Verdijk *et al.*, 1999). As the adjuvant activity of LPS resides in its lipid moiety, lipid A derivatives and analogs such as MPL and OM-197-MP-AC have been developed with the aim of reducing toxicity and pyrogenicity while maintaining the activity of the molecule. Although there are safety concerns when using LPS in clinical trials, an *ex vivo* treatment provides a unique opportunity for reducing contaminants below acceptable limits before administration of the vaccine.

An additional parameter to be considered in the design of protocols for generating therapeutic DCs is the duration of exposure to the maturation agent. It was demonstrated that final DC maturation is associated with a decreased ability to produce IL-12 during the interaction with CD4$^+$ T cells (Kalinski *et al.*, 1999). Terminally mature, 'exhausted' DCs preferentially induce Th2 cells (Langenkamp *et al.*, 2000), and only DCs at early maturation stages, which are actively secreting IL-12, are able to recruit and expand large numbers of naïve CD8$^+$ T cells *in vitro* in the absence of CD4$^+$ T cells (Kaiser *et al.*, 2003). In most current clinical studies, APCs are exposed *ex vivo* to maturation stimuli for at least 24 hours. We have shown that a short contact with a potent stimulus is sufficient to trigger a DC activation process that proceeds spontaneously upon further DC culture in the absence of any maturation agent (Boccaccio *et al.*, 2002; Kaiser *et al.*, 2003). Such 'maturing' DCs can be cryo-preserved, and, after thawing, they continue to mature and secrete IL-12.

In vivo maturation may also represent a viable alternative protocol: antigen-loaded, immature DCs can be injected into areas of skin that have been treated with an adjuvant (Nair *et al.*, 2003).

Antigens and loading methods

In the last few years, genomic and proteomic approaches have led to the molecular identification and patenting of many tumor-associated antigens (TAA) that may potentially be recognized by T cells on the surface of tumor cells. According to their pattern of expression in tumor and normal tissues, TAA have been divided into five main categories: tumor-specific shared antigens (cancer germ-line genes), differentiation antigens, antigens resulting from point mutations, antigens resulting from gene over-expression, and viral antigens. Early reviews focus especially on melanoma antigens (Van den Eynde and Boon, 1997), but new antigens are being identified in prostate, breast, colon and other cancers. Particularly attractive for the design of vaccination strategies are those antigens whose expression is shared by different tumors. However, it is not always known whether a T cell repertoire can be mobilized against these antigens, and *in vitro* immunogenicity studies with human cells are still warranted for several of them. The following basic criteria may help guide the selection of best suited targets for vaccination purposes:

1   expression in different tumor stages (e.g. primary as well as metastatic tumors);
2   limited expression in normal vital organs;
3   expression shared by different tumors;
4   relevant structure and function (involvement in cancer formation and dissemination may avoid development of escape mutants after vaccination);
5   immunogenicity.

Other criteria such as ease and yield of production or stability may be considered depending on the form of antigen (for example, recombinant protein versus plasmid or vector).

Altogether, however, it is still unclear what defines a good tumor rejection antigen, and the vast majority of new targets are still awaiting clinical validation.

Peptides

MHC class I peptides probably represent the simplest and safest antigenic formulation for DC loading. Analog peptides with higher affinity for the HLA molecules (Tourdot *et al.*, 2000), increased immunogenicity (Tangri *et al.*, 2001) or enhanced resistance to proteases (Calbo *et al.*, 2000) can be easily produced. In addition, peptides can be manufactured and GMP-formulated using simple processes. They can be loaded on HLA molecules directly, without any need for internalization and processing by the APCs. Up to 10% of MHC class I molecules can be complexed with a high affinity peptide (Langlade-Demoyen *et al.*, 1994). In addition, the immunoproteasome in mature DCs may generate epitopes that are optimal HLA-binders and capable to induce a CTL response, but which are not naturally presented by cancer cells, since the latter use the standard proteasome (Van den Eynde and Morel, 2001). Using peptides for loading, we can provide DCs with selected epitopes.

Main limitations in the use of peptides include the HLA restriction (which confines application to patients with certain HLA haplotypes only) and the single antigen-specificity of the response generated (which may favour the emergence of tumor variants (Jager *et al.*, 1997)). However, the use of multiple peptides represents a simple solution to circumvent these problems as it broadens the number of patients who can be treated while simultaneously reducing the risk of tumor escape. If autologous tumor cells are available, acid-eluted peptides offer the possibility of pulsing the DCs with a broad repertoire of HLA-matched tumor antigens (Storkus *et al.*, 1993; Yu *et al.*, 2001). However, class II-derived peptides, which are loaded in an acidic compartment, are generally not eluted by acid treatment.

It has been observed that vaccination with a mixture of antigens generates a response to the immunodominant antigen exclusively (Palmowski *et al.*, 2002a). Pre-existing immune responses to one of the peptides may prevent further immunization against the other epitopes when presented by the same APCs, a finding described with viral variants as the original antigenic sin (Singh *et al.*, 2002). The main mechanism for these observations seems to be competition at the level of APCs (for review see Kedl *et al.*, 2003). Experimental models indicate that responses to subdominant antigens may be rescued by immunization with separate APCs bearing single peptides (Grufman *et al.*, 1999). In addition, immunodominance could potentially be broken by immunization with an excess of APCs (Palmowski *et al.*, 2002b).

Currently, three main problems remain to be solved for peptide approaches:

1   the limited half-life of MHC–peptide complexes (Ojcius *et al.*, 1993; Wang and Wang, 2002);
2   the MHC polymorphism, in that each allele selects a different set of peptide ligands (Rammensee *et al.*, 1993);
3   the lack of CD4 help that is required for a high-quality, protective memory CD8[+] T cell response unless CD4 epitopes are used (Janssen *et al.*, 2003; Shedlock and Shen, 2003; Sun and Bevan, 2003).

Proteins

A feature considered unique to DCs is their ability to cross-present exogenous antigens (following either macropinocytosis, endocytosis or phagocytosis by immature DCs) on MHC class I molecules (Belz *et al.*, 2002). This pathway probably requires antigen transport to the cytosol and is largely TAP-dependent. A protein internalized by DCs could therefore provide both class I and class II epitopes necessary for a long-lasting memory immune response. Antigen delivery into the APCs may have the advantage of leading to a prolonged presentation when compared with non-processed, externally loaded peptides (Chow *et al.*, 2002; Wang and Wang, 2002). Also, instead of native proteins, polypeptides designed to contain overlapping regions of class I and class II epitopes can be used.

Cross-presentation, however, is a rather inefficient process when soluble, non-targeted antigens are used. Several methods have been tested experimentally for increasing the 'throughput' of loading and/or cross-presentation. There is evidence that immune complexes, internalized via Fc receptors, reach an intracellular pathway that eventually allows them to to deliver the antigen to the cytosol, thus favoring cross-presentation

(Regnault *et al.*, 1999; Wallace *et al.*, 2001; Nagata *et al.*, 2002). The targeting of mannose receptors is highly efficient for protein uptake, and antigens internalized through such a pathway seem to be presented by both MHC class II (Engering *et al.*, 1997) and MHC class I (Ramakrishna *et al.*, 2004) molecules. Other targeting approaches focus on heat-shock protein and GM-CSF receptors (Castellino *et al.*, 2000; Small *et al.*, 2000). Depending on the system, these targeting methods may simply provide a way to concentrate antigens on the DCs (which could be important when purity of APCs is low), or enhance and sustain cross-presentation by redirecting the antigen to a specific cellular pathway.

There are several other technologies in development for improving antigen delivery to APCs. Carriers such as liposomes (which can be targeted to specific receptors) or virosomes are able to fuse with the endosomal membrane and deliver the antigens to the cytoplasm (Bungener *et al.*, 2002). Osmotic loading and electroporation also allow delivery of a high amount of antigen to the cytosol (for a review see Zhou *et al.*, 2002). Peptides that spontaneously translocate across the membrane (also called 'Penetratins', e.g. HIV tat protein, or the third helix of the *Drosophila* Antennapedia homeodomain protein (Derossi *et al.*, 1998)) can be conjugated to tumor antigens and exploited for cytosol transport. Fusogenic peptides, derived from a viral protein mediating the fusion of the viral envelope with the target cell membrane, may be used in a similar fashion (Day *et al.*, 2003). Finally, detoxified recombinant toxins or toxin subunits, such as the B subunit of shiga toxin (Haicheur *et al.*, 2000), normally able to gain access to the cytosol, could potentially improve DC loading and and facilitate the induction of cytotoxic lymphocytes.

Whole tumor cells

Using antigens from whole tumor cells as opposed to well-defined proteins generates a broader T cell immune response. However, due to the presence of significant amount of normal tissue antigens in the preparations, the risk of inducing autoimmune pathologies is also higher.

Tumor cell-derived antigens are prepared in the form of lysates, necrotic, or apoptotic cells. Due to the ease of production, lysates are commonly used to load DCs. They are obtained by submitting tumor cells to freezing and thawing cycles, sonication, or mechanical disruption, followed by irradiation. A centrifugation step is sometimes performed to remove larger particles. Necrotic tumor cells may be prepared by similar methods or derived from apoptotic cells submitted to serum starvation (Berard *et al.*, 2000). Apoptosis can be induced by either UVB, γ-irradiation, or treatment with various pharmacological agents, such as actinomycin D, ceramide, mitomycin C, or lovastatin. Tumor cells of different origins may present different susceptibilities to apoptosis induction by these treatments.

The uptake of lysates by DCs occurs mainly by macropinocytosis, while apoptotic bodies are phagocytosed via αvβ5 integrins and CD36 molecules (Albert *et al.*, 1998). Several groups compared lysates, necrotic and apoptotic cell-based preparations with the aim of identifying the most effective formulation for cross-priming of cytotoxic lymphocytes. Some reports indicate that apoptotic tumor cells are superior to cell lysates (Hoffmann *et al.*, 2000; Schnurr *et al.*, 2002; Zhou *et al.*, 2003), others that they are equivalent (Kotera *et al.*, 2001; Lambert *et al.*, 2001). Based on the observation that necrotic but not apoptotic cells induce DC maturation, it was proposed that necrotic cells may provide a critical signal for the initiation of immunity (Sauter *et al.*, 2000).

Although these results are contradictory (possibly due to the fact that protocols for antigen preparation may differ), there is a consensus on the fact that cytotoxic lymphocytes can be induced with both antigenic preparations.

Some of the methods for improving antigen uptake discussed above are also applicable to whole tumor cells: for example, Dhodapkar and collegues demonstrated enhanced cross-presentation of cellular antigens upon uptake of antibody-opsonized myeloma cells by DCs. Interestingly, this was not due to a superior uptake, hence supporting the notion that a different intracellular pathway is responsible for increased cross-presentation of FcγR-targeted antigens (Dhodapkar et al., 2002).

While numerous trials have been conducted with DCs loaded with lysates from autologous tumors (Nestle et al., 1998; Geiger et al., 2001; Chang et al., 2002; Maier et al., 2003; Stift et al., 2003b), antigenic preparations based on apoptotic cells are still in early development (Berard et al., 2000; Dhodapkar et al., 2002). In this case, it is likely that the antigenic material is not completely internalized by DCs and difficult to eliminate, and thus final product characterization could become problematical.

Autologous tumor tissues are rarely available in adjuvant settings or for immunization of early stage cancer patients. In addition, the amount of antigenic material may vary from patient to patient, so that DC loading cannot be standardized and the amount of tumor antigens available may have an impact on clinical results. These problems can be solved by using either allogeneic tumor cell lines, or total tumor RNA (as discussed later). The use of allogeneic tumor cell lines as a source of tumor-associated antigens is an attractive strategy. The combination of lysates from several cell lines, possibly representative of distinct tumor stages, provides a broad variety of TAA. Safety concerns may be addressed by an extensive assessment of sterility, adventitious viral contaminants or residual tumorigenicity. Antigen composition, identity and stability criteria can also be defined and applied to the various allo-lysate batches, but not to auto-lysates. While the immunogenicity of DCs loaded with autologous tumor have been reported by numerous groups, experience with DCs loaded with allogeneic tumor is more sporadic (Stift et al., 2003a). We have completed a phase I/II clinical trial on 16 melanoma patients indicating feasibility and safety of the approach (Salcedo et al., in preparation).

Another technology that may allow vaccination against whole tumor antigens is hybrid cell vaccines. The fusion of autologous tumor cells with autologous or allogeneic APCs has been proposed as an efficient method to make antigenic tumor cells highly immunogenic, as such hybrids express a full repertoire of tumor antigens along with the antigen-presenting machinery of the APC. Cell fusion is classically performed with chemical reagents such as PEG or physical techniques as electrofusion (Gottfried et al., 2002; Hayashi et al., 2002; Krause et al., 2002). In addition, a genetic method, based on gene transfer of a viral fusogenic membrane glycoprotein into tumor cells, has recently been described (Phan et al., 2003b). Given the continuous source of endogenous tumor antigen, presentation via MHC class I is likely to be favored, when compared with loading with exogenous tumor lysate. However, interest in fusing tumor cells with DCs has been questioned (Celluzzi and Falo, 1998). Success rate in clinical trials is not yet well established and lack of reproducibility is a hurdle for commercialization.

As DCs acquire antigens from both apoptotic and living cells (Harshyne et al., 2003), delivery of DCs directly into a solid tumor following chemotherapy or radiotherapy represents an interesting strategy for 'in vivo loading', and this is being investigated in both mouse models (Candido *et al.*, 2001) and clinical trials (Triozzi *et al.*, 2000). *Ex vivo*-activated DCs are expected to take up apoptotic autologous tumor cells *in vivo*, prior to migrating to local lymph nodes and inducing an immune response. This approach is attractive because no antigen selection, formulation, or validation is required, and because the same product can be used for multiple clinical indications. However, it is limited to patients with accessible tumor mass. To reduce the risk that the immunosuppressive tumor microenvironment or the uptake of apoptotic bodies inhibit DC function, infused DCs have to be properly activated and irreversibly committed to maturation. Migration of intra-tumorally injected DCs to draining lymph nodes was not detected (Triozzi *et al.*, 2000), therefore it is important to demonstrate that this approach can elicit systemic immunity.

Nucleic acids

Recombinant DNA technologies provide an alternative for improving the efficiency of antigen presentation to CD8[+] T cells. Advantages include ease of production and cytosolic expression of protein, which favors prolonged class I presentation.

When using DNA-based vaccination strategies, the gene for the antigen of interest is cloned into a bacterial plasmid under the control of a eukaryotic or viral (e.g. CMV) promoter to ensure antigen expression by transfected DCs. Plasmids can be delivered via a viral vector or non-viral techniques, but the latter methods (i.e. electroporation or liposomes-mediated transfection) are usually rather inefficient (Arthur *et al.*, 1997). Improved delivery has been observed when DNA is complexed with the CL22 cationic peptide (Irvine *et al.*, 2000) or encapsulated in biodegradable hydrophilic microspheres (Walter *et al.*, 2001). Among viral vectors, adenovirus, herpes simplex virus, and vaccinia virus can infect DCs with transduction efficiencies that can be as high as 90% (Drexler *et al.*, 1999; Zhong *et al.*, 1999). Retroviruses have also been tested in preclinical studies but the efficiency of transfection is generally lower, due to the lack of cell division of monocytes and DCs (Ahuja, 2001). Importantly, *ex vivo* DC infection bypasses any pre-existing neutralizing immune response against the vector (for example, antibodies to adenovirus). The use of viral vectors in cellular vaccination is still limited by safety concerns related to both the potential toxicity of the vector itself and the influence of transduction on DC functions (e.g. in the case of random recombination of the vector sequence with the host genome). Reduction in DC viability, inhibition or induction of maturation, impairment of T cell stimulation abilities have been observed at high multiplicity of infection, even if these findings are not always consistent and may be subject to batch-related differences. Several experimental demonstrations of induction of antitumor immunity with DCs transduced with viral vectors have been reported (Drexler *et al.*, 1999; Kaplan *et al.*, 1999).

Bacterial vectors constitute an alternative tool for transduction, presenting the advantage of simultaneous DC loading and activation. For instance, virulence-attenuated or inactivated recombinant *Listeria* was shown to deliver antigens for class I presentation by DCs (Gentschev *et al.*, 2000).

DCs can also be transfected with the messenger RNA for the antigen(s) of choice. Feasibility of this approach has been demonstrated in recent clinical trials (Heiser *et al.*, 2002; Su *et al.*, 2003). Of particular interest is the possibility to transfect DCs with total tumor RNA (Heiser *et al.*, 2001), as it presents the advantage of targeting multiple autologous TAA and it is not restricted by autologous tumor availability. Unlimited amounts of RNA can be amplified by RT-PCR followed by *in vitro* transcription, starting from a few cells micro-dissected from frozen tissue sections (Boczkowski *et al.*, 2000). In addition, tumor-restricted RNA may be enriched by subtractive hybridization with RNA from normal tissue, thus decreasing the risk of generating autoimmunity. Transfection efficiency is usually optimized using electroporation, liposome carriers or micro-particles. The issue of a potential lack of cognate help in this setting was addressed by testing a chimeric hTERT/LAMP-1 construct targeting the RNA to the endosomal compartment (Su *et al.*, 2002).

Quality controls for cellular vaccines

Quality controls assess vaccine safety, identity, purity and activity. Although the basic principles of quality control for cellular vaccines are essentially the same as for standard drugs, few of the classical tests can be applied (e.g. drug sterility and endotoxin content). Methods and acceptance criteria for defining identity and potency of cellular vaccines are currently a matter of discussion. DCs can be obtained from distinct precursors, matured and loaded with different techniques: given these sources of variability, developing standard tests for investigating DC preparations is crucial.

DC purity is often defined based on morphology (evaluating the proportion of large, 'veiled' cells) (Triozzi *et al.*, 2000; Schuler-Thurner *et al.*, 2002). The analysis of surface marker expression by flow cytometry is, however, a preferred method to simultaneously assess identity, purity, and the state of activation of the cells, even in the absence of consensus on the markers to use. For example, DCs are identified on the basis of CD1a expression and lack of CD14. However, simple changes in culture conditions can modify the expression of these two markers without clear correlation with DC functionality (Loudovaris *et al.*, 2001; Guyre *et al.*, 2002). Various additional surface markers have been used to assess the purity and/or state of activation of DC preparations for clinical trials. These include HLA-DR (Fong *et al.*, 2001b), CD54 (Small *et al.*, 2000), or CD83 (Schuler-Thurner *et al.*, 2002) expressed by DCs in the absence of the lineage markers CD3, CD14, CD19, CD56. Acceptance criteria for purity need to be based on DC origin: while for monocyte-derived DCs it is feasible to reach purity levels higher than 80 or 90%, average purities for blood and CD34-derived DCs may range between 10 and 60%, depending on the method used to prepare the cells (Banchereau *et al.*, 2001; Fong *et al.*, 2001a; Small *et al.*, 2000).

An even more crucial need is to define a potency assay. A standardized measure of vaccine activity should allow the comparison between DCs prepared by different groups, and among subsequent versions of a single vaccine product during preclinical and clinical development. In addition, because cellular vaccines are often tested in small trials enrolling limited numbers of patients, a correct evaluation of clinical and immunological data is highly dependent on the establishment of the activity of the vaccine *in vitro*.

The most relevant measure of vaccine activity for cell-based vaccines is a test assessing priming of antigen-specific T cells. However, these priming assays are tedious and complex to perform, and may require sophisticated instrumentation. Assays conducted over several days, for example, are not applicable to the release of vaccines which rely upon fresh cells to be administered within hours from final formulation. The allogeneic mixed lymphocyte reaction (MLR) assay is currently being used by several groups as a quality control of DC activity (Small *et al.*, 2000; Banchereau *et al.*, 2001; Geiger *et al.*, 2001; Lau *et al.*, 2001; Yu *et al.*, 2001). In order to obtain a large single pool of responder cells, T cells can be expanded with various mitogenic stimuli, and then used to test multiple DC preparations. However, in MLR assays, the T cell proliferation index is influenced by the extent of HLA mismatch between stimulator cells (the vaccine) and responder cells, independently of the DC stimulatory activity. In addition, the response is not tumor antigen-specific. Although in principle antigen-specific T cell clones can be used as responder cells, they are hard to maintain in culture for prolonged periods of time and a reiterated procedure would be required. In addition, when using expanded T cell lines or clones, reactivation of memory responses rather than priming of naïve lymphocytes by DCs is measured.

The expression of CD54 has been used to evaluate both DC purity and potency, based upon cell sorting experiments demonstrating that all antigen-presenting activity resides in the CD54$^+$ population. It is thus conceivable to propose a potency assay combining a measure of antigen presence on DCs with one or several indirect measures of DC costimulatory activity (in an antigen-independent manner). Effective loading of DC with antigen can be confirmed for example with antibodies recognizing MHC–peptide complexes (Chames *et al.*, 2000; Cohen *et al.*, 2002; Lev *et al.*, 2002). However, the level of sensitivity required to detect only a few peptide–MHCs on DCs is rarely achieved. For protein or nucleic acid-based antigens, immunobiochemical assays demonstrating antigen presence within the cells may therefore be proposed. In addition, expression of surface molecules or secretion of a factor required for T cell stimulation may be used as an indirect assay of DC activity. Extensive preclinical studies correlating the expression a specific DC marker (e.g. a costimulatory molecule) or a cytokine (e.g. IL-12) with DC potency are still required.

Dose, route of injection and *in vivo* migration

It is essential for DC activity that these cells localize to the lymph nodes. Direct intranodal or intralymphatic administration is feasible (Nestle *et al.*, 1998; Maier *et al.*, 2003), but represents a more invasive and challenging protocol compared with subcutaneous, intradermal, or intravenous injection. Although it is well established that DC mobility and chemotactic responsiveness to the lymph node-derived CCR7 ligands (CCL19 and CCL21) is up-regulated during maturation, not all maturation factors are equivalent in this respect. For example, addition of prostaglandin E$_2$ or other activators of adenylate cyclase to the maturation stimuli appears to be important to 'switch-on' the chemokine receptor and generate migratory-type DCs. In addition, after maturation, peripheral blood DCs have been shown to be more responsive to CCL19 compared with monocyte-derived DCs (Luft *et al.*, 2002b; Scandella *et al.*, 2002).

Several *in vivo* studies have investigated the various homing compartments, as well as the kinetics and efficiency of migration of DCs administered via different routes. Administration through the intravenous route results in the distribution of DCs to the lung, liver, spleen and bone marrow, but not to lymph nodes or tumor sites (Mackensen *et al.*, 1999; Morse *et al.*, 1999a). Despite these findings, other reports indicate that intravenous administration of either monocyte or blood-derived DC results in the induction of an antigen-specific immune response, presumably after migration to secondary lymphoid organs (Lau *et al.*, 2001; Fong *et al.*, 2001a; Heiser *et al.*, 2002). Interestingly, Fong and colleagues observed that intravenously infused blood DCs induce Th2 polarized immune responses (characterized by T cells which do not secrete IFN-γ). The intradermal route is thought to be superior not only to the intravenous but also to the subcutaneous one (Morse *et al.*, 1999a; Butterfield *et al.*, 2003). It is nonetheless striking that, even upon intradermal administration, a very minor fraction of the injected cells is found in the draining lymph node. The migration capacity of mature DCs is superior to the one of immature DCs, of which only about 0.3–0.4% home to draining lymph nodes. Still, no more than 2% to 6% of the intradermally injected mature DCs localize to the lymph nodes (Thomas *et al.*, 1999; De Vries *et al.*, 2003). This corresponds to approximately 300,000 cells for a vaccine dose of ten million DCs. Importantly, classical dose–responses curves observed for drugs do not seem to apply to DC-based vaccines: a clear dose-effect cannot be demonstrated in most of the clinical studies addressing this issue (Banchereau *et al.*, 2001; Butterfield *et al.*, 2003). The number of APCs reaching the lymph node may not be limiting, as few cells could be sufficient to induce a specific immune response. On the other hand, it can be argued that relying upon high APC number may be critical to obviate the problem of immunodominance in the response, as discussed above (Palmowski *et al.*, 2002b).

Classical pharmacokinetics rules are also difficult to apply to cellular vaccines. Fast migration to draining lymphoid organs is important given the known limited stability of MHC–peptide complexes. In addition, since DCs have a limited life span, in the absence of a prompt response to chemokine gradients, the majority of these cells may die at the site of injection. Although most DCs attain the lymph node only 24 to 48 hours after intradermal inoculation (De Vries *et al.*, 2003), several groups have reported that the first DCs can be detected in the node within 10 to 20 minutes after injection (Thomas *et al.*, 1999).

Efficacy evaluation: the need for surrogate markers

For ethical reasons, most cellular vaccine trials have so far been conducted in advanced cancer patients for whom no alternative effective treatment is available. The vast majority of these patients exhibit large tumor masses and evidence for an impaired immune system. In these patient populations, some tumor regressions have been documented following treatment. Considering the relatively low rate of clinical responses observed with the products currently under development, in order to obtain meaningful data on clinical outcomes (e.g. evidence for tumor shrinkage, impact on time to progression or overall survival), the analysis on hundreds of patients over several years is required. This is not compatible with the need for a rapid evaluation of vaccine activity, which is essential to optimize the technology. The development of assays measuring surrogate biological markers of *in vivo* vaccine activity is thus very important. In addition, when such surrogate biological markers of efficacy become available, they may be used to facilitate prognosis and to adapt the therapeutic protocol depending on the predicted response of each patient.

In the last few years, monitoring cellular vaccine activity has focused on immune responses. Classical immunomonitoring assays are based on the measurement of T cell (e.g. delayed-type hypersensitivity, proliferation assays) and antibody responses. More recently, tools such as ELISPOT, MHC–peptide tetramers, Immunoscope have been developed to track and characterize antigen-specific T cells at a single cell level. These assays allow to look at specific effector functions and at the diversity of the repertoire generated, and overall to evaluate the quality of the immune response (Bercovici *et al.*, 2000). The ideal assay for measuring the immune response following immunization should be specific, sensitive enough to detect low frequency of antigen-specific T cells, quantitative, standardized, and the assessed parameter should correlate with clinical responses. In clinical studies where T cell responses were measured, a positive correlation with clinical responses has not always been observed (Rosenberg *et al.*, 1999). Although this may be due to the low immunogenicity of the vaccine, there is some evidence that the techniques available may not always measure accurately the immune response. Recent data suggest that, even if low levels of cytotoxic T cells appear to be able to initiate tumor rejection, their detection requires lengthy expansion, cloning, and sequencing of the lymphocyte cultures (Coulie *et al.*, 2001). In addition, the T cell responses measured may not be those associated with the clinical benefit. Monitoring of T cell responses is commonly performed on peripheral blood lymphocytes, but tumor-infiltrating lymphocytes may present different specificities and activities. Finally, epitope spreading seems to be a better predictor of clinical responses. Thus, immunomonitoring should not be limited to the antigenic composition of the vaccine (Butterfield *et al.*, 2003). Relevant immunomonitoring assays, although essential to better document the biological activity of the vaccine, may prove complex, difficult to standardize, and too expensive for routine testing on patients.

Although up to now monitoring was mostly focusing on T cells, it is known that other cellular components and soluble factors contribute to tumor eradication (Smyth *et al.*, 2001). Triggering tumor-specific T cells with the vaccine is crucial but not sufficient. A cascade of events should be initiated to amplify the immune response, leading to the establishment of protective immunity. In fact, general non-immune biological events associated with vaccination are important to monitor. Genomic profiling can be used in this regard to analyse gene expression at the RNA level. Normalization of the genomic profile has recently been found in patients treated with a DC-based vaccine and this correlated well with overall survival and time to disease progression in treated melanoma patients (Palucka *et al.*, 2003). Proteomic profiling involves the characterization of proteins present in a biological sample or cells (Kennedy, 2001), and is already used for diagnostic purposes for some types of cancer (Wulfkuhle *et al.*, 2003). Indeed, this method can identify proteins patterns that completely differ between cancer and non-cancer patients, or which helps distinguishing different stages of disease (Adam *et al.*, 2002).

Cost

If cell-based immunotherapy is to have any future and to be applicable to the benefit of large number of patients, cost issues have to be addressed. Most current cell preparation protocols are still cumbersome and significant savings should be made by simplifying and automating cell production. Two factors, however, suggest that cell-based immunotherapies may be cost effective in the near future: (i) the lack of toxicity observed so far (NB: the management of side-effects represents a major cost for chemo- and radiotherapies) and (ii) the simplicity and safety of cell-based immunotherapy which allows outpatient treatment. One of the major costs associated with DC vaccine production is the need to test each individual lot. The development of simple and cheap assays for batch release is thus critical to contain costs.

Tumor cells

Therapeutic cancer vaccination with tumor cells was pioneered by the group of Berd and Mastrangelo: since the 1980s, irradiated autologous tumor cells were injected, together with BCG and/or DNP-modification, to hundreds of melanoma patients in the course of multiple clinical trials (Berd and Mastrangelo, 1988a; Berd *et al.*, 1990; Berd *et al.*, 2001). This approach is now in advanced development (Lotem *et al.*, 2002; Berd *et al.*, 2002), but is feasible only in patients with resectable foci of metastatic disease.

The rationale for immunization with allogeneic tumor vaccines relies upon the observation that the expression of some tumor antigens is shared amoung tumors from various patients. Advantages are as follows: (i) a predetermined number of doses can be administered to all patients, (ii) the preparation does not vary from patient to patient and (iii) the vaccine can be used in maintenance therapies. In addition, immune response against alloantigens may provide help for the generation of tumor-specific responses. Some allogeneic tumor cell-based vaccines are in advanced clinical development in melanoma patients. One of these, termed Canvaxin™, contains three irradiated human melanoma cell lines expressing a total of 38 tumor antigens. The first injection of the vaccine is made together with BCG as an adjuvant. Canvaxin is now in phase III clinical evaluation. A similar therapy is being developed for prostate cancer. Melacine®, a lysate derived from mechanical disruption of two human melanoma cell lines, has been in clinical development for over 18 years and is now registered in Canada (Mitchell *et al.*, 1988). It is administered with DETOX™ (an adjuvant containing MPL® and mycobacterial cell wall components).

Tumor cells are not optimal APCs per se, and may contain immunosuppressive factors. To prevent these problems, autologous or allogeneic tumor cells have been genetically modified to express immunostimulatory cytokines or other biological response modifiers. Indeed, transduction of genes encoding cytokines into tumor cells may enhance tumor immunogenicity without causing the systemic toxicity that often results from administration of the molecule. Pilot trials have been conducted with genetically modified autologous tumor cells expressing either IL-7 (Moller *et al.*, 1998), IL-12 (Sun *et al.*, 1998), GM-CSF (Soiffer *et al.*, 1998), IFN-γ (Abdel-Wahab *et al.*, 1997), B7.1 (Antonia *et al.*, 2002). GVAX® is in development for several indications and consists of irradiated autologous tumor transduced with an adenovirus expressing GM-CSF (Dummer, 2001).

PERSPECTIVES: WHAT IS MISSING?

Regulation of immune responses: a role for enhancers?

Combination of cellular vaccines with cytokines (e.g. IL-2, IFN-γ, IFN-α) and other biological modifiers to enhance the immune response has been previously reported (Abdel-Wahab *et al.*, 1997; Shimizu *et al.*, 2000). Co-stimulatory signals may complement or modify activation signals provided to a lymphocyte through antigen receptors. For example, T cell priming is made possible by costimulation via CD28 (together with a battery of other molecules including OX40 and 4–1BB), and is downregulated by inhibitory signals delivered by molecules such as CTLA-4 and PD-1. Vaccination may therefore benefit from the association with agonists of costimulatory molecules or blockers of inhibitory molecules. However, even if T cell activation is enhanced by an agonist of costimulatory molecules, negative (e.g. CTLA-4) and regulatory (e.g. CD4$^+$CD25$^+$ cells) pathways may be dominant and result in suppression of the T cell response. Therefore, blocking inhibitory signals could be a very effective complement of vaccination with APCs. This strategy is currently tested in clinical trials of candidate cellular vaccines.

Anti-CTLA-4 blocking antibodies

CTLA-4 is expressed by T cells following activation and plays a critical role in the down-regulation of T cell responses. Upon binding to B7 molecules, it inhibits IL-2 production and cell cycle progression by mechanisms which are not yet completely clear (Krummel and Allison, 1996; Greenwald *et al.*, 2002). CTLA-4 is also constitutively expressed intracellularly at high levels in a subset of CD4$^+$CD25$^+$ regulatory T cells. Whether its expression in this cell subset is critical for suppression of T cells responses remains controversial (Levings *et al.*, 2001; Sutmuller *et al.*, 2001). By blocking delivery of the negative signal, anti-CTLA-4 antibodies can both extend T cell activation and modify the repertoire of T cells which are recruited (Chambers *et al.*, 2001). In animal models, treatment with anti-CTLA-4 antibodies alone was effective in reducing some tumors (Leach *et al.*, 1996; Kwon *et al.*, 1997; Yang *et al.*, 1997), but it failed as a single agent against poorly immunogenic tumors. Combination of CTLA-4 blockade with tumor vaccines augmented the antitumor activity, however this effect was often associated with autoimmunity (Hurwitz *et al.*, 1998; van Elsas *et al.*, 1999; Hurwitz *et al.*, 2000).

MDX-CTLA-4 is a human monoclonal antibody specific for the human CTLA-4 antigen. Three clinical studies have been conducted in metastatic melanoma patients with this blocking antibody as a single agent or in combination with peptides (Phan *et al.*, 2003a). Recently, MDX-CTLA4 was also infused into nine cancer patients which were previously immunized with peptide-pulsed DCs or autologous GM-CSF-secreting tumor cells (Hodi *et al.*, 2003). This treatment induced extensive tumor necrosis, with lymphocyte and granulocyte infiltration in the tumor of melanoma patients, and reduction or stabilization of CA-125 blood levels in patients ovarian carcinoma (who had been vaccinated with their autologous tumor). Infiltrates, but not tumor necrosis were observed in melanoma patients previously immunized with peptide-loaded DCs. Five out of seven melanoma patients developed T cell reactivity to normal melanocytes. Although the mechanisms underlying the ability of CTLA-4 blockade to increase tumor immunity and autoimmunity remain to be clarified, this strategy represents an interesting complement of cellular vaccines.

Depletion of regulatory T cells

Immunoregulatory mechanisms that physiologically protect against the development of autoimmunity may also prevent the host from mounting an immune response to autoantigens, such as tumor-associated antigens. A subset of CD4+ T cells which can inhibit proliferation of activated T cells and spontaneously express the IL-2 receptor α chain (CD25) has been identified in human PBMC (Levings *et al.*, 2001). Mechanisms of suppression are not yet fully clarified but both soluble factors and cell-to-cell contacts appear be involved. Enhanced frequencies (up to 33%) of CD4+CD25+ T cells with high levels of surface CTLA-4 are found among tumor-infiltrating lymphocytes of patients with various cancers, including non-small cell lung cancer, and such cells were shown to inhibit autologous T cell proliferation (Woo *et al.*, 2001; Woo *et al.*, 2002).

Although subsets of regulatory cells distinct from CD4+CD25+ T cells have also been described (Taniguchi *et al.*, 1996; Chang *et al.*, 2002), mouse studies suggest that both spontaneous antitumor immune responses (Onizuka *et al.*, 1999; Shimizu *et al.*, 1999) and immune responses induced by therapeutic cancer vaccination (Sutmuller *et al.*, 2001) are enhanced by depletion of CD4+CD25+ T cells with an anti-CD25 antibody administered 4 days before therapeutic vaccination. Regulatory T cell depleting agents with a short half-life will be cleared fast and should not interfere with the activated, CD25-expressing T cells generated by the vaccination protocol.

An IL-2–diphtheria toxin fusion protein (ONTAK®) is currently being tested in DC-based clinical studies. Although this strategy may potentially enhance antitumor responses induced by the vaccine, toxicity issues need to be carefully evaluated.

Cyclophosphamide and other chemotherapeutic drugs, used at a low dose prior to vaccination, have also been proposed to enhance primary and memory responses, due to their selective toxicity for suppressor cells and their precursors (Berd and Mastrangelo,

1988b). However, the precise target population has yet to be identified, as CD25-expressing T cells do not appear to be modulated by this treatment (Berd and Mastrangelo, 1988b).

High-dose chemotherapy induces lymphopenia, and as such could abrogate negative regulation mechanisms associated with T cell homeostasis. It could potentially prevent immune inertia and reduce antigen-specific competition among T cells, thereby facilitating the emergence of a new, more effective, tumor specific T cell repertoire (Dudley *et al.*, 2002).

CONCLUSIONS

Harnessing the immune system against cancer appears to be feasible. Careful biological monitoring of patients who respond to the treatment should provide directions on how to improve current vaccines. A global re-programming of the immune response against the tumor seems important to reach efficacy. Due to their composite nature, cellular vaccines may be better candidates to modulate broad antitumor responses. In particular, DCs have proven to be the most potent natural adjuvant of immune responses. Induction of cytotoxic and helper T cells, even if not sufficient by themselves to control tumor growth, should modify the overall equilibrium of the immune system. Activating NK cells and facilitating antitumor humoral responses by DC-based vaccines may also be critical to establish protective immunity. The lack of immediate toxicity associated with cellular vaccines is now well documented and will allow investigators to focus on patients with minimal residual disease, who are more likely to benefit from immunotherapy. Future developments in this field should capitalize on current knowledge at molecular and cellular levels of the immune system.

References

Abdel-Wahab, Z., Weltz, C., Hester, D., Pickett, N., Vervaert, C., Barber, J.R., Jolly, D., and Seigler, H.F. 1997. A Phase I clinical trial of immunotherapy with interferon-gamma gene-modified autologous melanoma cells: monitoring the humoral immune response. Cancer 80: 401–412.

Adam, B.L., Qu, Y., Davis, J.W., Ward, M.D., Clements, M.A., Cazares, L.H., Semmes, O.J., Schellhammer, P.F., Yasui, Y., Feng, Z., and Wright, G.L., Jr. 2002. Serum protein fingerprinting coupled with a pattern-matching algorithm distinguishes prostate cancer from benign prostate hyperplasia and healthy men. Cancer Res. 62: 3609–3614.

Ahuja, S.S. 2001. Genetic engineering of dendritic cells using retrovirus-based gene transfer techniques. Methods Mol. Biol 156: 79–87.

Albert, M.L., Pearce, S.F., Francisco, L.M., Sauter, B., Roy, P., Silverstein, R.L., and Bhardwaj, N. 1998. Immature dendritic cells phagocytose apoptotic cells via alphavbeta5 and CD36, and cross-present antigens to cytotoxic T lymphocytes. J. Exp. Med. 188: 1359–1368.

Antonia, S.J., Seigne, J., Diaz, J., Muro-Cacho, C., Extermann, M., Farmelo, M J., Friberg, M., Alsarraj, M., Mahany, J.J., Pow-Sang, J., *et al.* 2002. Phase I trial of a B7–1 (CD80) gene modified autologous tumor cell vaccine in combination with systemic interleukin 2 in patients with metastatic renal cell carcinoma. J. Urol. 167: 1995–2000.

Arthur, J.F., Butterfield, L.H., Roth, M.D., Bui, L.A., Kiertscher, S.M., Lau, R., Dubinett, S., Glaspy, J., McBride, W.H., and Economou, J.S. 1997. A comparison of gene transfer methods in human dendritic cells. Cancer Gene Ther. 4: 17–25.

Bai, L., Feuerer, M., Beckhove, P., Umansky, V., and Schirrmacher, V. 2002. Generation of dendritic cells from human bone marrow mononuclear cells: advantages for clinical application in comparison to peripheral blood monocyte derived cells. Int. J. Oncol. 20: 247–253.

Banchereau, J., Palucka, A.K., Dhodapkar, M., Burkeholder, S., Taquet, N., Rolland, A., Taquet, S., Coquery, S., Wittkowski, K.M., Bhardwaj, N., *et al.* 2001. Immune and clinical responses in patients with metastatic melanoma to CD34(+) progenitor-derived dendritic cell vaccine. Cancer Res. 61: 6451–6458.

Banchereau, J., and Steinman, R.M. 1998. Dendritic cells and the control of immunity. Nature 392: 245–252.

Belz, G.T., Carbone, F.R., and Heath, W.R. 2002. Cross-presentation of antigens by dendritic cells. Crit. Rev. Immunol. 22: 439–448.

Berard, F., Blanco, P., Davoust, J., Neidhart-Berard, E.M., Nouri-Shirazi, M., Taquet, N., RiMol.di, D., Cerottini, J.C., Banchereau, J., and Palucka, A.K. 2000. Cross-priming of naive CD8 T cells against melanoma antigens using dendritic cells loaded with killed allogeneic melanoma cells. J. Exp. Med. 192: 1535–1544.

Bercovici, N., Duffour, M.T., Agrawal, S., Salcedo, M., and Abastado, J.P. 2000. New methods for assessing T-cell responses. Clin. Diagn. Lab. Immunol. 7: 859–864.

Berd, D. 2002. M-Vax: an autologous, hapten-modified vaccine for human cancer. Expert Opin. Biol. Ther. 2: 335–342.

Berd, D., Maguire, H.C., Jr., McCue, P., and Mastrangelo, M.J. 1990. Treatment of metastatic melanoma with an autologous tumor-cell vaccine: clinical and immunologic results in 64 patients. J. Clin. Oncol. 8: 1858–1867.

Berd, D., and Mastrangelo, M.J. 1988a. Active immunotherapy of human melanoma exploiting the immunopotentiating effects of cyclophosphamide. Cancer Invest. 6: 337–349.

Berd, D., and Mastrangelo, M.J. 1988b. Effect of low dose cyclophosphamide on the immune system of cancer patients: depletion of CD4+, 2H4+ suppressor-inducer T-cells. Cancer Res. 48: 1671–1675.

Berd, D., Sato, T., Cohn, H., Maguire, H.C., Jr., and Mastrangelo, M.J. 2001. Treatment of metastatic melanoma with autologous, hapten-modified melanoma vaccine: regression of pulmonary metastases. Int. J. Cancer 94: 531–539.

Bernard, J., Ittelet, D., Christoph, A., Potron, G., Adjizian, J.C., Kochman, S., and Lopez, M. 1998. Adherent-free generation of functional dendritic cells from purified blood monocytes in view of potential clinical use. Hematol. Cell Ther. 40: 17–26.

Boccaccio, C., Jacod, S., Kaiser, A., Boyer, A., Abastado, J.P., and Nardin, A. 2002. Identification of a clinical-grade maturation factor for dendritic cells. J. Immunother. 25: 88–96.

Boczkowski, D., Nair, S.K., Nam, J.H., Lyerly, H.K., and Gilboa, E. 2000. Induction of tumor immunity and cytotoxic T lymphocyte responses using dendritic cells transfected with messenger RNA amplified from tumor cells. Cancer Res. 60: 1028–1034.

Bungener, L., Serre, K., Bijl, L., Leserman, L., Wilschut, J., Daemen, T., and Machy, P. 2002. Virosome-mediated delivery of protein antigens to dendritic cells. Vaccine 20: 2287–2295.

Butterfield, L.H., Ribas, A., Dissette, V.B., Amarnani, S.N., Vu, H.T., Oseguera, D., Wang, H.J., Elashoff, R.M., McBride, W.H., Mukherji, B., et al. 2003. Determinant spreading associated with clinical response in dendritic cell-based immunotherapy for malignant melanoma. Clin. Cancer Res. 9: 998–1008.

Bykovskaia, S.N., Shurin, G.V., Graner, S., Bunker, M.L., Olson, W., Thomas, R., Shurin, M.R., Marks, S., Storkus, W.J., and Shogan, J. 2002. Differentiation of immunostimulatory stem-cell- and monocyte-derived dendritic cells involves maturation of intracellular compartments responsible for antigen presentation and secretion. Stem Cells 20: 380–393.

Byl, B., Libin, M., Bauer, J., Martin, O.R., De Wit, D., Davies, G., Goldman, M., and Willems, F. 2003. OM197-MP-AC induces the maturation of human dendritic cells and promotes a primary T cell response. Int. Immunopharmacol. 3: 417–425.

Calbo, S., Guichard, G., Muller, S., Kourilsky, P., Briand, J.P., and Abastado, J.P. 2000. Antitumor vaccination using a major histocompatibility complex (MHC) class I-restricted pseudopeptide with reduced peptide bond. J. Immunother. 23: 125–130.

Campoli, M., Chang, C.C., and Ferrone, S. 2002. HLA class I antigen loss, tumor immune escape and immune selection. Vaccine 20 Suppl 4: A40–45.

Candido, K.A., Shimizu, K., McLaughlin, J.C., Kunkel, R., Fuller, J.A., Redman, B.G., Thomas, E.K., Nickoloff, B.J., and Mule, J.J. 2001. Local administration of dendritic cells inhibits established breast tumor growth: implications for apoptosis-inducing agents. Cancer Res. 61: 228–236.

Castellino, F., Boucher, P.E., Eichelberg, K., Mayhew, M., Rothman, J.E., Houghton, A.N., and Germain, R.N. 2000. Receptor-mediated uptake of antigen/heat shock protein complexes results in major histocompatibility complex class I antigen presentation via two distinct processing pathways. J. Exp. Med. 191: 1957–1964.

Caux, C., Dezutter-Dambuyant, C., Schmitt, D., and Banchereau, J. 1992. GM-CSF and TNF-alpha cooperate in the generation of dendritic Langerhans cells. Nature 360: 258–261.

Caux, C., Vanbervliet, B., Massacrier, C., Dezutter-Dambuyant, C., de Saint-Vis, B., Jacquet, C., Yoneda, K., Imamura, S., Schmitt, D., and Banchereau, J. 1996. CD34+ hematopoietic progenitors from human cord blood differentiate along two independent dendritic cell pathways in response to GM-CSF+TNF alpha. J. Exp. Med. 184: 695–706.

Cella, M., Salio, M., Sakakibara, Y., Langen, H., Julkunen, I., and Lanzavecchia, A. 1999. Maturation, activation, and protection of dendritic cells induced by double-stranded RNA. J. Exp. Med. 189: 821–829.

Celluzzi, C.M., and Falo, L.D., Jr. 1998. Physical interaction between dendritic cells and tumor cells results in an immunogen that induces protective and therapeutic tumor rejection. J. Immunol. 160: 3081–3085.

Chambers, C.A., Kuhns, M.S., Egen, J.G., and Allison, J.P. 2001. CTLA-4-mediated inhibition in regulation of T cell responses: mechanisms and manipulation in tumor immunotherapy. Annu. Rev. Immunol. 19: 565–594.

Chames, P., Hufton, S.E., Coulie, P.G., Uchanska-Ziegler, B., and Hoogenboom, H.R. 2000. Direct selection of a human antibody fragment directed against the tumor T-cell epitope HLA-A1-MAGE-A1 from a nonimmunized phage-Fab library. Proc. Natl. Acad. Sci. USA 97: 7969–7974.

Chang, A.E., Redman, B.G., Whitfield, J.R., Nickoloff, B.J., Braun, T.M., Lee, P.P., Geiger, J.D., and Mule, J.J. 2002. A phase I trial of tumor lysate-pulsed dendritic cells in the treatment of advanced cancer. Clin. Cancer Res. 8: 1021–1032.

Chen, B., Stiff, P., Sloan, G., Kash, J., Manjunath, R., Pathasarathy, M., Oldenburg, D., Foreman, K.E., and Nickoloff, B.J. 2001. Replicative response, immunophenotype, and functional activity of monocyte-derived versus CD34(+)-derived dendritic cells following exposure to various expansion and maturational stimuli. Clin. Immunol. 98: 280–292.

Chow, A., Toomre, D., Garrett, W., and Mellman, I. 2002. Dendritic cell maturation triggers retrograde MHC class II transport from lysosomes to the plasma membrane. Nature 418: 988–994.

Cohen, C.J., Hoffmann, N., Farago, M., Hoogenboom, H.R., Eisenbach, L., and Reiter, Y. 2002. Direct detection and quantitation of a distinct T-cell epitope derived from tumor-specific epithelial cell-associated mucin using human recombinant antibodies endowed with the antigen-specific, major histocompatibility complex-restricted specificity of T cells. Cancer Res. 62: 5835–5844.

Coulie, P.G., Karanikas, V., Colau, D., Lurquin, C., Landry, C., Marchand, M., Dorval, T., Brichard, V., and Boon, T. 2001. A monoclonal cytolytic T-lymphocyte response observed in a melanoma patient vaccinated with a tumor-specific antigenic peptide encoded by gene MAGE-3. Proc. Natl. Acad. Sci. USA 98: 10290–10295.

Coulie, P.G., Karanikas, V., Lurquin, C., Colau, D., Connerotte, T., Hanagiri, T., Van Pel, A., Lucas, S., Godelaine, D., Lonchay, C., et al. 2002. Cytolytic T-cell responses of cancer patients vaccinated with a MAGE antigen. Immunol. Rev. 188: 33–42.

Dauer, M., Obermaier, B., Herten, J., Haerle, C., Pohl, K., Rothenfusser, S., Schnurr, M., Endres, S., and Eigler, A. 2003. Mature dendritic cells derived from human monocytes within 48 hours: a novel strategy for dendritic cell differentiation from blood precursors. J. Immunol. 170: 4069–4076.

Day, F.H., Zhang, Y., Clair, P., Grabstein, K.H., Mazel, M., Rees, A.R., Kaczorek, M., and Temsamani, J. 2003. Induction of antigen-specific CTL responses using antigens conjugated to short peptide vectors. J. Immunol. 170: 1498–1503.

De Vries, I.J., Krooshoop, D.J., Scharenborg, N.M., Lesterhuis, W.J., Diepstra, J.H., Van Muijen, G.N., Strijk, S.P., Ruers, T.J., Boerman, O.C., Oyen, W.J., et al. 2003. Effective migration of antigen-pulsed dendritic cells to lymph nodes in melanoma patients is determined by their maturation state. Cancer Res. 63: 12–17.

Derossi, D., Chassaing, G., and Prochiantz, A. 1998. Trojan peptides: the penetratin system for intracellular delivery. Trends Cell Biol. 8: 84–87.

Dhodapkar, K.M., Krasovsky, J., Williamson, B., and Dhodapkar, M.V. 2002. Antitumor monoclonal antibodies enhance cross-presentation of cellular antigens and the generation of myeloma-specific killer T cells by dendritic cells. J. Exp. Med. 195: 125–133.

Dhodapkar, M.V., Steinman, R.M., Krasovsky, J., Munz, C., and Bhardwaj, N. 2001. Antigen-specific Inhibition of effector T cell function in humans after injection of immature dendritic cells. J. Exp. Med. 193: 233–238.

Di Pucchio, T., Lapenta, C., Santini, S.M., Logozzi, M., Parlato, S., and Belardelli, F. 2003. CD2+/CD14+ monocytes rapidly differentiate into CD83+ dendritic cells. Eur. J. Immunol. 33: 358–367.

Drexler, I., Antunes, E., Schmitz, M., Wolfel, T., Huber, C., Erfle, V., Rieber, P., Theobald, M., and Sutter, G. 1999. Modified vaccinia virus Ankara for delivery of human tyrosinase as melanoma-associated antigen: induction of tyrosinase- and melanoma-specific human leukocyte antigen A*0201-restricted cytotoxic T cells in vitro and in vivo. Cancer Res. 59: 4955–4963.

Dudley, M.E., Wunderlich, J.R., Robbins, P.F., Yang, J.C., Hwu, P., Schwartzentruber, D.J., Topalian, S.L., Sherry, R., Restifo, N.P., Hubicki, A.M., et al. 2002. Cancer regression and autoimmunity in patients after clonal repopulation with antitumor lymphocytes. Science 298: 850–854.

Dummer, R. 2001. GVAX (Cell Genesys). Curr. Opin. Investig. Drugs 2: 844–848.

Dunn, G.P., Bruce, A.T., Ikeda, H., Old, L.J., and Schreiber, R.D. 2002. Cancer immunoediting: from immunosurveillance to tumor escape. Nature Immunol. 3: 991–998.

Duperrier, K., Eljaafari, A., Dezutter-Dambuyant, C., Bardin, C., Jacquet, C., Yoneda, K., Schmitt, D., Gebuhrer, L., and Rigal, D. 2000. Distinct subsets of dendritic cells resembling dermal DCs can be generated in vitro from monocytes, in the presence of different serum supplements. J. Immunol. Methods 238: 119–131.

Engering, A.J., Cella, M., Fluitsma, D., Brockhaus, M., Hoefsmit, E.C., Lanzavecchia, A., and Pieters, J. 1997. The mannose receptor functions as a high capacity and broad specificity antigen receptor in human dendritic cells. Eur. J. Immunol. 27: 2417–2425.

Eue, I., Kumar, R., Dong, Z., Killion, J.J., and Fidler, I.J. 1998. Induction of nitric oxide production and tumoricidal properties in murine macrophages by a new synthetic lipopeptide JBT3002 encapsulated in liposomes. J. Immunother. 21: 340–351.

Fazekas de St Groth, B. 1998. The evolution of self-tolerance: a new cell arises to meet the challenge of self-reactivity. Immunol. Today 19: 448–454.

Ferlazzo, G., Klein, J., Paliard, X., Wei, W.Z., and Galy, A. 2000. Dendritic cells generated from CD34+ progenitor cells with flt3 ligand, c-kit ligand, GM-CSF, IL-4, and TNF-alpha are functional antigen-presenting cells resembling mature monocyte-derived dendritic cells. J. Immunother. 23: 48–58.

Fong, L., Brockstedt, D., Benike, C., Wu, L., and Engleman, E.G. 2001a. Dendritic cells injected via different routes induce immunity in cancer patients. J. Immunol. 166: 4254–4259.

Fong, L., Hou, Y., Rivas, A., Benike, C., Yuen, A., Fisher, G.A., Davis, M.M., and Engleman, E.G. 2001b. Altered peptide ligand vaccination with Flt3 ligand expanded dendritic cells for tumor immunotherapy. Proc. Natl. Acad. Sci. USA 98: 8809–8814.

Fujii, S., Shimizu, K., Fujimoto, K., Kiyokawa, T., Tsukamoto, A., Sanada, I., and Kawano, F. 2001. Treatment of post-transplanted, relapsed patients with hematological malignancies by infusion of HLA-matched, allogeneic-dendritic cells (DCs) pulsed with irradiated tumor cells and primed T cells. Leuk. Lymphoma 42: 357–369.

Gabrilovich, D.I., Corak, J., Ciernik, I.F., Kavanaugh, D., and Carbone, D.P. 1997. Decreased antigen presentation by dendritic cells in patients with breast cancer. Clin. Cancer Res. 3: 483–490.

Gagliardi, M.C., Sallusto, F., Marinaro, M., Langenkamp, A., Lanzavecchia, A., and De Magistris, M.T. 2000. Cholera toxin induces maturation of human dendritic cells and licences them for Th2 priming. Eur. J. Immunol. 30: 2394–2403.

Geiger, J.D., Hutchinson, R.J., Hohenkirk, L.F., McKenna, E.A., Yanik, G.A., Levine, J.E., Chang, A.E., Braun, T.M., and Mule, J.J. 2001. Vaccination of pediatric solid tumor patients with tumor lysate-pulsed dendritic cells can expand specific T cells and mediate tumor regression. Cancer Res. 61: 8513–8519.

Geissmann, F., Prost, C., Monnet, J.P., Dy, M., Brousse, N., and Hermine, O. 1998. Transforming growth factor beta1, in the presence of granulocyte/macrophage colony-stimulating factor and interleukin 4, induces differentiation of human peripheral blood monocytes into dendritic Langerhans cells. J. Exp. Med. 187: 961–966.

Gentschev, I., Dietrich, G., Spreng, S., Kolb-Maurer, A., Daniels, J., Hess, J., Kaufmann, S.H., and Goebel, W. 2000. Delivery of protein antigens and DNA by virulence-attenuated strains of *Salmonella typhimurium* and *Listeria monocytogenes*. J. Biotechnol. 83: 19–26.

Gottfried, E., Krieg, R., Eichelberg, C., Andreesen, R., Mackensen, A., and Krause, S.W. 2002. Characterization of cells prepared by dendritic cell-tumor cell fusion. Cancer Immun. 2: 15.

Goxe, B., Latour, N., Chokri, M., Abastado, J.P., and Salcedo, M. 2000. Simplified method to generate large quantities of dendritic cells suitable for clinical applications. Immunol. Invest. 29: 319–336.

Greenwald, R.J., Oosterwegel, M.A., van der Woude, D., Kubal, A., Mandelbrot, D.A., Boussiotis, V.A., and Sharpe, A.H. 2002. CTLA-4 regulates cell cycle progression during a primary immune response. Eur. J. Immunol. 32: 366–373.

Grufman, P., Sandberg, J.K., Wolpert, E.Z., and Karre, K. 1999. Immunization with dendritic cells breaks immunodominance in CTL responses against minor histocompatibility and synthetic peptide antigens. J. Leuk. Biol. 66: 268–271.

Guyre, C.A., Fisher, J.L., Waugh, M.G., Wallace, P.K., Tretter, C.G., Ernstoff, M.S., and Barth, R.J., Jr. 2002. Advantages of hydrophobic culture bags over flasks for the generation of monocyte-derived dendritic cells for clinical applications. J. Immunol. Methods 262: 85–94.

Haicheur, N., Bismuth, E., Bosset, S., Adotevi, O., Warnier, G., Lacabanne, V., Regnault, A., Desaymard, C., Amigorena, S., Ricciardi-Castagnoli, P., *et al.* 2000. The B subunit of Shiga toxin fused to a tumor antigen elicits CTL and targets dendritic cells to allow MHC class I-restricted presentation of peptides derived from exogenous antigens. J. Immunol. 165: 3301–3308.

Harshyne, L.A., Zimmer, M.I., Watkins, S.C., and Barratt-Boyes, S.M. 2003. A role for class a scavenger receptor in dendritic cell nibbling from live cells. J. Immunol. 170: 2302–2309.

Hayashi, T., Tanaka, H., Tanaka, J., Wang, R., Averbook, B.J., Cohen, P.A., and Shu, S. 2002. Immunogenicity and therapeutic efficacy of dendritic-tumor hybrid cells generated by electrofusion. Clin. Immunol. 104: 14–20.

Heiser, A., Coleman, D., Dannull, J., Yancey, D., Maurice, M.A., Lallas, C.D., Dahm, P., Niedzwiecki, D., Gilboa, E., and Vieweg, J. 2002. Autologous dendritic cells transfected with prostate-specific antigen RNA stimulate CTL responses against metastatic prostate tumors. J. Clin. Invest 109: 409–417.

Heiser, A., Maurice, M.A., Yancey, D.R., Coleman, D.M., Dahm, P., and Vieweg, J. 2001. Human dendritic cells transfected with renal tumor RNA stimulate polyclonal T-cell responses against antigens expressed by primary and metastatic tumors. Cancer Res. 61: 3388–3393.

Herbst, B., Kohler, G., Mackensen, A., Veelken, H., Mertelsmann, R., and Lindemann, A. 1997. CD34$^+$ peripheral blood progenitor cell and monocyte derived dendritic cells: a comparative analysis. Br. J. Haematol. 99: 490–499.

Hilkens, C.M., Kalinski, P., de Boer, M., and Kapsenberg, M.L. 1997. Human dendritic cells require exogenous interleukin 12-inducing factors to direct the development of naive T-helper cells toward the Th1 phenotype. Blood 90: 1920–1926.

Hinkel, A., Tso, C.L., Gitlitz, B.J., Neagos, N., Schmid, I., Paik, S.H., deKernion, J., Figlin, R., and Belldegrun, A. 2000. Immunomodulatory dendritic cells generated from nonfractionated bulk peripheral blood mononuclear cell cultures induce growth of cytotoxic T cells against renal cell carcinoma. J. Immunother. 23: 83–93.

Hodi, F.S., Mihm, M.C., Soiffer, R.J., Haluska, F.G., Butler, M., Seiden, M.V., Davis, T., Henry-Spires, R., MacRae, S., Willman, A., et al. 2003. Biologic activity of cytotoxic T lymphocyte-associated antigen 4 antibody blockade in previously vaccinated metastatic melanoma and ovarian carcinoma patients. Proc. Natl. Acad. Sci. USA 100: 4712–4717.

Hoffmann, T.K., Meidenbauer, N., Dworacki, G., Kanaya, H., and Whiteside, T.L. 2000. Generation of tumor-specific T-lymphocytes by cross-priming with human dendritic cells ingesting apoptotic tumor cells. Cancer Res. 60: 3542–3549.

Hurwitz, A.A., Foster, B.A., Kwon, E.D., Truong, T., Choi, E.M., Greenberg, N.M., Burg, M.B., and Allison, J.P. 2000. Combination immunotherapy of primary prostate cancer in a transgenic mouse model using CTLA-4 blockade. Cancer Res. 60: 2444–2448.

Hurwitz, A.A., Yu, T.F., Leach, D.R., and Allison, J.P. 1998. CTLA-4 blockade synergizes with tumor-derived granulocyte-macrophage colony-stimulating factor for treatment of an experimental mammary carcinoma. Proc. Natl. Acad. Sci. USA 95: 10067–10071.

Irvine, A.S., Trinder, P.K., Laughton, D.L., Ketteringham, H., McDermott, R.H., Reid, S.C., Haines, A.M., Amir, A., Husain, R., Doshi, R., et al. 2000. Efficient nonviral transfection of dendritic cells and their use for in vivo immunization. Nature Biotechnol. 18: 1273–1278.

Ismaili, J., Rennesson, J., Aksoy, E., Vekemans, J., Vincart, B., Amraoui, Z., Van Laethem, F., Goldman, M., and Dubois, P.M. 2002. Monophosphoryl lipid A activates both human dendritic cells and T cells. J. Immunol. 168: 926–932.

Jager, E., Ringhoffer, M., Altmannsberger, M., Arand, M., Karbach, J., Jager, D., Oesch, F., and Knuth, A. 1997. Immunoselection in vivo: independent loss of MHC class I and melanocyte differentiation antigen expression in metastatic melanoma. Int. J. Cancer 71: 142–147.

Janssen, E.M., Lemmens, E.E., Wolfe, T., Christen, U., von Herrath, M.G., and Schoenberger, S.P. 2003. CD4$^+$ T cells are required for secondary expansion and memory in CD8$^+$ T lymphocytes. Nature 421: 852–856.

Jeannin, P., Renno, T., Goetsch, L., Miconnet, I., Aubry, J.P., Delneste, Y., Herbault, N., Baussant, T., Magistrelli, G., Soulas, C., et al. 2000. OmpA targets dendritic cells, induces their maturation and delivers antigen into the MHC class I presentation pathway. Nature Immunol. 1: 502–509.

Jonuleit, H., Giesecke-Tuettenberg, A., Tuting, T., Thurner-Schuler, B., Stuge, T.B., Paragnik, L., Kandemir, A., Lee, P.P., Schuler, G., Knop, J., and Enk, A.H. 2001. A comparison of two types of dendritic cell as adjuvants for the induction of melanoma-specific T-cell responses in humans following intranodal injection. Int. J. Cancer 93: 243–251.

Kaiser, A., Bercovici, N., Abastado, J.P., and Nardin, A. 2003. Naive CD8$^+$ T cell recruitment and proliferation are dependent on stage of dendritic cell maturation. Eur. J. Immunol. 33: 162–171.

Kalinski, P., Schuitemaker, J.H., Hilkens, C.M., and Kapsenberg, M.L. 1998. Prostaglandin E2 induces the final maturation of IL-12-deficient CD1a+CD83+ dendritic cells: the levels of IL-12 are determined during the final dendritic cell maturation and are resistant to further modulation. J. Immunol. 161: 2804–2809.

Kalinski, P., Schuitemaker, J.H., Hilkens, C.M., Wierenga, E.A., and Kapsenberg, M.L. 1999. Final maturation of dendritic cells is associated with impaired responsiveness to IFN-γamma and to bacterial IL-12 inducers: decreased ability of mature dendritic cells to produce IL-12 during the interaction with Th cells. J. Immunol. 162: 3231–3236.

Kaplan, J.M., Yu, Q., Piraino, S.T., Pennington, S.E., Shankara, S., Woodworth, L.A., and Roberts, B.L. 1999. Induction of antitumor immunity with dendritic cells transduced with adenovirus vector-encoding endogenous tumor-associated antigens. J. Immunol. 163: 699–707.

Kedl, R.M., Kappler, J.W., and Marrack, P. 2003. Epitope dominance, competition and T cell affinity maturation. Curr. Opin. Immunol. 15: 120–127.

Kennedy, S. 2001. Proteomic profiling from human samples: the body fluid alternative. Toxicol Lett. 120: 379–384.

Kiertscher, S.M., Luo, J., Dubinett, S.M., and Roth, M.D. 2000. Tumors promote altered maturation and early apoptosis of monocyte-derived dendritic cells. J. Immunol. 164: 1269–1276.

Kotera, Y., Shimizu, K., and Mule, J.J. 2001. Comparative analysis of necrotic and apoptotic tumor cells as a source of antigen(s) in dendritic cell-based immunization. Cancer Res. 61: 8105–8109.

Kourilsky, P., and Fazilleau, N. 2001. Self peptides and the peptidic self. Int. Rev. Immunol. 20: 575–591.

Krause, S.W., Neumann, C., Soruri, A., Mayer, S., Peters, J.H., and Andreesen, R. 2002. The treatment of patients with disseminated malignant melanoma by vaccination with autologous cell hybrids of tumor cells and dendritic cells. J. Immunother. 25: 421–428.

Krummel, M.F., and Allison, J.P. 1996. CTLA-4 engagement inhibits IL-2 accumulation and cell cycle progression upon activation of resting T cells. J. Exp. Med. 183: 2533–2540.

Kwon, E.D., Hurwitz, A.A., Foster, B.A., Madias, C., Feldhaus, A.L., Greenberg, N.M., Burg, M.B., and Allison, J.P. 1997. Manipulation of T cell costimulatory and inhibitory signals for immunotherapy of prostate cancer. Proc. Natl. Acad. Sci. USA 94: 8099–8103.

Lambert, L.A., Gibson, G.R., Maloney, M., and Barth, R.J., Jr. 2001. Equipotent generation of protective antitumor immunity by various methods of dendritic cell loading with whole cell tumor antigens. J. Immunother. 24: 232–236.

Langenkamp, A., Messi, M., Lanzavecchia, A., and Sallusto, F. 2000. Kinetics of dendritic cell activation: impact on priming of TH1, TH2 and nonpolarized T cells. Nature Immunol. 1: 311–316.

Langlade-Demoyen, P., Levraud, J.P., Kourilsky, P., and Abastado, J.P. 1994. Primary cytotoxic T lymphocyte induction using peptide-stripped autologous cells. Int. Immunol. 6: 1759–1766.

Lau, R., Wang, F., Jeffery, G., Marty, V., Kuniyoshi, J., Bade, E., Ryback, M.E., and Weber, J. 2001. Phase I trial of intravenous peptide-pulsed dendritic cells in patients with metastatic melanoma. J. Immunother. 24: 66–78.

Leach, D.R., Krummel, M.F., and Allison, J.P. 1996. Enhancement of antitumor immunity by CTLA-4 blockade. Science 271: 1734–1736.

Lev, A., Denkberg, G., Cohen, C.J., Tzukerman, M., Skorecki, K.L., Chames, P., Hoogenboom, H.R., and Reiter, Y. 2002. Isolation and characterization of human recombinant antibodies endowed with the antigen-specific, major histocompatibility complex-restricted specificity of T cells directed toward the widely expressed tumor T-cell epitopes of the telomerase catalytic subunit. Cancer Res. 62: 3184–3194.

Levings, M.K., Sangregorio, R., and Roncarolo, M.G. 2001. Human CD25(+)CD4(+) T regulatory cells suppress naive and memory T cell proliferation and can be expanded in vitro without loss of function. J. Exp. Med. 193: 1295–1302.

Lin, C.L., Lo, W.F., Lee, T.H., Ren, Y., Hwang, S.L., Cheng, Y.F., Chen, C.L., Chang, Y.S., Lee, S.P., Rickinson, A.B., and Tam, P.K. 2002. Immunization with Epstein-Barr Virus (EBV) peptide-pulsed dendritic cells induces functional CD8+ T-cell immunity and may lead to tumor regression in patients with EBV-positive nasopharyngeal carcinoma. Cancer Res. 62: 6952–6958.

Liyanage, U.K., Moore, T.T., Joo, H.G., Tanaka, Y., Herrmann, V., Doherty, G., Drebin, J.A., Strasberg, S.M., Eberlein, T.J., Goedegebuure, P.S., and Linehan, D.C. 2002. Prevalence of regulatory T cells is increased in peripheral blood and tumor microenvironment of patients with pancreas or breast adenocarcinoma. J. Immunol. 169: 2756–2761.

Lopez, J.A., Bioley, G., Turtle, C.J., Pinzon-Charry, A., Ho, C.S., Vuckovic, S., Crosbie, G., Gilleece, M., Jackson, D.C., Munster, D., and Hart, D.N. 2003. Single step enrichment of blood dendritic cells by positive immunoselection. J. Immunol. Methods 274: 47–61.

Lotem, M., Peretz, T., Drize, O., Gimmon, Z., Ad El, D., Weitzen, R., Goldberg, H., Ben David, I., Prus, D., Hamburger, T., and Shiloni, E. 2002. Autologous cell vaccine as a post operative adjuvant treatment for high-risk melanoma patients (AJCC stages III and IV. The new American Joint Committee on Cancer. Br. J. Cancer 86: 1534–1539.

Loudovaris, M., Hansen, M., Suen, Y., Lee, S.M., Casing, P., and Bender, J.G. 2001. Differential effects of autologous serum on CD34(+) or monocyte-derived dendritic cells. J. Hematother. Stem Cell Res. 10: 569–578.

Luft, T., Jefford, M., Luetjens, P., Hochrein, H., Masterman, K.A., Maliszewski, C., Shortman, K., Cebon, J., and Maraskovsky, E. 2002a. IL-1 beta enhances CD40 ligand-mediated cytokine secretion by human dendritic cells (DC): a mechanism for T cell-independent DC activation. J. Immunol. 168: 713–722.

Luft, T., Jefford, M., Luetjens, P., Toy, T., Hochrein, H., Masterman, K.A., Maliszewski, C., Shortman, K., Cebon, J., and Maraskovsky, E. 2002b. Functionally distinct dendritic cell (DC) populations induced by physiologic stimuli: prostaglandin E(2) regulates the migratory capacity of specific DC subsets. Blood 100: 1362–1372.

Luft, T., Luetjens, P., Hochrein, H., Toy, T., Masterman, K.A., Rizkalla, M., Maliszewski, C., Shortman, K., Cebon, J., and Maraskovsky, E. 2002c. IFN-α enhances CD40 ligand-mediated activation of immature monocyte-derived dendritic cells. Int. Immunol. 14: 367–380.

Mackensen, A., Krause, T., Blum, U., Uhrmeister, P., Mertelsmann, R., and Lindemann, A. 1999. Homing of intravenously and intralymphatically injected human dendritic cells generated in vitro from CD34+ hematopoietic progenitor cells. Cancer Immunol. Immunother. 48: 118–122.

Maier, T., Tun-Kyi, A., Tassis, A., Jungius, K.P., Burg, G., Dummer, R., and Nestle, F.O. 2003. Vaccination of cutaneous T-cell lymphoma patients using intranodal injection of autologous tumor lysate pulsed dendritic cells. Blood 7: 2338–2344.

Masterson, A.J., Sombroek, C.C., De Gruijl, T.D., Graus, Y.M., van der Vliet, H.J., Lougheed, S.M., van den Eertwegh, A.J., Pinedo, H.M., and Scheper, R.J. 2002. MUTZ-3, a human cell line model for the cytokine-induced differentiation of dendritic cells from CD34+ precursors. Blood 100: 701–703.

Mellman, I., and Steinman, R.M. 2001. Dendritic cells: specialized and regulated antigen processing machines. Cell 106: 255–258.

Mitchell, M.S., Kan-Mitchell, J., Kempf, R.A., Harel, W., Shau, H.Y., and Lind, S. 1988. Active specific immunotherapy for melanoma: phase I trial of allogeneic lysates and a novel adjuvant. Cancer Res. 48: 5883–5893.

Mohamadzadeh, M., Berard, F., Essert, G., Chalouni, C., Pulendran, B., Davoust, J., Bridges, G., Palucka, A.K., and Banchereau, J. 2001. Interleukin 15 skews monocyte differentiation into dendritic cells with features of Langerhans cells. J. Exp. Med. 194: 1013–1020.

Moller, P., Sun, Y., Dorbic, T., Alijagic, S., Makki, A., Jurgovsky, K., Schroff, M., Henz, B.M., Wittig, B., and Schadendorf, D. 1998. Vaccination with IL-7 gene-modified autologous melanoma cells can enhance the anti-melanoma lytic activity in peripheral blood of patients with a good clinical performance status: a clinical phase I study. Br. J. Cancer 77: 1907–1916.

Morse, M.A., Coleman, R.E., Akabani, G., Niehaus, N., Coleman, D., and Lyerly, H.K. 1999a. Migration of human dendritic cells after injection in patients with metastatic malignancies. Cancer Res. 59: 56–58.

Morse, M.A., Lyerly, H.K., and Li, Y. 1999b. The role of IL-13 in the generation of dendritic cells in vitro. J. Immunother. 22: 506–513.

Mortarini, R., Anichini, A., Di Nicola, M., Siena, S., Bregni, M., Belli, F., Mol.la, A., Gianni, A.M., and Parmiani, G. 1997. Autologous dendritic cells derived from CD34+ progenitors and from monocytes are not functionally equivalent antigen-presenting cells in the induction of melan-A/Mart-1(27–35)-specific CTLs from peripheral blood lymphocytes of melanoma patients with low frequency of CTL precursors. Cancer Res. 57: 5534–5541.

Nagata, Y., Ono, S., Matsuo, M., Gnjatic, S., Valmori, D., Ritter, G., Garrett, W., Old, L.J., and Mellman, I. 2002. Differential presentation of a soluble exogenous tumor antigen, NY-ESO-1, by distinct human dendritic cell populations. Proc. Natl. Acad. Sci. USA 99: 10629–10634.

Nair, S., McLaughlin, C., Weizer, A., Su, Z., Boczkowski, D., Donnull, J., Vieweg, J., and Gilboa, E. 2003. Injection of immature dendritic cells into adjuvant-treated skin obviates the need for ex vivo maturation. J. Immunol. 171: 6275–6282.

Nestle, F.O., Alijagic, S., Gilliet, M., Sun, Y., Grabbe, S., Dummer, R., Burg, G., and Schadendorf, D. 1998. Vaccination of melanoma patients with peptide- or tumor lysate-pulsed dendritic cells. Nature Med. 4: 328–332.

Ojcius, D.M., Godeau, F., Abastado, J.P., Casanova, J.L., and Kourilsky, P. 1993. Real-time measurement of antigenic peptide binding to empty and preloaded single-chain major histocompatibility complex class I molecules. Eur. J. Immunol. 23: 1118–1124.

Onizuka, S., Tawara, I., Shimizu, J., Sakaguchi, S., Fujita, T., and Nakayama, E. 1999. Tumor rejection by in vivo administration of anti-CD25 (interleukin 2 receptor alpha) monoclonal antibody. Cancer Res. 59: 3128–3133.

Palmowski, M., Salio, M., Dunbar, R.P., and Cerundolo, V. 2002a. The use of HLA class I tetramers to design a vaccination strategy for melanoma patients. Immunol. Rev. 188: 155–163.

Palmowski, M.J., Choi, E.M., Hermans, I.F., Gilbert, S.C., Chen, J.L., Gileadi, U., Salio, M., Van Pel, A., Man, S., Bonin, E., et al. 2002b. Competition between CTL narrows the immune response induced by prime-boost vaccination protocols. J. Immunol. 168: 4391–4398.

Palucka, A. K., Paczesny, S., Dhodapkar, M., Steinman, R., Fay, J., and Banchereau, J. 2003. Dendritic cells as melanoma vaccines. Paper presented at: Dendritic cells: interfaces with immunobiology and medicine. Keystone: Colorado.

Paquette, R.L., Hsu, N.C., Kiertscher, S.M., Park, A.N., Tran, L., Roth, M.D., and Glaspy, J.A. 1998. Interferon-alpha and granulocyte-macrophage colony-stimulating factor differentiate peripheral blood monocytes into potent antigen-presenting cells. J. Leuk. Biol. 64: 358–367.

Peiper, M., Goedegebuure, P.S., and Eberlein, T.J. 1997. Generation of peptide-specific cytotoxic T lymphocytes using allogeneic dendritic cells capable of lysing human pancreatic cancer cells. Surgery 122: 235–241; discussion 241–242.

Penna, G., and Adorini, L. 2000. 1 Alpha,25-dihydroxyvitamin D3 inhibits differentiation, maturation, activation, and survival of dendritic cells leading to impaired alloreactive T cell activation. J. Immunol. 164: 2405–2411.

Peshwa, M.V., Benike, C., Dupuis, M., Kundu, S.K., Engleman, E.G., Merigan, T.C., and van Schooten, W.C. 1998. Generation of primary peptide-specific CD8[+] cytotoxic T-lymphocytes in vitro using allogeneic dendritic cells. Cell Transplant. 7: 1–9.

Phan, G.Q., Yang, J.C., Sherry, R.M., Hwu, P., Topalian, S.L., Schwartzentruber, D.J., Restifo, N.P., Haworth, L.R., Seipp, C.A., Freezer, L.J., et al. 2003a. Cancer regression and autoimmunity induced by cytotoxic T lymphocyte-associated antigen 4 blockade in patients with metastatic melanoma. Proc. Natl. Acad. Sci. USA 100: 8372–8377.

Phan, V., Errington, F., Cheong, S.C., Kottke, T., Gough, M., Altmann, S., Brandenburger, A., Emery, S., Strome, S., Bateman, A., et al. 2003b. A new genetic method to generate and isolate small, short-lived but highly potent dendritic cell–tumor cell hybrid vaccines. Nature Med. 9: 1215–1219.

Ramakrishna, V., Treml, J.F., Vitale, L., Connolly, J.E., O'Neill, T., Smith, P.A., Jones, C.L., He, L.Z., Goldstein, J., Wallace, P.K., Keler, T., and Endres, M.J. 2004. Mannose receptor targeting of tumor antigen pmel17 to human dendritic cells directs anti-melanoma T cell responses via multiple HLA molecules. J. Immunol. 172: 2845–2852.

Rammensee, H.G., Falk, K., and Rotzschke, O. 1993. Peptides naturally presented by MHC class I molecules. Annu. Rev. Immunol. 11: 213–244.

Regnault, A., Lankar, D., Lacabanne, V., Rodriguez, A., Thery, C., Rescigno, M., Saito, T., Verbeek, S., Bonnerot, C., Ricciardi-Castagnoli, P., and Amigorena, S. 1999. Fcgamma receptor-mediated induction of dendritic cell maturation and major histocompatibility complex class I-restricted antigen presentation after immune complex internalization. J. Exp. Med. 189: 371–380.

Romani, N., Gruner, S., Brang, D., Kampgen, E., Lenz, A., Trockenbacher, B., Konwalinka, G., Fritsch, P.O., Steinman, R.M., and Schuler, G. 1994. Proliferating dendritic cell progenitors in human blood. J. Exp. Med. 180: 83–93.

Rosenberg, S.A., Yang, J.C., Schwartzentruber, D.J., Hwu, P., Marincola, F.M., Topalian, S.L., Restifo, N.P., Sznol, M., Schwarz, S.L., Spiess, P.J., et al. 1999. Impact of cytokine administration on the generation of antitumor reactivity in patients with metastatic melanoma receiving a peptide vaccine. J. Immunol. 163: 1690–1695.

Sallusto, F., and Lanzavecchia, A. 1994. Efficient presentation of soluble antigen by cultured human dendritic cells is maintained by granulocyte/macrophage colony-stimulating factor plus interleukin 4 and downregulated by tumor necrosis factor alpha. J. Exp. Med. 179: 1109–1118.

Santini, S.M., Lapenta, C., Logozzi, M., Parlato, S., Spada, M., Di Pucchio, T., and Belardelli, F. 2000. Type I interferon as a powerful adjuvant for monocyte-derived dendritic cell development and activity in vitro and in Hu-PBL-SCID mice. J. Exp. Med. 191: 1777–1788.

Sauter, B., Albert, M.L., Francisco, L., Larsson, M., Somersan, S., and Bhardwaj, N. 2000. Consequences of cell death: exposure to necrotic tumor cells, but not primary tissue cells or apoptotic cells, induces the maturation of immunostimulatory dendritic cells. J. Exp. Med. 191: 423–434.

Scandella, E., Men, Y., Gillessen, S., Forster, R., and Groettrup, M. 2002. Prostaglandin E2 is a key factor for CCR7 surface expression and migration of monocyte-derived dendritic cells. Blood 100: 1354–1361.

Schadendorf, D., Paschen, A., and Sun, Y. 2000. Autologous, allogeneic tumor cells or genetically engineered cells as cancer vaccine against melanoma. Immunol. Lett. 74: 67–74.

Schnurr, M., Scholz, C., Rothenfusser, S., Galambos, P., Dauer, M., Robe, J., Endres, S., and Eigler, A. 2002. Apoptotic pancreatic tumor cells are superior to cell lysates in promoting cross-priming of cytotoxic T cells and activate NK and gammadelta T cells. Cancer Res. 62: 2347–2352.

Schule, J., Bergkvist, L., Hakansson, L., Gustafsson, B., and Hakansson, A. 2002. Down-regulation of the CD3-zeta chain in sentinel node biopsies from breast cancer patients. Breast Cancer Res. Treat. 74: 33–40.

Schuler-Thurner, B., Schultz, E.S., Berger, T.G., Weinlich, G., Ebner, S., Woerl, P., Bender, A., Feuerstein, B., Fritsch, P.O., Romani, N., and Schuler, G. 2002. Rapid induction of tumor-specific type 1 T helper cells in metastatic melanoma patients by vaccination with mature, cryopreserved, peptide-loaded monocyte-derived dendritic cells. J. Exp. Med. 195: 1279–1288.

Shedlock, D.J., and Shen, H. 2003. Requirement for CD4 T cell help in generating functional CD8 T cell memory. Science 300: 337–339.

Shimizu, J., Yamazaki, S., and Sakaguchi, S. 1999. Induction of tumor immunity by removing CD25$^+$CD4$^+$ T cells: a common basis between tumor immunity and autoimmunity. J. Immunol. 163: 5211–5218.

Shimizu, K., Fields, R.C., Redman, B.G., Giedlin, M., and Mule, J.J. 2000. Potentiation of Immunologic responsiveness to dendritic cell-based tumor vaccines by recombinant interleukin 2. Cancer J. Sci. Am. 6 Suppl. 1: S67–75.

Shortman, K., and Liu, Y.J. 2002. Mouse and human dendritic cell subtypes. Nature Rev. Immunol. 2: 151–161.

Singh, R.A., Rodgers, J.R., and Barry, M.A. 2002. The role of T cell antagonism and original antigenic sin in genetic immunization. J. Immunol. 169: 6779–6786.

Small, E.J., Fratesi, P., Reese, D.M., Strang, G., Laus, R., Peshwa, M.V., and Valone, F.H. 2000. Immunotherapy of hormone-refractory prostate cancer with antigen-loaded dendritic cells. J. Clin. Oncol. 18: 3894–3903.

Smyth, M.J., Godfrey, D.I., and Trapani, J.A. 2001. A fresh look at tumor immunosurveillance and immunotherapy. Nature Immunol. 2: 293–299.

Soiffer, R., Lynch, T., Mihm, M., Jung, K., Rhuda, C., SchMol.linger, J.C., Hodi, F.S., Liebster, L., Lam, P., Mentzer, S., et al. 1998. Vaccination with irradiated autologous melanoma cells engineered to secrete human granulocyte-macrophage colony-stimulating factor generates potent antitumor immunity in patients with metastatic melanoma. Proc. Natl. Acad. Sci. USA 95: 13141–13146.

Somasundaram, R., Jacob, L., Swoboda, R., Caputo, L., Song, H., Basak, S., Monos, D., Peritt, D., Marincola, F., Cai, D., et al. 2002. Inhibition of cytolytic T lymphocyte proliferation by autologous CD4$^+$/CD25$^+$ regulatory T cells in a colorectal carcinoma patient is mediated by transforming growth factor-beta. Cancer Res. 62: 5267–5272.

Steinman, R.M., and Cohn, Z.A. 1973. Identification of a novel cell type in peripheral lymphoid organs of mice. I. Morphology, quantitation, tissue distribution. J. Exp. Med. 137: 1142–1162.

Steinman, R.M., Hawiger, D., Liu, K., Bonifaz, L., Bonnyay, D., Mahnke, K., Iyoda, T., Ravetch, J., Dhodapkar, M., Inaba, K., and Nussenzweig, M. 2003. Dendritic cell function in vivo during the steady state: a role in peripheral tolerance. Ann. N. Y. Acad. Sci. 987: 15–25.

Stift, A., Friedl, J., Dubsky, P., Bachleitner-Hofmann, T., Benkoe, T., Brostjan, C., Jakesz, R., and Gnant, M. 2003a. In vivo induction of dendritic cell-mediated cytotoxicity against allogeneic pancreatic carcinoma cells. Int. J. Oncol. 22: 651–656.

Stift, A., Friedl, J., Dubsky, P., Bachleitner-Hofmann, T., Schueller, G., Zontsich, T., Benkoe, T., Radelbauer, K., Brostjan, C., Jakesz, R., and Gnant, M. 2003b. Dendritic cell-based vaccination in solid cancer. J. Clin. Oncol. 21: 135–142.

Storkus, W.J., Zeh, H.J., 3rd, Maeurer, M.J., Salter, R.D., and Lotze, M.T. 1993. Identification of human melanoma peptides recognized by class I restricted tumor infiltrating T lymphocytes. J. Immunol. 151: 3719–3727.

Su, Z., Dannull, J., Heiser, A., Yancey, D., Pruitt, S., Madden, J., Coleman, D., Niedzwiecki, D., Gilboa, E., and Vieweg, J. 2003. Immunological and clinical responses in metastatic renal cancer patients vaccinated with tumor RNA-transfected dendritic cells. Cancer Res. 63: 2127–2133.

Su, Z., Vieweg, J., Weizer, A.Z., Dahm, P., Yancey, D., Turaga, V., Higgins, J., Boczkowski, D., Gilboa, E., and Dannull, J. 2002. Enhanced induction of telomerase-specific CD4(+) T cells using dendritic cells transfected with RNA encoding a chimeric gene product. Cancer Res. 62: 5041–5048.

Suen, Y., Lee, S.M., Aono, F., Hou, S., Loudovaris, M., Ofstein, G., and Bender, J.G. 2001. Comparison of monocyte enrichment by immuno-magnetic depletion or adherence for the clinical-scale generation of DC. Cytotherapy 3: 365–375.

Sun, J.C., and Bevan, M.J. 2003. Defective CD8 T cell memory following acute infection without CD4 T cell help. Science 300: 339–342.

Sun, Y., Jurgovsky, K., Mol.ler, P., Alijagic, S., Dorbic, T., Georgieva, J., Wittig, B., and Schadendorf, D. 1998. Vaccination with IL-12 gene-modified autologous melanoma cells: preclinical results and a first clinical phase I study. Gene Ther. 5: 481–490.

Suss, G., and Shortman, K. 1996. A subclass of dendritic cells kills CD4 T cells via Fas/Fas-ligand-induced apoptosis. J. Exp. Med. 183: 1789–1796.

Sutmuller, R.P., van Duivenvoorde, L.M., van Elsas, A., Schumacher, T.N., Wildenberg, M.E., Allison, J.P., Toes, R.E., Offringa, R., and Melief, C.J. 2001. Synergism of cytotoxic T lymphocyte-associated antigen 4 blockade and depletion of CD25(+) regulatory T cells in antitumor therapy reveals alternative pathways for suppression of autoreactive cytotoxic T lymphocyte responses. J. Exp. Med. 194: 823–832.

Tangri, S., Ishioka, G.Y., Huang, X., Sidney, J., Southwood, S., Fikes, J., and Sette, A. 2001. Structural features of peptide analogs of human histocompatibility leukocyte antigen class I epitopes that are more potent and immunogenic than wild-type peptide. J. Exp. Med. 194: 833–846.

Taniguchi, M., Makino, Y., Cui, J., Masuda, K., Kawano, T., Sato, H., Kondo, E., and Koseki, H. 1996. V alpha 14+ NK T cells: a novel lymphoid cell lineage with regulatory function. J. Allergy Clin. Immunol. 98: S263–269.

Thomas, R., Chambers, M., Boytar, R., Barker, K., Cavanagh, L.L., MacFadyen, S., Smithers, M., Jenkins, M., and Andersen, J. 1999. Immature human monocyte-derived dendritic cells migrate rapidly to draining lymph nodes after intradermal injection for melanoma immunotherapy. Melanoma Res. 9: 474–481.

Tourdot, S., Scardino, A., Saloustrou, E., Gross, D.A., Pascolo, S., Cordopatis, P., Lemonnier, F.A., and Kosmatopoulos, K. 2000. A general strategy to enhance immunogenicity of low-affinity HLA-A2. 1-associated peptides: implication in the identification of cryptic tumor epitopes. Eur. J. Immunol. 30: 3411–3421.

Triozzi, P.L., Khurram, R., Aldrich, W.A., Walker, M.J., Kim, J.A., and Jaynes, S. 2000. Intratumoral injection of dendritic cells derived in vitro in patients with metastatic cancer. Cancer 89: 2646–2654.

Van den Eynde, B.J., and Boon, T. 1997. Tumor antigens recognized by T lymphocytes. Int. J. Clin. Lab. Res. 27: 81–86.

Van den Eynde, B.J., and Morel, S. 2001. Differential processing of class-I-restricted epitopes by the standard proteasome and the immunoproteasome. Curr. Opin. Immunol. 13: 147–153.

van Elsas, A., Hurwitz, A.A., and Allison, J.P. 1999. Combination immunotherapy of B16 melanoma using anti-cytotoxic T lymphocyte-associated antigen 4 (CTLA-4) and granulocyte/macrophage colony-stimulating factor (GM-CSF)-producing vaccines induces rejection of subcutaneous and metastatic tumors accompanied by autoimmune depigmentation. J. Exp. Med. 190: 355–366.

Verdijk, R.M., Mutis, T., Esendam, B., Kamp, J., Melief, C.J., Brand, A., and Goulmy, E. 1999. Polyriboinosinic polyribocytidylic acid (poly(I: C)) induces stable maturation of functionally active human dendritic cells. J. Immunol. 163: 57–61.

Wallace, P.K., Tsang, K.Y., Goldstein, J., Correale, P., Jarry, T.M., Schlom, J., Guyre, P.M., Ernstoff, M.S., and Fanger, M.W. 2001. Exogenous antigen targeted to FcgammaRI on myeloid cells is presented in association with MHC class I. J. Immunol. Methods 248: 183–194.

Walter, E., Dreher, D., Kok, M., Thiele, L., Kiama, S.G., Gehr, P., and Merkle, H.P. 2001. Hydrophilic poly(DL-lactide-co-glycolide) microspheres for the delivery of DNA to human-derived macrophages and dendritic cells. J. Control Release 76: 149–168.

Wang, R.F., and Wang, H.Y. 2002. Enhancement of antitumor immunity by prolonging antigen presentation on dendritic cells. Nature Biotechnol. 20: 149–154.

Woo, E.Y., Chu, C.S., Goletz, T.J., Schlienger, K., Yeh, H., Coukos, G., Rubin, S.C., Kaiser, L.R., and June, C.H. 2001. Regulatory CD4(+)CD25(+) T cells in tumors from patients with early-stage non-small cell lung cancer and late-stage ovarian cancer. Cancer Res. 61: 4766–4772.

Woo, E.Y., Yeh, H., Chu, C.S., Schlienger, K., Carroll, R.G., Riley, J.L., Kaiser, L.R., and June, C.H. 2002. Cutting edge: Regulatory T cells from lung cancer patients directly inhibit autologous T cell proliferation. J. Immunol. 168: 4272–4276.

Wulfkuhle, J.D., Liotta, L.A., and Petricoin, E.F. 2003. Proteomic applications for the early detection of cancer. Nature Rev. Cancer 3: 267–275.

Yang, Y.F., Zou, J.P., Mu, J., Wijesuriya, R., Ono, S., Walunas, T., Bluestone, J., Fujiwara, H., and Hamaoka, T. 1997. Enhanced induction of antitumor T-cell responses by cytotoxic T lymphocyte-associated molecule-4 blockade: the effect is manifested only at the restricted tumor-bearing stages. Cancer Res. 57: 4036–4041.

Yu, J.S., Wheeler, C.J., Zeltzer, P.M., Ying, H., Finger, D.N., Lee, P.K., Yong, W.H., Incardona, F., Thompson, R.C., Riedinger, M.S., et al. 2001. Vaccination of malignant glioma patients with peptide-pulsed dendritic cells elicits systemic cytotoxicity and intracranial T-cell infiltration. Cancer Res. 61: 842–847.

Zhong, L., Granelli-Piperno, A., Choi, Y., and Steinman, R.M. 1999. Recombinant adenovirus is an efficient and non-perturbing genetic vector for human dendritic cells. Eur. J. Immunol. 29: 964–972.

Zhou, Y., Bosch, M.L., and Salgaller, M.L. 2002. Current methods for loading dendritic cells with tumor antigen for the induction of antitumor immunity. J. Immunother. 25: 289–303.

Zhou, Y., McEarchern, J.A., Howard, E., Pestano, G., Salgaller, M.L., and Bosch, M.L. 2003. Dendritic cells efficiently acquire and present antigen derived from lung cancer cells and induce antigen-specific T-cell responses. Cancer Immunol. Immunother. 52: 413–422.

Chapter 7

Veterinary Applications of the Canarypox Vaccine Vector Technology – Recent Developments for Vaccines in Domestic Mammalian Species

Jean-Christophe Audonnet, Jules Minke and Hervé Poulet

Abstract

One of the most significant changes in the field of veterinary vaccines in the past few years has been the introduction of several recombinant vaccines based on the canarypox vector platform. The commercial success of this platform seems paradoxical when one looks at the published vaccine literature on 'canarypox' or 'ALVAC'. Out of the approximately 150 references that can be found (as of February 2004) on the PubMed database, only 12 are directly related to veterinary vaccine applications. Yet the innovative canarypox platform has clearly found commercial viability for a number of veterinary targets, mainly for companion animals (cats, dogs and horses), whereas the very same platform has not delivered new products for human vaccines. The registration of canarypox-based veterinary vaccines, both in Europe and in North America, reflects in fact the excellent properties of this vector (e.g. proven safety in the target species, ability to be combined with existing vaccine formulations, ability to be integrated into a marketing strategy and proven efficacy against infectious challenges in target species) as well as the advantages of the technology when compared with classical vaccines used in the field.

INTRODUCTION

Poxviruses, and more specifically vaccinia, have been used as vectors for the first demonstration of the expression of a protective immunogen in an heterologous vector. The Raboral® vaccine (vaccinia Copenhagen thymidine kinase-negative strain recombinant expressing the rabies glycoprotein G) exemplifies the success of poxviruses as vaccine vectors. This vaccine was developed and originally used in Europe for the oral vaccination of red foxes in the wild. It has greatly contributed to the elimination of sylvatic rabies from large areas of Western Europe (Belgium, France and Luxembourg) and is now successfully used in the US and Canada for vaccination of raccoons, coyotes and grey foxes (for more details, see Pastoret and Brochier, 1996; Mackowiak *et al.,* 1999).

The extraordinary capacity to express genes *in vivo* using a non-replicative vector was observed for the first time in 1988 (Taylor *et al.,* 1988) with an experimental fowlpox construct expressing rabies. Following this pioneer work with a fowlpox–rabies recombinant virus, two avipox recombinant constructs (fowlpox and canarypox) were compared side by side: the immunogenicity and protection data, both in mice and cats, showed that the canarypox vector had superior characteristics over the fowlpox virus vector for inducing a protective immune response at relatively low doses in dogs (Taylor *et al.*, 1991). Although these immunological differences are still not fully understood, the natural host restriction of canarypox (non-replicative in mammalian species) was immediately recognized as a key factor for the development of a new range of vaccines, relying upon this virus as a new vaccine platform for veterinary species. In addition, its high safety profile and its ability to express foreign genes *in vivo*, thereby eliciting both humoral and cellular responses without the need for adjuvant, have been the driving factors for the generation of a number of commercial applications.

In 2004, the canarypox virus is widely used as a vaccine vector, essentially in companion animals. Several vaccine products based on this platform have been registered, and new products should continue to be introduced in the coming years. This review presents an overview of the new vaccine tools based on ALVAC, available to veterinarians and their customers.

CANARYPOX-BASED RECOMBINANT VACCINES FOR CATS

ALVAC–rabies vaccine

Rabies was the model used to demonstrate the biological features of canarypox as a potential vector in mammalian species (see above), but it has also been the first canarypox construct developed for the feline vaccine range. The recombinant virus vCP65 was further assessed in a number of species including primates (Taylor *et al.*, 1995) and a safety clinical trial was conducted in humans (Fries *et al.*, 1996). This very same recombinant canarypox virus expressing the rabies glycoprotein G met in fact a new need for rabies vaccination in cats. The putative association of adjuvanted vaccines and occurrence of fibrosarcomas (Backer, 1998) led to a perceived risk linked to the administration of adjuvanted vaccines in cats. The ALVAC–rabies vCP65 recombinant virus proved to be the ideal solution for addressing concerns of veterinarians and cat owners, and it was licensed in the USA for use in cats in 1999, under the brand name of Purevax®. This vaccine, which induces a long-lasting immunity after only one injection, is unique in the veterinary market since it is the first non-adjuvanted rabies vaccine for cats. Because it is adjuvant-free, this vaccine captured rapidly a significant share of the rabies vaccine market and several millions of doses are used each year in the USA and Canada.

ALVAC–feline leukemia virus vaccine

A recombinant canarypox expressing the envelope glycoprotein (env), the capsid proteins (gag) and part of the polymerase (pol) genes of the feline leukemia virus subgroup A, has been registered in the European Union in 2001. This vaccine, which is not adjuvanted, has been proven safe and efficacious in preventing infection, and is encountering a large success on the market. The ALVAC–FeLV construct (vCP97) was initially shown to protect cats against FeLV (Tartaglia *et al.*, 1993), when administered twice subcutaneously at a titre of $10^{8.0}$ pfu/dose.

To further characterize the efficacy of ALVAC–FeLV and define the formulation of the commercial vaccine, a dose–response model was established in a challenge system complying with the European Pharmacopeia, and excellent efficacy of the vaccine was confirmed in kittens even at doses lower than the standard commercial dose (Poulet *et al.*, 2003).

Importantly, protection with ALVAC–FeLV in this model was demonstrated not only against a virulent challenge performed via the oronasal route (natural route of infection), but also using the natural conditions of a severe 'in-contact' challenge. In one experiment where ALVAC–FeLV vaccinated cats or control cats were housed together with persistently infected cats for 25 weeks, ALVAC–FeLV vaccination protected 83% of the animals whereas 78% of the controls became infected (Gruffydd-Jones *et al.*, submitted).

Finally, ALVAC–FeLV was shown to induce at least one year of protective immunity, confirming the ability of the canarypox vector to induce a long-lasting immunity (Poulet *et al.*, 2003).

Although protective efficacy has been convincingly demonstrated in several independent studies, the mechanisms of protection induced by ALVAC–FeLV immunization are not understood. This is rather linked to the complexity of the FeLV model than to the characteristics of the vector itself. As for most of the other FeLV vaccines, vaccination with ALVAC–FeLV does not induce detectable levels of anti-gp70 antibodies, and seroconversion occurs only a few weeks after challenge in those cats that were protected. Some cats however are protected in the absence of any antibody response suggesting that protection could be mediated by other mechanisms, such as cytotoxic T cells (Flynn *et al.*, 2002). Additional evidence that part of the immunity induced by ALVAC–FeLV is cell-mediated comes from the observation that this immunity appears to be very solid. No latent infection could indeed be detected in most ALVAC–FeLV vaccinated and challenged cats, and the repeated administration of high doses of corticosteroïds failed to reactivate FeLV infection in ALVAC–FeLV vaccinated cats that had been transiently infected after challenge (Poulet *et al.*, 2003).

These very good performances of ALVAC–FeLV are achieved in the absence of any adjuvant, ensuring an excellent local tolerance and minimum inflammatory reactions. This advantage, already underlined for the ALVAC–rabies vaccine construct is highly significant in feline vaccinology, as chronic inflammation at the injection site might indeed be a factor facilitating post-vaccinal fibrosarcomas in cats (Backer, 1998; Brearley, 2003).

The compatibility between ALVAC–FeLV and other feline vaccines is key for a full commercial use in the field. ALVAC–FeLV does not alter the efficacy of the other antigens demonstrated by serology and virulent challenge. Conversely, other feline vaccines do not interfere with the efficacy of the canarypox-FeLV vaccine, as illustrated by the similar performance of the monovalent and combined ALVAC–FeLV in a study evaluating the duration of immunity (Poulet *et al.*, 2003). This full compatibility between ALVAC and other antigens, either live or inactivated, is another advantage of this vector. As a consequence, ALVAC–FeLV has been registered in 2002 for use in a range of combined feline vaccines (Eurifel® FeLV, and Eurifel® RCCP-FeLV), expanding its commercial reach into the field.

ALVAC–feline IL-2 therapeutic vaccine

The relatively high occurrence of fibrosarcomas in cats (Backer, 1998) led to a feasibility clinical trial in cats with a recombinant canarypoxvirus expressing the feline interleukin 2 (feIL-2). A series of seven injections of the recombinant vector performed over 8 weeks, after the surgical removal of the tumor and initiated during the iridium brachytherapy, could induce a 54% reduction in the rate of recurrence of the tumor. In this experiment, the canarypox vector expressing the feIL-2 showed a slightly better efficacy than the highly attenuated vaccinia strain NYVAC expressing the human IL-2 (Jourdier *et al.*, 2003). The high acceptance of canarypox as a vector for cat vaccines such as ALVAC–rabies and ALVAC–FeLV could lead to the development of the ALVAC–feIL-2 construct as a therapeutic vaccine for cats with fibrosarcomas, and potentially other tumor targets in the future. Further studies are needed in order to determine the optimal immunization regimen (vaccine dose and frequency of injections) since the experimental schedule used for the reported trial was quite arbitrary. Therefore, a better definition of the immunization schedule which will ensure the strongest therapeutic impact against recurrence of fibrosarcomas is needed before commercial development of this innovative product can be initiated.

This study also clearly documented the absence of replication *in vivo* of canarypox virus, confirming the excellent safety profile of this vector. In dogs with melanomas, no virus could be reisolated, even a few hours after administration of high doses in the tumor bed or in other tissues. This represents of course a key advantage when using ALVAC recombinants in immunocompromised animals, such as those suffering from malignant tumors. It supports convincingly the vector's safety for pets and other veterinary species.

The cancer market for pets is currently not as mature as in human health and it is difficult to predict when this new application of the canarypox vaccine platform will reach commercialization. However, this efficient immunotherapy could find its place along the classical ways of intervention in the veterinary oncology clinics which are expanding in North America and now in Europe.

CANARYPOX-BASED RECOMBINANT VACCINES FOR DOGS AND FERRETS

ALVAC–canine distemper virus vaccine for dogs

A recombinant canarypox construct expressing the HA and F genes from a canine distemper virus (CDV) was actually the first licensed canarypox-vectored vaccine in the US, ever (Recombitek® CDV and Recombitek® range of vaccines). Since 2003, this ALVAC–CDV vaccine is also registered as a monovalent product for ferrets (see below). This construct was developed following an initial work, done with a recombinant canarypox/measles, which demonstrated good efficacy in dogs against a canine distemper challenge (Taylor *et al.*, 1992). It is interesting to note that, in this model, the canarypox virus was equivalent to a replicative vaccinia/measles recombinant. ALVAC–CDV was developed specifically for dogs as a a safe and more efficient alternative to live CDV vaccines. Indeed, some live attenuated strains are either over or underattenuated and have been linked respectively with lack of immune responses, or with rare episodes of reversion to virulence in part of the vaccinated dog population. Efficacy of ALVAC–CDV was tested in SPF dogs, immunized twice 3 weeks apart with a low dose of the vaccine (40 times less than the average commercial dose). The vaccinated dogs and non-vaccinated control dogs were then submitted to a severe intracranial challenge with the Snyder-Hill strain. All 26 vaccinated animals in this experiment were completely protected (i.e. no morbidity, no mortality) whereas the seven control dogs displayed 100% morbidity and 86% mortality rates (Pardo *et al.*, 1997). Moreover, the stability of this recombinant vectored vaccine allowed it to be combined with the other classical live attenuated vaccines for hepatitis (CAV 2), parvovirosis (CPV) parainfluenza (CPI 2), and coronavirus (CCV) included in the immunization programs of dogs. A full range of vaccine combinations including ALVAC–CDV is now available in North America and Brazil.

ALVAC–CDV for ferrets

The ALVAC–CDV construct was also developed as a monovalent vaccine for ferrets. Unknown to the general public, ferrets have become quite important numerically as pets, especially in the USA, and a similar trend is observed in Europe. Ferrets are exquisitely susceptible to CDV and breeders are immunized on a regular basis in order to ensure high levels of antibodies in infant ferrets. Moreover, live attenuated vaccine strains can retain some level of virulence for ferrets if the antibody levels are too low. Stephensen C. *et al.* (1997) evaluated the efficacy of NYVAC (vaccinia-derived vector)–CDV and ALVAC–CDV recombinants in juvenile ferrets in comparison with a live attenuated CDV strain. All animals were immunized twice with 10^8 pfu administered intramuscularly 4 weeks apart. Protection against viremia and clinical signs induced by an intranasal CDV virulent challenge was complete in all ferrets immunized with either NYVAC–CDV or ALVAC–CDV. However, protection against clinical signs was only partial in ferrets receiving the live attenuated CDV vaccine strain. Interestingly, ALVAC–CDV performed as well as the NYVAC–CDV recombinant vaccine (Stephensen *et al.*, 1997) in those challenge experiments.

Administration of NYVAC–CDV and ALVAC–CDV by mucosal routes (intranasal and intraduodenal) was also evaluated (Welter *et al.*, 1999). NYVAC-CDV, when administered either through the intranasal or intraduodenal routes, could induce seroneutralizing (SN) antibody titers equivalent to the ones induced by the intramuscular (i.m.) route. ALVAC–CDV, on the other hand, could not induce significant SN titers by the intraduodenal route, and elicited antibody titers which only reached the level of 'i.m. titers' after a second intranasal administration. Protection against a CDV challenge via the nasal route was however excellent for both groups immunized intranasally. In contrast, neither NYVAC–CDV nor ALVAC–CDV conferred protection when administered by the intraduodenal route. The excellent protective activity of ALVAC–recombinants demonstrated in ferrets by the intranasal route in this study has not been confirmed so far in other species.

Finally, the activity and efficacy of NYVAC–CDV and ALVAC–CDV constructs were assessed in infant ferrets with or without maternal antibody protection (Welter *et al.*, 2000). The results on the actual inhibitory impact of the anti-CDV maternal antibodies on the activity of both recombinant poxviruses were ambiguous and not conclusive. Upon challenge, animals with either NYVAC–CDV or ALVAC–CDV exhibited a delayed onset of clinical signs when compared with the control group, but did not survive to the challenge as did the animals vaccinated with the attenuated CDV vaccine.

Interestingly, the ALVAC–CDV recombinant vaccine is also active in other wildlife animals (Wimsatt *et al.*, 2003). In Siberian polecats, the highest level of protection against challenge (80%) was achieved with a high dose of the vaccine (10^8 pfu) administered through the oropharyngeal route, whereas smaller doses ($10^{5.5}$ pfu and $10^{5.0}$ pfu) administered subcutaneously conferred respectively only 50% and 60% protection rates. These data, although not as convincing as in dogs, nevertheless suggest that this vaccine can be used in wildlife and endangered species.

ALVAC–CDV fulfilled all requirement for USDA registration, and was licensed as a commercial vaccine for ferrets in 2003, also under the brand name Recombitek® CDV.

CANARYPOX-BASED RECOMBINANT VACCINES FOR HORSES

ALVAC–equine influenza vaccine

Equine influenza is an economically important and highly contagious infectious disease of the horse. All major outbreaks of the past 20 years have been caused by influenza A viruses of the H3N8 subtype. Prevention and control of equine influenza depend heavily on vaccination and management regimens. Current inactivated influenza vaccines for horses only provide incomplete protection lasting a few months at best. In contrast to natural influenza infections, killed vaccines do not stimulate significant cytotoxic T-cell responses or mucosal immunity. These qualitative differences between the immune responses induced by infection and vaccination with killed vaccines have fuelled development of second generation vaccines. Recently a new equine flu vaccine (registered under the ProteqFlu™ brand name) containing two recombinant canarypox viruses expressing the hemagglutinin (HA) genes of the two epidemiologically relevant H3N8 equine influenza strains was commercialized in the European Union. This is the first recombinant vaccine, as well as the first live influenza vaccine, licensed for use in horses in Europe. Although this vaccine is efficacious in the absence of an adjuvant, early studies showed that the addition of a Carbomer adjuvant greatly enhanced the efficacy of the constructs, allowing to significantly reduce the minimum protective dose (Minke *et al.*, 2000). The immune enhancing properties of Carbomer adjuvant in the horse was confirmed using other canarypox virus constructs expressing genes from the equine herpes virus (Audonnet *et al.*, 1998) and West Nile virus (unpublished). This observation is of particular interest since it supports the combined use of ALVAC–influenza with conventional killed antigens, which generally need an adjuvant. The efficacy of the vaccine was extensively tested in challenge experiments, in which horses were exposed to a virus aerosol generated by nebulization (mimicking the natural intranasal route of infection). The onset of immunity thus induced was rapid, and sterile immunity was obtained 2 weeks following the second vaccination. Partial protection persisted for over 10 months after the second dose as evidenced by a significant reduction in both duration and severity of clinical symptoms and virus excretion after experimental infection. Protection was demonstrated against an homologous challenge, but also against a heterologous challenge (Edlund-Toulemond *et al.*, 2005). The usefulness of this vaccine was recently confirmed in the face of an outbreak of influenza H3N8 in South Africa (unpublished). The vaccine was massively used in a 'ring vaccination' program and was successful in containing the epidemic.

ALVAC–West Nile virus vaccine

West Nile virus (WNV) is an enveloped, positive stranded RNA virus. The virus has been isolated in Asia, Africa and some parts of Europe and is transmitted by mosquitoes. Birds are the main vertebrate hosts, but the virus can also occasionally cause encephalitis in horses and humans. The West Nile virus first appeared in the United States in 1999 in New York, where it was associated with a small number of illnesses in horses and humans. Since then, the virus has spread across most of continental United States and into Canada, and the virus is now considered to be endemic in North America. In 2002, more than 14,000 horses were diagnosed with West Nile virus infection, out of which approximately one-third perished, a trend which persisted for the 2003 season. There is currently no effective treatment, and control relies on mosquito management and vaccination of horses. A recombinant canarypox virus, expressing the prM-E polyprotein (a 1999 New York isolate), has proven to be effective against a live WNV-infected mosquito challenge, a method that approximates natural exposure in the field (Minke *et al.,* 2004). A single dose study documented protection with this vaccine as early as 26 days post-vaccination (Siger *et al.*, 2004). The construct not only induced fast protection, but also a long-lasting immunity for at least 1 year following the initial vaccination regimen of two injections. Interestingly, protection 1 year after immunization occurred in the absence of detectable neutralizing antibodies. As for the ALVAC–FeLV and ALVAC–CDV constructs previously described, the requirement for significant levels of neutralizing antibodies at the time of exposure may not be critical as long as vaccination properly primes the immune system, thereby facilitating a rapid recall. It should be noted that this ALVAC construct was evaluated in horses in combination with the Carbopol adjuvant. Previous studies conducted with ALVAC–equine influenza virus and ALVAC–equine herpes virus constructs (see previous paragraph) have shown that efficacy of the vaccine construct was in fact enhanced when combined with Carbopol. Although Carbopol is a well-known adjuvant for other classical vaccine antigens in horses, its activity when combined with recombinant canarypox-vectored vaccines is nevertheless quite remarkable. The immunological mechanisms underlying carbopol activity in horses are however not well understood. Following extensive safety testing in target and non-target species, this vaccine (Recombitek® WNV) was licensed in 2003 for use in horses by the USDA, adding another component to the current series of commercial canarypox vaccines.

Interestingly, the same canarypox vaccine construct, when administered in the absence of any adjuvant, induced a significant level protection to cats against challenge with West Nile virus-infected mosquitoes (unpublished). It could therefore represent a good option for veterinarians if West Nile virus is confirmed to infect pets.

CONCLUSION

As a result of its exquisite safety, the canarypox vector platform is the most successful recombinant vaccine technology in veterinary medicine as of today. The use of a non-replicative vector is the perfect way to combine the safety of an inactivated vaccine and the efficacy of a modified live vaccine. Following its initial validation using the rabies virus model, the application of the non-replicative vector vaccine concept has been extended to other disease targets. It has most particularly been successfully proven in the veterinary vaccine field. The advantages of this vaccine technology have been confirmed by end-users, as canarypox-based vaccines bring well-documented benefits to the animals. Although not fully explained today, the canarypox virus displays unique properties in terms of immunogenicity and lack of induction of inhibiting anti-vector immunity. This makes it as a preferred vector candidate for new vaccine development for animals. It is expected that many more new vaccines will be added to the existing range of preventative veterinary vaccines, potentially extending the use of this non-replicative vector to the field of cancer immunotherapy. One can only hope that the canarypox vector will find also useful applications in the mid-term future as a platform for human vaccines.

References

Audonnet, J.C., Mumford, J., Jessett, D., Pardo, M.C., Taylor, J., Tartaglia, J., and Minke, J. Safety and efficacy of a canarypox-EHV recombinant vaccine in horse. In: Equine Infectious Diseases VIII. Eds. Wernery U., Wade J.F., Mumford J.A. and Kaaden O.R. R and W Publications, Newmarket, UK, pp. 418–419.

Backer, R.J. 1998. Feline fibrosarcomas in vaccination sites. Feline Practice 26: 18–20.

Brearley, M.J. 2001. Vaccine-associated feline fibrosarcomas. Vet. Rec. 148: 580.

Edlund-Toulemonde, C., Daly, J., Sindle, T., Guigal, P.M., Audinnet, J.C., and Minke, J.M. 2005. Efficacy of a recombinant equine influenza vaccine (ProTeqFlu[TM]) against challenge with an American lineage H3N8 influenza virus responsible for the 2003 outbreak in the UK. Vet. Record (in press).

Flynn, J.N., Dunham, S.P., Watson, V., and Jarrett, O. 2002. Longitudinal analysis of feline leukemia virus-specific cytotoxic T lymphocytes: correlation with recovery from infection. J. Virol. 76: 2306–2315.

Fries, L.F., Tartaglia, J., Taylor, J., Kauffman, E.K., Meignier, B., Paoletti, P., and Plotkin, S. 1996. Human safety and immunogenicity of a canarypox-rabies glycoproteins recombinant vaccine: an alternative poxvirus vector system. Vaccine 14: 428–434.

Jourdier, T.M., Moste, C., Bonnet, M.C., Delisle, F., Tafani, J.P., Devauchelle, P., and Moingeon, P. 2003. Local immunotherapy of spontaneous feline fibrosarcomas using recombinant poxviruses expressing interleukin 2 (IL2). Gene Ther. 10: 2126–2132.

Leveque, N.W. 1998. Symposium devoted to vaccine-associated feline sarcomas. J. Am. Vet Med. Assoc. 213: 785.

Mackowiak, M., Maki, J., Motes-Kreimeyer, L., Harbin, T., and Van Kampen, K. 1999. Vaccination of wildlife against rabies: successful use of a vectored vaccine obtained by recombinant technology. Adv. Vet. Med. 41: 571–583.

Minke, J., Audonnet, J.C., Jessett, D.M., Fischer, L., Guigal, P.M., Coupier, H., Pardo, M.C., Taylor, J., Tartaglia, J., and Mumford, J. 2000. Canarypox as a vector for influenza and EHV-1 genes: challenges and rewards. In: 2nd International Veterinary Vaccines and Diagnostics Conference, Oxford, UK, p. 36.

Minke, J., Siger, L., Karaca, K., Austgen, L., Gordy, P., Bowen, R., Glaser, A., Loosmore, S., Audonnet, J.C., and Nordgren, B. 2004. Recombinant canarypoxvirus vaccine carrying the prM/E genes of West Nile virus–mosquito challenge. Arch. Virol. 18 (suppl.): 221–231.

Pardo, M.C., Baumann, J.E., and Mackowiak, M. 1997. Protection of dogs against canine distemper by vaccination with a canarypox virus recombinant expressing canine distemper virus fusion and hemagglutinin glycoproteins. Am. J. Vet. Res. 58: 833–836.

Pastoret, P.P., and Brochier, B. 1996. The development and use of a vaccinia-rabies recombinant oral vaccine for the control of wildlife rabies: a link between Jenner and Pasteur. Epidemiol. Infect. 116: 235–240.

Poulet, H., Brunet, S., Boularand, C., Guiot, A.L., Leroy, V., Tartaglia, J., Minke, J., Audonnet, J.C., and Desmettre, P. 2003. Efficacy of a canarypox virus-vectored vaccine against feline leukaemia. Vet. Rec. 153: 141–145.

Siger, L., Bowen, R.A., Karaca, K., Murray, M.J., Gordy, P.W., Loosmore, S., Audonnet, J.C.F., Nordgren, R.M., and Minke, J.M. 2004. Assessment of the efficacy of a single dose of a recombinant vaccine against West Nile virus in response to a natural challenge with West Nile virus-infected mosquitoes in horses. Am. J. Vet. Res. 11: 1459–1462.

Stephensen, C., Welter, J., Thaker, S.R., Taylor, J., Tartaglia, J., and Paoletti, E. 1997. Canine distemper virus (CDV) infection in ferrets as a model for testing Morbillivirus vaccine strategies: NYVAC- and ALVAC-based CDV recombinants protect against symptomatic infection. J. Virol. 71: 1506–1513.

Tartaglia, J., Jarrett, O., Neil, J.C., Desmettre, P., and Paoletti, E. 1993. Protection of cats against feline leukemia virus by vaccination with a canarypox virus recombinant, ALVAC–FL. J. Virol. 67: 2370–2375.

Taylor, J., Weinberg, R., Languet, B., Desmettre, P., and Paoletti, E. 1988. Recombinant fowlpox virus inducing protective immunity in non-avian species. Vaccine 6: 497.

Taylor, J., Trimarchi, C., Weinberg, R., Languet, B., Guillemin, F., Desmettre, P., and Paoletti, E. 1991. Efficacy studies on a canarypox-rabies recombinant virus. Vaccine 9: 190–193.

Taylor, J., Weinberg, R., Tartaglia, J., Richardson, C., Alkhatib, G., Briedis, D., Appel, M., Norton, E., and Paoletti, E. 1992. Nonreplicating viral vectors as potential vaccines: Recombinant canarypox virus expressing measles virus fusion (F) and hemagglutinin (HA) glycoproteins. Virology 187: 321–328.

Welter, J., Taylor, J., Tartaglia, J., Paoletti, J., and Stephensen, C. 1999. Mucosal vaccination with recombinant poxvirus vaccines protects ferrets against symptomatic CDV infection. Vaccine 17: 308–318.

Welter, J., Taylor, J., Tartaglia, J., Paoletti, E., and Stephensen, C. 2000. Vaccination against canine distemper virus infection in infant ferrets with and without maternal antibody protection using recombinant attenuated poxvirus vaccines. J. Virol. 74: 6358–6367.

Wimsatt, J., Biggins, D., Innes, K., Taylor, B., and Garell, D. 2003. Evaluation of oral and subcutaneous delivery of an experimental canarypox recombinant canine distemper vaccine in the Siberian polecat (*Mustela eversmanni*). J. Zoo. Wildl. Med. 34: 25–35.

Chapter 8

Immunological Aspects of Vaccine Safety: Where Do We Go?

Paul-Henri Lambert and Michel Goldman

Abstract

All vaccines carry some risk of adverse events, but fortunately vaccine-related toxicity is usually rare, mild and transient. Some questions are often raised regarding the potential immunological impact of vaccination. It is likely that in some exceptional circumstances, an inappropriate vaccine-induced response to a targeted pathogen may occasionally lead to the enhancement of natural disease. Vaccine-induced immune complex mediated manifestations (e.g. vasculitis) are rarely reported and usually considered as the consequence of immunization. Many fewer data indicate that vaccines may influence the quality of the immune response to other antigens or to allergens and there is no reason to believe that they could induce a kind of 'immunological overload'. There is so far very little evidence that autoimmune diseases might be induced or triggered by vaccination. Despite their excellent safety record, vaccines often remain the target of unsubstantiated allegations of undesirable immunological effects. Although these are not justified, it is essential to consider immunological safety as a first priority in vaccine development, even in the earliest stages of research.

INTRODUCTION

Vaccines are among the most effective tools in preventive medicine and their safety record is probably exceeding that of any drug introduced in clinical practice. However, despite the remarkable achievements of vaccines in protecting populations from major infectious threats, there is an increasing rampant public skepticism about vaccination safety. The fact that vaccines are mostly used in healthy individuals is considerably amplifying the visibility of any perceived adverse effect, particularly when the target disease burden has decreased to very low levels (Wilson and Marcuse, 2001; Halsey, 2003). This is contrasting with the extreme rarity of severe adverse events following routine vaccination. Indeed, most of common adverse effects of vaccines are related to mild, transient and often local inflammatory reactions. Within this context, appropriate consideration of safety issues is of rising importance in the development of new vaccines and of novel vaccination strategies.

During vaccine development, particular attention has always been given to short term inflammatory or toxic effects of inactivated or subunit vaccine formulations and to the potential pathogenicity of live attenuated vaccines. Another area that is drawing increasing concern is the medium or long-term immunological safety of new vaccines. Along that line, one should question whether undesirable immunological manifestations could occur as a result of specific vaccine-induced responses or of non-specific effects of vaccination.

VACCINE-INDUCED RESPONSES AND IMMUNOLOGICAL SAFETY

An inappropriate vaccine-induced response to a targeted pathogen may occasionally lead to the enhancement of natural disease

Although inducing a strong immune response is an essential aim of vaccination, vaccine-induced responses can also be harmful. The best-documented examples are with respiratory syncytial virus (RSV), measles, and dengue infections.

Disease enhancement was initially seen in the context of clinical trials of a low immunogenicity formalin-inactivated RSV vaccine that were conducted in infants and children in 1966–1967. During subsequent RSV exposure, no significant protection was observed and, more strikingly, 80% of RSV vaccinees (vs 5% in control group) needed hospitalization and a few deaths were recorded (Kim *et al.*, 1969). There was an intense inflammatory cellular infiltrate comprising mononuclear cells, eosinophils and polymorphonuclear cells in the lungs of vaccinated children suggesting an immunopathological cause of enhanced disease. Although it has not been possible to exactly delineate the cause of disease enhancement in man, animal models strongly suggest that it was due to strong and perhaps unbalanced T cell priming rather than infection-enhancing or sensitizing antibody (Openshaw *et al.*, 2001). Early inactivated measles vaccines were also shown to occasionally enhance pathology during subsequent infection (Fulginiti *et al.*, 1967).

Epidemiological studies indicate that a potential risk of immunologically mediated disease enhancement should also be considered in the development of dengue vaccines. Indeed, whereas primary infections with dengue virus type 2 or 4 are largely subclinical, symptomatic dengue, including dengue hemorrhagic fever and deaths have been shown to occur in patients that were previously exposed, up to 20 years before, to dengue virus type 1 (Vaughn, 2000).

Therefore, defining the correlates of protection and of disease enhancement in man is critical to the rational development of effective and protective vaccines.

Vaccine-induced immune complex-mediated manifestations

About 20 cases of vaculitis, often with a leucoclastic pattern, have been reported within 1–2 weeks following an influenza vaccination. In these cases both small and medium sized vessels were involved, but there was no direct evidence of a causal relationship. Skin lesions were predominant but there was also evidence of systemic involvement, including proteinuria, compatible with an immune-complex mediated pathogenesis (Mader *et al.*, 1993; Tavadia *et al.*, 2003). Similar isolated case reports do suggest that vasculitis may be associated with other viral vaccines, e.g. hepatitis B, but so far such associations have not been confirmed by relevant epidemiological studies.

Effects on the quality of the immune response to other antigens/allergens? Can vaccines lead to an 'immunological overload'?

In most industrialized countries, the pediatric immunization schedule has grown in parallel with the availability of new children's vaccines. This has resulted in a significant increase in the number of vaccine doses (up to 20 in the USA) given to a child by 2 years of age. This has raised questions in the general public as to whether too many immunizations might weaken the maturing immune system or influence its qualitative development (e.g. favor allergic types of responses). This issue has been recently reviewed by the

Immunization Safety Committee of the US Institute of Medicine (see Immunization Safety Review: Multiple Immunizations and Immune Dysfunction, Kathleen Stratton, Christopher B. Wilson and Marie C. McCormick, Editors, Immunization Safety Review Committee, Board on Health Promotion and Disease Prevention – 2002). It was concluded from presently available data that multiple immunizations did not appear to increase the risk of heterologous infections (other than those targeted by the vaccines), nor of allergic diseases.

Interference can exist between different vaccines that may influence positively or negatively the specific responses to one or several antigens. For example, negative interference was observed in infants who received either DTP or the PRP-T *Haemophilus* vaccine alone or together with a vaccine containing pneumococcal polysaccharide antigens conjugated to TT or diphtheria toxoid (Dagan *et al.*, 1998). The anti-*H. influenzae* type b polysaccharide polyribosylribitol phosphate (PRP) antibody response decreased significantly when the PRP-T conjugate was administered together with DTP and the tetravalent PncT conjugates. This decrease was dose dependent and also affected the anti-tetanus antibody response. Notably, this suppression was carrier specific, since it was more accentuated with increasing loads of TT and was not observed after simultaneous administration of PRP-T with pneumococcal polysaccharide conjugated to diphtheria toxoid. It is reassuring that although the simultaneous administration of PncT and PRP-T conjugates may decrease the anti-PRP antibody response, the levels of anti-PRP antibodies induced by such combined vaccines still exceeded the concentrations needed for protection against invasive Hib disease. Clear evidence for the induction of memory toward the polysaccharide antigens was obtained.

When BCG was given to neonates at the time of administration of hepatitis B or polio vaccines, it was found that BCG enhanced immune responses to these antigens. However, it was striking that antibody, TH1 cytokine (e.g. interferon gamma) and TH2 cytokine (e.g. IL-13) cellular responses were all increased without any particular polarization (Ota *et al.*, 2002).

Induction or triggering of autoimmune diseases?
It is estimated that as much as 5% of the population in Western countries suffers from autoimmune disorders. Quite often, the first manifestations of the autoimmune process occur during childhood or in young adults, as in type 1 juvenile diabetes or multiple sclerosis. Because the increase in the incidence of these disorders over the recent years was concomitant of the implementation of vaccination programmes, it is not surprising that the question of a potential interaction between vaccines and autoimmune diseases is being raised with insistence. Mechanisms leading to autoimmune responses and to their occasional translation into autoimmune diseases are now better understood. Autoimmune responses result from the combined effects of antigen-specific stimulations of the immune system and of an antigen-non-specific activation of antigen-presenting cells in the context of a genetically determined predisposition. Most often such responses are not followed by any clinical manifestations unless additional events favor disease expression, e.g. a localized inflammatory process at tissue level.

The role of infections has been occasionally demonstrated either as an etiologic factor or as a triggering event in autoimmune diseases. It is on the basis of such observations that questions are raised regarding the potential risk of autoimmune responses and of autoimmune diseases following vaccination. Is there a significant risk that some vaccines may induce autoimmune responses through the introduction of microbial epitopes that cross-react with host antigens? Can adjuvant-containing vaccines trigger the clinical expression of an underlying autoimmune process through a 'non-specific' activation of antigen-presenting cells and the release of inflammatory cytokines? Until now, answers to these questions have been largely based on epidemiological studies, with limitations due to the difficulty in assessing the frequency of relatively rare events during clinical trials or post-marketing surveillance. Understanding the mechanisms by which autoimmune responses are generated and how they may or may not lead to autoimmune diseases is therefore of paramount importance in defining the real risk of vaccine-associated autoimmune reaction. During the course of vaccine development, it is now becoming conceivable that a comprehensive and multidisciplinary approach would help to reduce to a minimum the risk that a new vaccine would induce autoimmune manifestations. Later, once the new vaccine is largely used in public health programmes, systems should be in place to readily assess observations or allegations of unexpected autoimmune adverse effects. Although in the last few years there has been a dramatic increase in the number of such allegations, it is somewhat reassuring to see that autoimmune adverse effects were only demonstrated in very few instances.

Herein, we summarize the current knowledge on autoimmune pathology caused by infection or vaccination and we propose a rational approach to minimize the risk of autoimmunity associated with new vaccines under development.

Mechanisms of autoimmunity induction

Activation and clonal expansion of autoreactive lymphocytes represent critical steps in the pathogenesis of autoimmune diseases. Infections might be responsible for these key events through several non-mutually exclusive mechanisms including molecular mimicry, enhanced presentation of self-antigens, bystander activation, polyclonal B cell activation, and impaired T cell regulation (Wucherpfennig, 2001).

The molecular mimicry hypothesis is based on sequence homologies between microbial peptides and self-antigen epitopes. This concept was initially established in an experimental model where immunization with a hepatitis B virus polymerase peptide containing a 6 amino-acid sequence of rabbit myelin basic protein elicited an autoimmune T cell response leading to autoimmune encephalomyelitis (Fujinami and Oldstone, 1985). The demonstration that a viral infection in itself can lead to autoimmune pathology caused by molecular mimicry was established in a murine model of herpes simplex keratitis, where pathogenic autoreactive T cell clones were shown to cross-react with a peptide from the UL6 protein of the herpes simplex virus (Zhao et al., 1998). Evidence that a viral infection can induce pathogenic autoreactive T cells was also provided in a model of Theiler's murine encephalomyelitis virus encoding a mimic peptide (Olson et al., 2001). Autoimmunity dependent on CD8+ T lymphocytes might also involve molecular mimicry as shown in the model of inflammatory bowel disease induced in immunodeficient mice by CD8+ T cell clones directed against mycobacterial heat shock protein hsp60 and cross-reacting with the hsp60 self antigen (Steinhoff et al., 1999). Whatever these experimental data suggest, there is still uncertainty as to whether molecular mimicry is a key mechanism in the pathogenesis of autoimmunity (Benoist and Mathis, 2001). As a matter of fact, molecular mimicry in itself is probably not sufficient to trigger autoimmune pathology.

Infection can promote processing and presentation of self-antigens by several mechanisms. First, cellular damages induced by microbes can result in the release of sequestered self-antigens that stimulate autoreactive T cells, as clearly demonstrated in autoimmune diabetes induced by coxsackievirus B4 infection in mice (Horwitz *et al.*, 2002). Second, the local inflammatory reaction elicited in tissues by microbes promotes dendritic cell maturation which represents a key step in the induction phase of immune responses. Indeed, microbial products engage Toll-like receptors on dendritic cells, resulting in upregulation of the membrane expression of major histocompatibility complex and costimulatory molecules and secretion of cytokines promoting T cell activation including interleukin 12 (Medzhitov and Janeway, 2002). Third, a T cell response directed at a single self-peptide can diversify during an inflammatory reaction, by a process of 'epitope spreading' which has been well documented in murine models of encephalomyelitis (Wucherpfennig, 2001).

The release of cytokines such as interleukin 12 can promote bystander activation of memory T cells and thereby trigger autoimmune reactions. Indeed, Shevach *et al.* established in murine models of encephalomyelitis that quiescent autoreactive T cells can differentiate into pathogenic Th1 effectors in the presence of microbial products or synthetic CpG-containing oligodeoxynucleotides inducing IL-12 synthesis (Segal *et al.*, 2000; Segal *et al.*, 1997). Recent data suggest that it is actually IL-23, a cytokine containing the IL-12p40 chain, which might be the pathogenic cytokine in such settings (Watford and O'Shea, 2003). Likewise, the group of Fujinami demonstrated that viral infection can elicit relapses of autoimmune encephalomyelitis in primed animals in a non-antigen specific manner (Theil *et al.*, 2001).

Hypergammaglobulinemia and autoantibody responses can occur as a consequence of the activation of B cells independent of the specificity of their membrane receptor. Recent observations in a model of lymphocytic choriomeningitis virus infection demonstrated that this process might occur as a consequence of B cell receptor-independent antigen uptake, followed by the presentation of viral peptides to CD4$^+$ T cells which upon activation provide helper signals to B cells (Hunziker *et al.*, 2003).

Beside their pathogenic role as direct effectors of autoimmune pathology, antibodies promote or enhance autoreactive T cell responses in several ways. Indeed, antibodies can facilitate capture of self-antigen by antigen-presenting cells and as a consequence the activation of autoreactive T cells (Tung *et al.*, 2001; von Herrath and Bach, 2002). Furthermore, they might induce inflammation in the targeted tissue and thereby promote local release of self antigens, epitope spreading and recruitment of activated T cells (von Herrath and Bach, 2002). These and other mechanisms probably explain the impact of maternal antibodies on the development of autoimmune pathology in early life as documented in experimental models of type 1 diabetes and autoimmune ovarian disease (Greeley *et al.*, 2002; Setiady *et al.*, 2003).

There is growing evidence that regulatory T cells are instrumental in controlling autoreactive T cells both in neonates and adults (Shevach, 2000). Indeed, depletion of regulatory CD4$^+$ CD25$^+$ T cells promotes autoimmunity, although in adult animals this maneuver is not sufficient by itself and requires administration of self antigen (McHugh and Shevach, 2002). Infectious agents can influence T cell regulatory circuits in several ways. On one hand, the engagement of Toll-like receptors on dendritic cells by microbial products induces the production of interleukin 6, which inhibits the suppressive effects of regulatory T cells (Pasare and Medzhitov, 2003), providing thereby an additional mechanism promoting effector T cell responses upon dendritic cell activation. On the other hand, regulatory T cells themselves express Toll-like receptors and respond to bacterial products by increasing their suppressor activity (Caramalho *et al.*, 2003). Elucidation of the factors which determine the net result of these interactions in the course of infections *in vivo* will certainly represent an area of intense investigation in the near future.

Autoimmune pathology in the course of infectious diseases

In the clinics, rheumatic fever caused by an anti-streptococcal immune response that cross-reacts with cardiac myosin represents the prototype of autoimmune disease of infectious origin (Cunningham *et al.*, 1997). Another well-documented example is the Guillain–Barré syndrome occurring in the course of *Campylobacter jejuni* infection and mediated by antibacterial lipopolysaccharide antibodies cross-reacting with human gangliosides (Rees *et al.*, 1995). More recently, antibodies directed against the Tax protein of the human T-lymphotropic virus type 1 (HTLV-1) and cross-reacting with the heterogeneous nuclear ribonucleoprotein-A1 (hnRNP-A1) self-antigen were demonstrated in HTLV-1-associated myelopathy/tropical spastic paraparesis (Levin *et al.*, 2002). As far as T cell-mediated autoimmunity is concerned, cross-reactivity between microbial peptides and self-antigens has been documented in several disorders including type I diabetes, multiple sclerosis and antibiotic-resistant Lyme arthritis (Rose and Mackay, 2000; Davidson and Diamond, 2001). From a clinical perspective a clear-cut relation between the onset of autoimmune pathology and viral infection has only been firmly established for type 1 diabetes consecutive to congenital rubella (Clarke *et al.*, 1984; Robles and Eisenbarth, 2001).

Infection-associated autoimmunity in humans also occurs in the context of polyclonal B cell activation. This is the case in chronic hepatitis C virus infection which causes mixed cryoglobulinemia (Casato *et al.*, 1991) and in HIV infection which is sometimes associated with autoantibody-induced thrombocytopenia (Nardi *et al.*, 2001).

As a whole, the role of infections as etiological agents of human autoimmune disease has been demonstrated in only a few instances. However, their involvement in the exacerbation of a pre-existing autoimmune disorder is rather well established. For example, in multiple sclerosis, epidemiological data strongly suggest that relapses of the disease can be triggered by bacterial or viral infections (Andersen *et al.*, 1993; Rapp *et al.*, 1995).

THE RISK OF VACCINE-ASSOCIATED AUTOIMMUNITY

Isolated case reports and increased attention in the media to possible side-effects of vaccines has dramatically modified the perception in the medical community and the public of the risk of autoimmunity elicited by vaccination despite the lack of epidemiological support for such a concern. Indeed, there are only few examples of autoimmune pathology that could be firmly attributed to vaccination (see below). Interestingly, autoimmune reactions were observed only rarely after administration of vaccines against infections known to be associated with autoimmunity (Chen *et al.*, 2001). The case of the vaccine against Lyme disease is especially relevant as this vaccine contained the self-mimic OspA antigen thought to be involved in arthritis consecutive to the infection with *Borrelia burgdorferi*. This supports the concept that the development of autoimmune pathology most often requires the tissue damage and the long-lasting inflammatory reaction which occur during natural infections but not after vaccination.

VACCINE-ATTRIBUTABLE AUTOIMMUNE DISEASES

Guillain–Barré syndrome and influenza vaccine

Guillain–Barré syndrome (GBS, polyradiculoneuritis) was associated with the 1976–1977 vaccination campaign against swine influenza using the A/New Jersey/8/76 swine-flu vaccine (Schonberger *et al.*, 1979). The estimated attributable risk of vaccine-related GBS in the adult population was just under one case per 100,000 vaccinations and the period of increased risk in swine-flu vaccinated versus non-vaccinated individuals was concentrated primarily within the 5-week period after vaccination (relative risk: 7.60). Although these original Centers for Disease Control study demonstrated a statistical association and suggested a causal relation between the two events, controversy has persisted for several years. The causal relation was reassessed and confirmed in a later study focusing on cases observed in Michigan and Minnesota (Safranek *et al.*, 1991). The relative risk of developing Guillain–Barré syndrome in the vaccinated population of these two states, as compared with swine-flu non-vaccinated individuals, during the 6 weeks following vaccination was 7.10, whereas the excess cases of Guillain–Barré syndrome during the first 6 weeks attributed to the vaccine was 8.6 per million vaccinees in Michigan and 9.7 per million vaccinees in Minnesota. The pathogenic mechanisms involved are still unknown. With subsequent influenza vaccines, no significant increase in the development of Guillain–Barré syndrome was noted (Lasky *et al.*, 1998) and it is currently assumed that the risk of developing the Guillain–Barré syndrome following vaccination (one additional case per million persons vaccinated) is substantially less than the risk for severe influenza and influenza-related complications (Chen *et al.*, 2001).

Measles–mumps–rubella vaccine and thrombocytopenia

Another example of confirmed autoimmune adverse effect of vaccination is idiopathic thrombocytopenia (ITP) that may occur after measles–mumps–rubella (MMR) vaccination (Oski and Naiman, 1966; Beeler *et al.*, 1996; Jonville-Bera *et al.*, 1996; Vlacha *et al.*, 1996; Miller *et al.*, 2001). The reported frequency of clinically apparent ITP after this vaccine is around 1 in 30,000 vaccinated children. In one study (Miller *et al.*, 2001), the relative incidence in the 6-week post-immunization risk period has been estimated at 3.27 (95% CI: 1.49 to 7.16) when compared with the control period. In about two-thirds of the patients, platelet counts under 20,000/μL have been recorded. The clinical course of MMR-related ITP is usually transient but it is not infrequently associated with bleeding and, as shown in a study conducted in Finland, it can occasionally be severe (Nieminen *et al.*, 1993). In this latter study, there was an increase in platelet-associated immunoglobulins in 10 out of 15 patients whereas circulating antiplatelet autoantibodies, specific for platelet glycoprotein IIb/IIIa, were detected in 5 out of 15 patients. These findings are compatible with an autoimmune mechanism triggered by the immune response to MMR vaccination. However, it should be noted that the risk for thrombocytopenia following natural rubella (1/3000) or measles (1/6000) infections is much greater than after vaccination (Chen *et al.*, 2001). Patients with a history of previous immune thrombocytopenic purpura are prone to develop this complication and in these individuals the risk of vaccination should be weighed against that of being exposed to the corresponding viral diseases (Pool *et al.*, 1997).

VACCINE-RELATED ALLEGATIONS OF AUTOIMMUNE ADVERSE EFFECTS

Hepatitis B and multiple sclerosis

The possible association of hepatitis B (HB) vaccination with the development of multiple sclerosis (MS) was primarily questioned in France, following the report of 35 cases of primary demyelinating events occurring at one Paris hospital between 1991 and 1997, within eight weeks of recombinant HB vaccine injection (Gout et al., 1997; Tourbah et al., 1999). The neurological manifestations were similar to those observed in MS. There were inflammatory changes in the cerebrospinal fluid and high signal intensity lesions were observed in the cerebral white matter on T2-weighted magnetic resonance imaging. After a mean follow-up of 3 years, half of them became clinically definite MS. These neurological manifestations occurred in individuals considered at higher risk for MS: a preponderance of women, mean age near 30 years, over-representation of the DR2 HLA antigen and a positive family history of MS. These observations rapidly called the attention of the French pharmaco-vigilance system and from 1993 through 1999, several hundred cases with similar demographic and clinical characteristics were identified. It is essential to note that this episode occurred in a very special context. In France, close to 25 million people received the HB vaccine during this period, of which 18 million were adults, and this represented about 40% of the population of the country. No cases were reported in children under three years of age. Since these initial reports, at least 10 studies aiming at defining the significance of such observations have now been completed. There was no significant association between hepatitis B vaccination and the occurrence of demyelinating events or MS in any of these studies.

Two recent studies bear particular weight in confirming the lack of a significant association between hepatitis B vaccination and the occurrence of MS. Confavreux et al. (2001) conducted a case–crossover study in patients included in the European Database for Multiple Sclerosis who had a relapse between 1993 and 1997. The index relapse was the first relapse confirmed by a visit to a neurologist and preceded by a relapse-free period of at least 12 months. Exposure to vaccination in the 2-month risk period immediately preceding the relapse was compared with that in the four previous 2-month control periods for the calculation of relative risks. Of 643 patients with relapses of multiple sclerosis, 2.3% had been vaccinated during the preceding 2-month risk period as compared with 2.8 to 4.0% who were vaccinated during one or more of the four control periods. The relative risk of relapse associated with exposure to any vaccination during the previous 2 months was 0.71 (95% CI, 0.40 to 1.26). There was no increase in the specific short-term risk of relapse associated with hepatitis B. Another recent study (Ascherio et al., 2001) also excluded a possible link between hepatitis B (HB) vaccine and multiple sclerosis. These authors conducted a nested case–control study in two large cohorts of nurses in the United States, those in the Nurses' Health Study (which has followed 121,700 women since 1976) and those in the Nurses' Health Study II (which has followed 116,671 women since 1989). For each woman with multiple sclerosis, five healthy women and one woman with breast cancer were selected as controls. The analyses included 192 women with multiple sclerosis and 645 matched controls. The multivariate relative risk of multiple sclerosis associated with exposure to the hepatitis B vaccine at any time before the onset of the disease was 0.9 (95% CI, 0.5 to 1.6). The relative risk associated with hepatitis B vaccination within two years before the onset of the disease was 0.7 (95% CI, 0.3 to 1.8). The results were similar in analyses restricted to women with multiple sclerosis that began after the introduction of the recombinant hepatitis B vaccine. These reassuring data are consistent with the fact that, since the integration of hepatitis B vaccine into national childhood immunization schedules in over 125 countries, it has been used in more than 500 million persons and has proved to be among the safest vaccines yet developed.

Vaccination and diabetes

Type-1 diabetes (formerly known as insulin-dependent diabetes mellitus, IDDM, or juvenile diabetes) results from autoimmune destruction of pancreatic β-cells in genetically susceptible individuals exposed to environmental risk factors. The incidence is particularly high in some geographic areas, e.g. Finland and Sardinia, where it can reach 40 cases per 100,000. During the last decades, there has been a regular increase in the incidence of type 1 diabetes in most countries of the world. In a recent European multicenter study covering the period 1989–1994, the annual rate of increase in incidence was found to be 3·4%, with a particularly rapid rate of increase in children under 4 years of age (6.3%) (2000). In this context, it is not surprising that the potential role of childhood vaccines as a triggering event for this disease has been questioned. This possibility has been evaluated in a few epidemiologic studies. A case–control study conducted in Sweden in the mid-1980s did not observe any significant effect of vaccination against tuberculosis, smallpox, tetanus, pertussis or rubella on odd-risk for diabetes (Blom *et al.*, 1991). However, some authors (Classen and Classen, 1999a; Classen and Classen, 1999b) have hypothesized that the timing of vaccination may be of importance and that certain vaccines (e.g. *Haemophilus influenzae* type b, Hib), if given at 2 months of life or later may increase the risk of type 1 diabetes. This was not confirmed by a 10-year follow-up study of over 100,000 Finnish children involved in a clinical trial of Hib vaccine (Karvonen *et al.*, 1999). A recent study conducted in four large health maintenance organizations (HMOs) in the USA did not observe any association between administration of routine childhood vaccines and the risk of type 1 diabetes. There was no influence of the timing of hepatitis B or Hib vaccination on the diabetes risk (DeStefano *et al.*, 2001). Therefore, at this stage, there are no serious indications of any significant influence of current childhood vaccines on the occurrence of type 1 diabetes.

Overall, the risk of induction or exacerbation of autoimmune disease associated with current vaccines is very low. As several vaccine-preventable infections are well known to negatively influence the course of autoimmune diseases (e.g. multiple sclerosis or systemic lupus erythematosus), vaccination is strongly recommended in such cases (e.g. influenza vaccination in patients with multiple sclerosis).

Aluminum and macrophagic myofasciitis

A novel potential culprit appeared after publication of reports on a new disease entity named macrophagic myofasciitis (MMF). MMF is a poorly defined syndrome characterized by myalgias, arthralgias, and fatigue (Gherardi *et al.*, 2001). It is claimed to be sometimes associated with central nervous system lesions reminiscent of multiple sclerosis (Authier *et al.*, 2001). Muscle biopsies in MMF patients showed infiltration with inflammatory cells including macrophages loaded with intracytoplasmic inclusions corresponding to aluminum. A causal relation was then proposed between the occurrence of MMF and previous administration of vaccines containing aluminum salt as adjuvant (Gherardi *et al.*, 2001). However, there is no evidence so far of a direct link between the persistence of aluminum in a tiny (2 mm) muscle lesion and the observation of systemic manifestations.

Results of ongoing controlled studies will determine the real significance of these observations.

Multiple vaccinations and allergies

Finally, one should also mention unsubstantiated claims about immune disorders putatively attributed to the administration of a large number of vaccines in childhood. Indeed, children are now required to receive 23 or more vaccine doses by the age of 6 in the United States (Wilson and Marcuse, 2001). Whereas the fear of immune deficiency is not supported by a reasonable rationale, the hygiene hypothesis is used to support the theory that excessive immunizations in childhood might favor the development of atopic dermatitis, asthma and other related allergic disorders (Wilson and Marcuse, 2001). Although this is still a matter of debate, a recent study is reassuring as it demonstrates that high vaccination coverage does not favor but on the contrary transiently suppresses atopy in early childhood (Gruber *et al.*, 2003).

New vaccines and autoimmunity: approaches toward early risk assessment

Although available data are reassuring, we must remain vigilant as the risk of autoimmunity associated with some of the new generation vaccines might be increased as compared with current vaccines. A number of new adjuvants that are being developed aim at inducing strong cytotoxic and inflammatory Th1-type immune responses against viruses or other intracellular pathogens. Such agents may occasionally favor the expression of underlying autoimmune diseases or induce autoimmune responses in exceptional cases where the vaccine antigens contain immunodominant epitopes that cross-react with self-antigens. Indeed, a recent study indicates that inflammatory signals can drive organ-specific autoimmunity to a self-antigen that is tolerogenic under normal conditions (Vezys and Lefrancois, 2002). Special attention should certainly be given to adjuvants acting as strong inducers of IL-12 or IL-23 synthesis (Segal *et al.*, 1997; Segal *et al.*, 2000; Watford and O'Shea, 2003). Cancer vaccines based on dendritic cells pulsed with tumor antigens might result in autoimmunity induction as well (Ludewig *et al.*, 2000; Bondanza *et al.*, 2003). Whereas autoimmunity features might not be rare after dendritic cell vaccination, the development of clinical autoimmune pathology might depend on the genetic background as suggested by a recent study comparing lupus-prone and normal mice (Bondanza *et al.*, 2003). The administration of agents targeting regulatory T cells such as anti-CTLA4 antibody to enhance cancer vaccines also appears to be associated with a significant risk of autoimmunity induction as observed both in experimental and clinical settings (van Elsas *et al.*, 2001; Hodi *et al.*, 2003).

During the course of vaccine development, only a comprehensive and multidisciplinary strategy may help to reduce the theoretical risk that a new vaccine would induce autoimmune manifestations. This may include a search for potential molecular and immunological mimicry between vaccine antigens and host components through an intelligent combination of bioinformatics and immunological studies. One should keep in mind that, by itself, an identified mimicry is of little pathogenic significance. Information should be gathered on the relative ability of such epitopes to bind to human major histocompatibility complex molecules, to be processed by human antigen-presenting cells and to be recognized by autoreactive T cells. New vaccine formulations and adjuvants should be assessed for their capability to induce or enhance autoimmune pathology in relevant animal models. When the stage of clinical development is reached, appropriate immunological investigations (e.g. autoimmune serology) may be systematically included in phase I-II-III trials. On an *ad hoc* basis, clinical surveillance of potential autoimmune adverse effects may have to be included in the monitoring protocol. Such surveillance has to be extended through the post-marketing stage if specific rare events must be ruled out.

CONCLUSION

All vaccines carry some risk of adverse events, but fortunately vaccine-related toxicity is usually rare, mild and transient. Despite their excellent safety record, vaccines will remain the target of unsubstantiated accusations by antivaccine movements developing their activities on the basis of decreased public's trust in the medical establishment, vaccine manufacturers and health authorities. In this context, it is essential to consider safety as a first priority in vaccine development, even in the earliest stages of research. Furthermore, the public's questions on vaccine safety should be considered seriously and addressed properly, even if based on poorly documented allegations. Depending on the issue raised and its potential impact, well-designed and well-conducted epidemiological investigations might be necessary to gather objective data. Dissemination of the available information by appropriate means is essential to restore the public's trust in vaccines. The long-term challenge is to modify the perception of vaccination-associated risks, so that individuals everywhere benefit from the protection provided by carefully developed vaccines.

References

Andersen, O., Lygner, P.E., Bergstrom, T., Andersson, M,. and Vahlne, A. 1993. Viral infections trigger multiple sclerosis relapses: a prospective seroepidemiological study. J. Neurol. 240: 417–422.

Ascherio, A., Zhang, S.M., Hernan, M.A., Olek, M.J., Coplan, P.M., Brodovicz, K., and Walker, A.M. 2001. Hepatitis B vaccination and the risk of multiple sclerosis. N. Engl. J. Med. 344: 327–332.

Authier, F.J., Cherin, P., Creange, A., Bonnotte, B., Ferrer, X., Abdelmoumni, A., Ranoux, D., Pelletier, J., Figarella-Branger, D., Granel, B., Maisonobe, T., Coquet, M., Degos, J.D., and Gherardi, R.K. 2001. Central nervous system disease in patients with macrophagic myofasciitis. Brain 124: 974–983.

Beeler, J., Varricchio, F., and Wise, R. 1996. Thrombocytopenia after immunization with measles vaccines: review of the vaccine adverse events reporting system 1990 to 1994. Pediatr. Infect. Dis. J. 15: 88–90.

Benoist, C., and Mathis, D. 2001. Autoimmunity provoked by infection: how good is the case for T cell epitope mimicry? Nature Immunol. 2: 797–801.

Blom, L., Nystrom, L., and Dahlquist, G. 1991. The Swedish childhood diabetes study. Vaccinations and infections as risk determinants for diabetes in childhood. Diabetologia 34: 176–181.

Bondanza, A., Zimmermann, V.S., Dell'Antonio, G., Dal Cin, E., Capobianco, A., Sabbadini, M.G., Manfredi, A.A., and Rovere-Querini, P. 2003. Cutting edge: dissociation between autoimmune response and clinical disease after vaccination with dendritic cells. J. Immunol. 170: 24–27.

Caramalho, I., Lopes-Carvalho, T., Ostler, D., Zelenay, S., Haury, M., and Demengeot, J. 2003. Regulatory T cells selectively express toll-like receptors and are activated by lipopolysaccharide. J. Exp. Med. 197: 403–411.

Casato, M., Taliani, G., Pucillo, L.P., Goffredo, F., Lagana, B., and Bonomo, L. 1991. Cryoglobulinaemia and hepatitis C virus. Lancet 337: 1047–1048.

Chen, R.T., Pless, R., and Destefano, F. 2001. Epidemiology of autoimmune reactions induced by vaccination. J. Autoimmun. 16: 309–318.

Clarke, W.L., Shaver, K.A., Bright, G.M., Rogol, A.D., and Nance, W.E. 1984. Autoimmunity in congenital rubella syndrome. J. Pediatr. 104: 370–373.

Classen, J.B., and Classen, D.C. 1999a. Association between type 1 diabetes and hib vaccine causal relation is likely. BMJ. 319: 1133.

Classen, J.B., and Classen, D.C. 1999b. Immunization in the first month of life may explain decline in incidence of IDDM in The Netherlands. Autoimmunity 31: 43–45.

Confavreux, C., Suissa, S., Saddier, P., Bourdes, V., and Vukusic, S. 2001. Vaccinations and the risk of relapse in multiple sclerosis. Vaccines in Multiple Sclerosis Study Group. N. Engl. J. Med. 344: 319–326.

Cunningham, M.W., Antone, S.M., Smart, M., Liu, R., and Kosanke, S. 1997. Molecular analysis of human cardiac myosin-cross-reactive B- and T-cell epitopes of the group A streptococcal M5 protein. Infect. Immun. 65: 3913–3923.

Dagan, R., Eskola, J., Leclerc, C., and Leroy, O. 1998. Reduced response to multiple vaccines sharing common protein epitopes that are administered simultaneously to infants. Infect. Immun. 66: 2093–2098.

Davidson, A., and Diamond, B. 2001. Autoimmune diseases. N. Engl. J. Med. 345: 340–350.

DeStefano, F., Mullooly, J.P., Okoro, C.A., Chen, R.T., Marcy, S.M., Ward, J.I., Vadheim, C.M., Black, S.B., Shinefield, H.R., Davis, R.L., and Bohlke, K. 2001. Childhood vaccinations, vaccination timing, and risk of type 1 diabetes mellitus. Pediatrics 108: E112.

EURODIAB ACE Study Group. 2000. Variation and trends in incidence of childhood diabetes in Europe. Lancet 355: 873–876.

Fujinami, R.S., and Oldstone, M.B. 1985. Amino acid homology between the encephalitogenic site of myelin basic protein and virus: mechanism for autoimmunity. Science 230: 1043–1045.

Fulginiti, V.A., Eller, J.J., Downie, A.W., and Kempe, C.H. 1967. Altered reactivity to measles virus. Atypical measles in children previously immunized with inactivated measles virus vaccines. JAMA 202: 1075–1080.

Gherardi, R.K., Coquet, M., Cherin, P., Belec, L., Moretto, P., Dreyfus, P.A., Pellissier, J.F., Chariot, P., and Authier, F.J. 2001. Macrophagic myofasciitis lesions assess long-term persistence of vaccine-derived aluminium hydroxide in muscle. Brain 124: 1821–1831.

Gout, O., Théodorou, I., Liblau, R., et al. 1997. Central nervous system demyelination after recombinant hepatitis B vaccination report of 25 cases. Neurology 48.

Greeley, S.A., Katsumata, M., Yu, L., Eisenbarth, G.S., Moore, D.J., Goodarzi, H., Barker, C.F., Naji, A., and Noorchashm, H. 2002. Elimination of maternally transmitted autoantibodies prevents diabetes in nonobese diabetic mice. Nature Med. 8: 399–402.

Gruber, C., Illi, S., Lau, S., Nickel, R., Forster, J., Kamin, W., Bauer, C.P., Wahn, V., and Wahn, U. 2003. Transient suppression of atopy in early childhood is associated with high vaccination coverage. Pediatrics 111: e282–288.

Halsey, N. 2003. Vaccine safety: Real and perceived issues. In: The Vaccine Book. B. Bloom and P.-H. Lambert eds. Elsevier Science, pp. 371–389.

Hodi, F.S., Mihm, M.C., Soiffer, R.J., Haluska, F.G., Butler, M., Seiden, M.V., Davis, T., Henry-Spires, R., MacRae, S., Willman, A., Padera, R., Jaklitsch, M.T., Shankar, S., Chen, T.C., Korman, A., Allison, J.P., and Dranoff, G. 2003. Biologic activity of cytotoxic T lymphocyte-associated antigen 4 antibody blockade in previously vaccinated metastatic melanoma and ovarian carcinoma patients. Proc. Natl. Acad. Sci. USA 100: 4712–4717.

Horwitz, M.S., Ilic, A., Fine, C., Rodriguez, E., and Sarvetnick, N. 2002. Presented antigen from damaged pancreatic beta cells activates autoreactive T cells in virus-mediated autoimmune diabetes. J. Clin. Invest. 109: 79–87.

Hunziker, L., Recher, M., Macpherson, A.J., Ciurea, A., Freigang, S., Hengartner, H., and Zinkernagel, R.M. 2003. Hypergammaglobulinemia and autoantibody induction mechanisms in viral infections. Nature Immunol. 4: 343–349.

Jonville-Bera, A.P., Autret, E., Galy-Eyraud, C., and Hessel, L. 1996. Thrombocytopenic purpura after measles, mumps and rubella vaccination: a retrospective survey by the French regional pharmacovigilance centres and pasteur-merieux serums et vaccins. Pediatr. Infect. Dis. J. 15: 44–48.

Karvonen, M., Cepaitis, Z., and Tuomilehto, J. 1999. Association between type 1 diabetes and Haemophilus influenzae type b vaccination: birth cohort study. BMJ. 318: 1169–1172.

Kim, H.W., Canchola, J.G., Brandt, C.D., Pyles, G., Chanock, R.M., Jensen, K., and Parrott, R.H. 1969. Respiratory syncytial virus disease in infants despite prior administration of antigenic inactivated vaccine. Am. J. Epidemiol. 89: 422–434.

Lasky, T., Terracciano, G.J., Magder, L., Koski, C.L., Ballesteros, M., Nash, D., Clark, S., Haber, P., Stolley, P.D., Schonberger, L.B., and Chen, R.T. 1998. The Guillain–Barre syndrome and the 1992–1993 and 1993–1994 influenza vaccines. N. Engl. J. Med. 339: 1797–1802.

Levin, M.C., Lee, S.M., Kalume, F., Morcos, Y., Dohan, F.C., Jr., Hasty, K.A., Callaway, J.C., Zunt, J., Desiderio, D., and Stuart, J.M. 2002. Autoimmunity due to molecular mimicry as a cause of neurological disease. Nature Med. 8: 509–513.

Ludewig, B., Ochsenbein, A.F., Odermatt, B., Paulin, D., Hengartner, H., and Zinkernagel, R.M. 2000. Immunotherapy with dendritic cells directed against tumor antigens shared with normal host cells results in severe autoimmune disease. J. Exp. Med. 191: 795–804.

Mader, R., Narendran, A., Lewtas, J., Bykerk, V., Goodman, R.C., Dickson, J.R., and Keystone, E.C. 1993. Systemic vasculitis following influenza vaccination – report of 3 cases and literature review. J. Rheumatol. 20: 1429–1431.

McHugh, R.S., and Shevach, E.M. 2002. Cutting edge: depletion of CD4+CD25+ regulatory T cells is necessary, but not sufficient, for induction of organ-specific autoimmune disease. J. Immunol. 168: 5979–5983.

Medzhitov, R., and Janeway, C.A., Jr. 2002. Decoding the patterns of self and nonself by the innate immune system. Science 296: 298–300.

Miller, E., Waight, P., Farrington, C.P., Andrews, N., Stowe, J., and Taylor, B. 2001. Idiopathic thrombocytopenic purpura and MMR vaccine. Arch Dis. Child. 84: 227–229.

Nardi, M., Tomlinson, S., Greco, M.A., and Karpatkin, S. 2001. Complement-independent, peroxide-induced antibody lysis of platelets in HIV-1-related immune thrombocytopenia. Cell 106: 551–561.

Nieminen, U., Peltola, H., Syrjala, M.T., Makipernaa, A., and Kekomaki, R. 1993. Acute thrombocytopenic purpura following measles, mumps and rubella vaccination. A report on 23 patients. Acta Paediatr. 82: 267–270.

Olson, J.K., Croxford, J.L., Calenoff, M.A., Dal Canto, M.C., and Miller, S.D. 2001. A virus-induced molecular mimicry model of multiple sclerosis. J. Clin. Invest. 108: 311–318.

Openshaw, P.J., Culley, F.J., and Olszewska, W. 2001. Immunopathogenesis of vaccine-enhanced RSV disease. Vaccine 20 Suppl 1: S27–31.

Oski, F.A., and Naiman, J.L. 1966. Effect of live measles vaccine on the platelet count. N. Engl. J. Med. 275: 352–356.

Ota, M.O., Vekemans, J., Schlegel-Haueter, S.E., Fielding, K., Sanneh, M., Kidd, M., Newport, M.J., Aaby, P., Whittle, H., Lambert, P.H., McAdam, K.P., Siegrist, C.A., and Marchant, A. 2002. Influence of *Mycobacterium bovis* bacillus Calmette–Guerin on antibody and cytokine responses to human neonatal vaccination. J. Immunol. 168(2): 919–925.

Pasare, C. and Medzhitov, R. 2003. Toll pathway-dependent blockade of CD4+CD25+ T cell-mediated suppression by dendritic cells. Science 299: 1033–1036.

Pool, V., Chen, R., and Rhodes, P. 1997. Indications for measles-mumps-rubella vaccination in a child with prior thrombocytopenia purpura. Pediatr. Infect. Dis. J. 16: 423–424.

Rapp, N.S., Gilroy, J., and Lerner, A.M. 1995. Role of bacterial infection in exacerbation of multiple sclerosis. Am. J. Phys. Med. Rehabil. 74: 415–418.

Rees, J.H., Soudain, S.E., Gregson, N.A., and Hughes, R.A. 1995. *Campylobacter jejuni* infection and Guillain–Barre syndrome. N. Engl. J. Med. 333: 1374–1379.

Robles, D.T., and Eisenbarth, G.S. 2001. Type 1A diabetes induced by infection and immunization. J. Autoimmun. 16: 355–362.

Rose, N.R., and Mackay, I.R. 2000. Molecular mimicry: a critical look at exemplary instances in human diseases. Cell Mol. Life Sci. 57: 542–551.

Safranek, T.J., Lawrence, D.N., Kurland, L.T., Culver, D.H., Wiederholt, W.C., Hayner, N.S., Osterholm, M.T., O'Brien, P., and Hughes, J.M. 1991. Reassessment of the association between Guillain–Barre syndrome and receipt of swine influenza vaccine in 1976–1977: results of a two-state study. Expert Neurology Group. Am. J. Epidemiol. 133: 940–951.

Schonberger, L.B., Bregman, D.J., Sullivan-Bolyai, J.Z., Keenlyside, R.A., Ziegler, D.W., Retailliau, H.F., Eddins, D.L., and Bryan, J.A. 1979. Guillain–Barre syndrome following vaccination in the National Influenza Immunization Program, United States, 1976 – 1977. Am. J. Epidemiol. 110: 105–123.

Segal, B.M., Chang, J.T., and Shevach, E.M. 2000. CpG oligonucleotides are potent adjuvants for the activation of autoreactive encephalitogenic T cells in vivo. J. Immunol. 164: 5683–5688.

Segal, B.M., Klinman, D.M., and Shevach, E.M. 1997. Microbial products induce autoimmune disease by an IL-12-dependent pathway. J. Immunol. 158: 5087–5090.

Setiady, Y.Y., Samy, E.T., and Tung, K.S. 2003. Maternal autoantibody triggers de novo T cell-mediated neonatal autoimmune disease. J. Immunol. 170: 4656–4664.

Shevach, E.M. 2000. Regulatory T cells in autoimmmunity. Annu. Rev. Immunol. 18: 423–449.

Steinhoff, U., Brinkmann, V., Klemm, U., Aichele, P., Seiler, P., Brandt, U., Bland, P.W., Prinz, I., Zugel, U., and Kaufmann, S.H. 1999. Autoimmune intestinal pathology induced by hsp60-specific CD8 T cells. Immunity 11: 349–358.

Tavadia, S., Drummond, A., Evans, C.D., and Wainwright, N.J. 2003. Leucocytoclastic vasculitis and influenza vaccination. Clin. Exp. Dermatol. 28: 154–156.

Theil, D.J., Tsunoda, I., Rodriguez, F., Whitton, J.L., and Fujinami, R.S. 2001. Viruses can silently prime for and trigger central nervous system autoimmune disease. J. Neurovirol. 7: 220–227.

Tourbah, A., Gout, O., Liblau, R., Lyon-Caen, O., Bougniot, C., Iba-Zizen, M.T., and Cabanis, E.A, 1999. Encephalitis after hepatitis B vaccination: recurrent disseminated encephalitis or MS? Neurology 53: 396–401.

Tung, K.S., Agersborg, S.S., Alard, P., Garza, K.M., and Lou, Y.H. 2001. Regulatory T-cell, endogenous antigen and neonatal environment in the prevention and induction of autoimmune disease. Immunol. Rev. 182: 135–148.

Vaccine Safety Advisory Committee. 1999. Vaccine safety. Wkly Epidemiol Rec. 74: 337–340.

van Elsas, A., Sutmuller, R.P., Hurwitz, A.A., Ziskin, J., Villasenor, J., Medema, J.P., Overwijk, W.W., Restifo, N.P., Melief, C.J., Offringa, R., and Allison, J.P. 2001. Elucidating the autoimmune and antitumor effector mechanisms of a treatment based on cytotoxic T lymphocyte antigen-4 blockade in combination with a B16 melanoma vaccine: comparison of prophylaxis and therapy. J. Exp. Med. 194: 481–489.

Vaughn, D.W. 2000. Invited commentary: Dengue lessons from Cuba. Am J. Epidemiol. 152: 800–803.

Vezys, V., and Lefrancois, L. 2002. Cutting edge: inflammatory signals drive organ-specific autoimmunity to normally cross-tolerizing endogenous antigen. J. Immunol. 169: 6677–6680.

Vlacha, V., Forman, E.N., Miron, D., and Peter, G. 1996. Recurrent thrombocytopenic purpura after repeated measles-mumps-rubella vaccination. Pediatrics 97: 738–739.

von Herrath, M., and Bach, J.F. 2002. Juvenile autoimmune diabetes: a pathogenic role for maternal antibodies? Nature Med. 8: 331–333.

Watford, W.T., and O'Shea, J.J. 2003. Autoimmunity: A case of mistaken identity. Nature 421: 706–708.

Wilson, C.B., and Marcuse, E.K. 2001. Vaccine safety – vaccine benefits: science and the public's perception. Nature Rev. Immunol. 1: 160–165.

Wucherpfennig, K.W. 2001. Mechanisms for the induction of autoimmunity by infectious agents. J. Clin. Invest. 108: 1097–1104.

Zhao, Z.S., Granucci, F., Yeh, L., Schaffer, P.A., and Cantor, H. 1998. Molecular mimicry by herpes simplex virus-type 1: autoimmune disease after viral infection. Science 279: 1344–1347.

Chapter 9

Vaccines Against Nosocomial Infections

Philippe Moingeon and Jeffrey Almond

Abstract

Nosocomial infections (NI) are associated with opportunistic pathogens, usually transmitted in hospital settings to immunosuppressed or highly exposed individuals (e.g. patients undergoing surgery, or hospitalized in intensive care units). The most frequently encountered pathogens include *Staphylococcus aureus, S. epidermidis*, enterococci *(E. faecium, E. faecalis), Clostridium difficile, Escherichia coli, Pseudomonas aeruginosa, Legionella pneumophila* and the yeast, *Candida albicans*. The burden of nosocomial infection is significantly increasing in the context of growing antimicrobial resistance among such pathogens. Attempts to develop vaccines, and for some of the targets, passive immunotherapies are discussed in the present review. Such innovative immunoprophylactic or therapeutic approaches are facilitated by the identification of new potential targets from genomics studies. In addition, the molecular analysis of biofilm formation is yielding important information regarding virulence factors for some of these pathogens. This can potentially be used for vaccine design.

This manuscript reports in part on presentations and discussions made during the International Symposium on Immunological approaches against nosocomial infections, organized by the Mérieux foundation and held at Les Pensières, Veyrier-du-Lac, France, 19–21 November, 2003.

THE BURDEN OF NOSOCOMIAL INFECTION

In the United States (1992), the estimated direct costs of extra treatment due to nosocomial infections (NI) and extra days of hospitalization were $4.5 billion dollars per year (Wenzel, 1995; Iorsi *et al.*, 2002; NNIS report, 2003). The number of extra days of hospitalization can be as high as 8 million per year. In Europe, costs due to extra treatment and extra days of hospitalization are estimated to be in the same range, keeping in mind that only a fraction of nocosomial infections are reported (Vegni *et al.*, 2004). In the UK alone, more than 300,000 hospitalized patients per annum acquire an infection, with an estimated extra cost for hospitals of £930 million (Plowman *et al.*, 2001). Nosocomial infections cause a significant increase in the duration of hospitalization (by 7 to 30 days) and high mortality rates (23% to 50% for bloodstream infection and 14 to 71% to pneumonia) (Kmietowicz, 2000). The overall cost per patient affected by NI was estimated in 1998 to be in the range of $15,000 to 35,000 (Spencer, 1998; Roberts *et al.*, 2003).

Pathogens causing NI include bacteria such as *Staphylococcus aureus*, *S. epidermidis*, enterococci (*E. faecium, E. faecalis*), *Clostridium difficile, Escherichia coli, Pseudomonas aeruginosa* and *Legionella pneumophila*. Nosocomial infections, however, are not limited to bacteria: fungi (e.g. *Candida albicans*) are also frequently involved in hospital-acquired infections. Rotavirus infections are normally acquired in the community, but this virus may also be involved in nosocomial infections (with up to 43% of children discharges from hospital with a diagnosis of diarrhea having acquired their infection during hospitalization). NB: the development of specific vaccines against rotavirus is treated in a separate chapter.

The main risk factors associated with the acquisition of a nosocomial infection are: prolonged hospitalization, age, invasive or surgical procedures, and recent antimicrobial therapy (Vincent, 2003). Burn patients who have breaches in their skin barrier as well as patients in intensive care units are particularly at risk. Also, antimicrobial resistance in hospitalized patients is becoming a major issue. Gram-positive pathogens, notably methicillin- or vancomycin-resistant *Staphylococcus areus* or enterococci are particularly problematic. Resistance has also increased in Gram-negative pathogens, including *Enterobacteriaceae*, *Pseudomonas* and other opportunists. Resistance to cephalosporins, carbapenems, and quinolones is also of growing concern (D. Goldman, 2003; Vincent, 2003). The number of new anti microbials being developed is limited with only a few new drugs having been approved for treatment of resistant Gram-positive microorganisms, and virtually none for the Gram-negatives. In this context new approaches to control NI are being developed, based on the modulation of immune defenses.

VIRULENCE FACTORS OF OPPORTUNISTIC PATHOGENS

General comments

Opportunistic pathogens are often commensal organisms, which can be acquired in hospitals, potentially leading to severe infections, for example in patients with altered mucosal surfaces (e.g. invasive catheters), impaired immune defenses (e.g. HIV infection), or receiving antibiotherapy (Walker *et al.*, 2004). Like many bacterial pathogens, the bacteria involved in nosocomial infections utilize strategies to escape from host immune effectors, often by manipulating the surface antigens that are primary targets of antibody-mediated opsonic killing. We will specifically focus on virulence factors from *Staphylococcus aureus*, as well as the molecular mechanisms involved in quorum sensing and biofilm formation. These features are important in pathogens involved in NI.

Staphylococcus aureus virulence factors

Partly due to its increasing role in NI, *Staphylococcus aureus* is recognized worldwide as a major health threat. The genome of *Staphylococcus aureus* has been sequenced recently. The *Staphylococcus aureus* chromosome is composed of two domains: a first one occupies more than 90% of the chromosome, and carries well-conserved housekeeping genes. Substantial polymorphisms are observed in the rest of the chromosome among various *Staphylococcus aureus* strains, with DNA sequences either absent, or present as distinct allelic forms (Hiramatsu, 2003). Some of these variable sequences can be transmitted or acquired by cell-to-cell horizontal transfer, and are called genomic islands (Gislands). Most of the genes associated with pathogenicity and antibiotic resistance are present within Gislands at several chromosomal loci (Hiramatsu, 2003). For example, the mec A gene, responsible for methicillin and β-lactam resistance was likely acquired from other commensal bacteria. A major concern is a worldwide emergence of either hospital or community acquired methicillin-resistant *Staphylococcus aureus* strains expressing both *luk-PV*, encoding Panton–Valentine leukocidin, and *mecA* genes. The Panton–Valentine leukocidin (PVL) is an exotoxin which belongs to the pore-forming toxin family. *In vitro*, PVL was shown to induce lysis of host immune cells such as human neutrophils, monocytes and macrophages (Genestier *et al.*, 2003). PVL induces the opening of Ca^{2+} channels and the formation of pores in the membrane of target cells. Other virulence factors are involved in biofilm formation in staphylococci. Their potential role in virulence is being analysed as discussed below.

Wall teichoic acid (WTA), a surface-exposed polymer comprising ribitol phosphate units was shown to be important in mediating interaction of *Staphylococcus aureus* with epithelial cells. As such, WTA represents an important factor for nasal colonization (Weidenmaier *et al.*, 2004).

Factors involved in biofilm formation

Biofilms represent communities of micororganisms developing on natural or artificial surfaces. The capacity to form biofilms is linked to the coordinated expression of multiple genes within the community, directed by small diffusible molecules called quorum sensors (Prince, 2002). Generally speaking, surface receptors and adhesisns involved in early phase infection represent major virulence factors that could be targeted by vaccines. Bacterial conjugation, which facilitates the horizontal transfer of genetic material between donor and recipient bacteria involves plasmids encoding factors inducing planktonic bacteria to form biofilms (Ghigo, 2001). Also, additional bacterial conjugation is favored within biofilms. The genetic and molecular basis of biofilm formation in staphylococci is being better characterized. The ability to form a biofilm is linked to two properties: the adherence of cells to a surface and their ability to accumulate into multilayered cell clusters. On a molecular basis, this involves the production of a slime substance termed PIA, a polysaccharide composed of β-1,6-linked *N*-acetylglucosamines with partly de-acetylated residues, in which the cells are embedded and protected against the host's immune defenses and against antibiotic treatment (Gotz, 2002). High-density oligonucleotide microarrays are being used to investigate global gene expression patterns in the course of biofilm formation.

Two quorum-sensing (QS) systems involving diffusible homoserine lactones, known as the *las* and *rhl* systems, have been identified in *Pseudomonas aeruginosa*. These QS systems have been shown to be important in the production of many of *Pseudomonas aeruginosa*'s virulence factors (e.g. proteases, pyocyanin, hemolysin). In addition, QS has been shown to be involved in biofilm development of *Pseudomonas aeruginosa* (Iglewski, 2003), by allowing the expression of genes facilitating persistence of bacteria in the lung and enabling antibodies to escape.

Under conditions of low bacterial density, planktonic growth predominates, and thus, in the normal host, inhaled bacteria are cleared by innate defenses of airways (Prince, 2002).

Uropathogenic *Escherichia coli* tend to form biofilms within the superficial umbrella cells of the bladder. Four distinct bacterial morphologies have been identified with respect to growth rate, bacterial length, colony organization and motility, in biofilm maturation (Suei Hung, 2003). In a first phase, intracellular bacteria are non-motile, rod shaped, and grow as loosely organized colonies. Subsequently, bacteria mature in a coccoid form as intracellular biofilms, in a highly organized, tightly packed colony that ultimately fills most of the cytoplasm. In the third phase bacteria switch to a motile rod-shaped phenotype allowing detachment from the biofilm and escape from the host cell. During the last phase, the bacteria establish filaments, in response to a TLR4-mediated innate defense mechanism (Suei Hung, 2003). This filamentation step appears to represent a mechanism through which bacteria evade infiltrating polymorphonuclear leukocytes (PMNs).

MAIN TARGETS FOR PROPHYLACTIC AND IMMUNOTHERAPEUTICS AGAINST NOSOCOMIAL INFECTIONS

Main targets for prophylactic or therapeutic vaccines or for passive immunotherapy using specific monoclonal antibodies are summarized in Table 9.1. Some of the targets are discussed below.

Staphylococcus aureus

Staphylococcus aureus is the most common cause of bacteremia in hospitalized patients. Those at particular risk are immunocompromised patients with implants or prostheses and those undergoing surgery (Lowy, 1998). Endocarditis, osteomyelitis, and septic arthritis are among the serious diseases caused by this pathogen. Because of its ability to colonize and high pathogenicity, methicillin resistant *Staphylococcus aureus* has become the most frequent nosocomial pathogen worldwide. An ideal vaccine against *Staphylococcus aureus* should induce antibodies to prevent bacterial adherence, promote opsonophagocytic killing by leukocytes, and neutralize toxic exoproteins produced by the bacterium. Ongoing efforts to design an *Staphylococcus aureus* vaccine have targeted known virulence factors and include staphylococcal surface proteins, polysaccharides, exoproteins, and expressed toxins.

Staphylococcus aureus possesses capsular polysaccharides functioning as an antiphagocytic barrier thereby promoting virulence. Currently eight capsular types have been identified, although types 5 and 8 constitute >80% of the clinical isolates worldwide. A conjugate vaccine associating these two CPs covalently bound to a carrier protein (non-toxic recombinant *Pseudomonas aeruginosa* exotoxin A), has been developed. This conjugate vaccine is highly immunogenic in mice and rabbits, eliciting antibodies with high opsonic activity. Moreover, active immunization with this vaccine protects mice in a *Staphylococcus aureus* lethal challenge model. In humans a double-blind placebo-controlled phase III efficacy trial involving 1800 patients with renal disease undergoing haemodialysis has been conducted. This study demonstrated a 57% reduction in bacteriemia in vaccinees, with no significant safety problems (Shinefield *et al.*, 2002). *Staphylococcus aureus* bacteriemia was prevented for up to 10 months following a single immunization (Fattom *et al.*, 2003). A second generation vaccine could include type 336, which represents a further 11% of *Staphylococcus aureus* clinical strains. Animals passively immunized with IgG antibodies generated by the conjugate vaccines and challenged with the appropriate organism are also protected. Another polysaccharide expressed both by *Staphylococcus aureus* and *S. epidermidis in vivo* was shown to broadly protect against both pathogens (McKenney *et al.*, 1999). These data strongly suggest that vaccine-induced protection against *Staphylococcus aureus* infection can rely upon antibody-mediated mechanisms and that the CP-specific antibodies could serve as a surrogate marker for protection *in vivo*. Noteworthy is the fact that a high number of virulent clinical isolates of both coagulase negative and *Staphylococcus aureus* strains express a polymer of β-1-6-linked N-acetyl glucosamine (PNAG) residues. In animals, immunization against PNAG is shown to confer protective immunity (Maira-Litran *et al.*, 2003).

Although *Staphylococcus aureus* capsular polysaccharide (CP) is a leading target for both active and passive immunotherapy, it should be noted that CP production is highly influenced by environmental conditions (with low expression during the exponential phase of bacterial growth). Also, although most strains produce either CP5 or CP8, still some staphylococcal isolates from humans are nontypeable (Lee, 2003). Thus, protein-based vaccines based on toxoids are also being developed. Balaban *et al.* (1998) showed that pathogenicity is largely due to production of bacterial toxin regulated by an RNA molecule RNAIII. The *Staphylococcus aureus* proteins RAP and RIP activate, and inbihit, respectively, RNAIII activity. Mice vaccinated with RAP or treated with RIP are protected from *Staphylococcus aureus* pathology. Other candidate protein vaccines target cell surface adhesins, that facilitate adherence and colonization by attaching to extracellular matrix components of host tissues or to serum conditioned implanted biomaterials. In preclinical models, a humanized monoclonal antibody recognizing ClfA (clumping factor A), a highly conserved fibrinogen-binding adhesin, prevents bacterial adherence to immobilized fibrinogen, promotes opsonization by neutrophils, and protects against staphylococcal infections. A phase I dose escalation study in healthy volunteers has established safety for this antibody administered passively (Patti, 2003). In mice, administration of a DNA vaccine encoding the fibrin-binding region A of Clf A induced antibodies blocking binding of the pathogen to fibrinogen and facilitating phagocytosis by macrophages, even if mice were not protected against challenge (Brouillette *et al.*, 2002).

A humanized mouse chimeric monoclonal antibody (BSYX-A110) that targets lipoteichoic acid, a major cell wall component of gram positive bacteria has been developed (Fisher, 2003). This antibody is highly opsonic, binds broadly across staphylococcal species and enhances survival in *S. epidermidis* and *Staphylococcus aureus* sepsis models. Such an antibody could be administered in a small fluid volume to low-birthweight infants with a high risk of late-onset hospital-acquired sepsis. This antibody was shown to be safe in healthy adult volunteers and is currently being tested in neonates (Fisher, 2003).

Pseudomonas aeruginosa

Pseudomonas aeruginosa causes significant mortality due to sepsis or pneumonia in patients with burns, malignancy, immunodeficiency, immunosuppression or malnutrition. It is also the major cause of chronic lung infection in cystic fibrosis (CF) patients, leading to chronic inflammation associated with progressive loss of lung function. Aminoglycoside resistance is frequently observed in clinical isolates (Yokoyama *et al.*, 2003). Altogether, *Pseudomonas aeruginosa* accounts for more than 10% of nosocomial, hospital acquired infections of immunocompromised patients and burn victims (Lang, 2003). In this context a prophylactic vaccine against *Pseudomonas aeruginosa* is highly desirable (Holder *et al.*, 2004).

Three different structures have been considered as vaccine candidates (Pier, 2003): the lipopolysaccharide, capsular polysaccharides and proteins. At least 31 different chemotypes of LPS have been described. Protein targets for vaccines include secreted proteins (exoprotein A, alkaline protease and elastase) and cell surface proteins (OprF protein, Oprl lipoprotein, type III translocation protein, pili and flagellar proteins). The completion of the genome sequence should allow the identification of additional protein-based vaccine candidates. Collectively, immunization in mice with CPS, LPS, Exoprotein A, Opr F, OprI and flagellar antigens are protective. CF patients with high levels of opsonic antibodies to the CPS are less likely to be colonized by *P. aeruginosa*. A prophylactic conjugate vaccine, composed of the O-polysaccharides of the eight most

Table 9.1 Infectious pathogens involved in nosocomial infections as targets for vaccines and immunotherapeutics

Pathogens	Disease burden	Vaccine development	Reference
Rotavirus	Rotavirus (RV) is a major cause of acute gastroenteritis in infants and young children and is responsible for 20–50% of hospitalizations for diarrhea worldwide. Approximately 440,000 deaths occur among children each year, primarily in developing countries	Current efforts to develop a rotavirus vaccine have focused on live oral attenuated strains of human or animal rotaviruses (e.g. rhesus vaccine that was licensed in the United States was used extensively for 9 months and then withdrawn due to problems of intussusception). Two vaccines are now in phase III clinical trials with 60,000 children per trial. One is a human attenuated serotype 1 strain by passage. The other is a pentavalent vaccine based on a bovine rotavirus strain and four reassortant human strains. Remaining questions relate to how well the vaccines function against the diversity of serotypes, how efficacious they are for children in developing countries, and whether either causes intussusception as a rare serious adverse event	Steele *et al.* (Chapter 11)
Staphylococcus aureus, *Staphylococcus epidermidis*	Bacteremia in immunocompromised patients. Endocarditis, osteomyeltis, septic arthritis.	Type-specific serum CP antibodies facilitate opsonophagocytosis of *S. aureus*, the major immune mechanism for clearance of this pathogen from the bloodstream. An ideal vaccine against *S. aureus* should induce antibodies to prevent bacterial adherence, promote opsonophagocytic killing by leukocytes, and neutralize toxic exoproteins produced by the bacterium. Ongoing efforts to design an *S. aureus* vaccine have targeted known virulence factors of this organism and include staphylococcal surface proteins, polysaccharides, exoproteins, and toxins elaborated by this pathogen. Possible target for passive immunotherapy (using MABs against capsular polysaccharides or lipoteicoic acid)	Shinefield *et al.* (2002)
Pseudomonas aeruginosa	Chronic lung infection (in CF patients) causes up to 10% of nosocomial infections in immunocompromised patients	In a phase II study in patients with cystic fibrosis (CF), a conjugate vaccine comprising O polysaccharides from 8 most frequent serotypes complexed to exotoxin A was shown to decrease infection rates and slow down lung colonization. This vaccine is undergoing phase III clinical evaluation. Other approaches showing encouraging results in mice are based on live attenuated *P. aeruginosa*, subunit vaccines targeting the outer membrane protein F or exotoxin A, as well as passive immunotherapy with antibodies against PCRV	Holder *et al.* (2004), Pier (2003)
Clostridium difficile	Infectious diarrhea, pseudomembranous colitis	A vaccine based on the two exotoxins, toxin A and toxin B, has been tested in phase I, and shown to elicit protective IgG levels against toxin A and B. Production of antibodies against toxin A following natural exposure to *C. difficile* is associated with protection from disease. *C. difficile* is a potential target for passive immunotherapy, using mono or polyclonal (IVIG) antibodies to the toxins	Giannasca *et al.* (2004)

Organism	Disease	Description	References
Streptococcus pyogenes (group A *Streptococcus*)	Puerperal fever, acute pharyngitis, impetigo, rheumatic fever and streptococcal toxic shock syndrome	The most extensively studied virulence factor of *S. pyogenes* is the surface M protein (a coiled coil alpha-helical surface protein), which inhibits phagocytosis and occurs in many sequence variants, allowing classification of clinical *S. pyogenes* isolates into ~120 M-types. It is commonly believed that the antiphagocytic property of M protein requires the N-terminal region, but the molecular function of this extremely variable region has remained unclear. Opsonic antibodies against the N terminus of the protein lead to serotypic immunity only	Brandt *et al.* (1998), Lindahl (2003)
Uropathogenic *E. coli*	Cystitis and pyelonephritis, mostly in female, with a high recurrence rate	Vaccines tested in humans are based on inactivated bacteria, mixtures of membrane glycoproteins (UroVaxom) or subunits (Fim H, P fimbriae)	Schmidhammer *et al.* (2002)
Enterococci (*E. faecium, E. fecalis*)	Bacteremia, endocarditis, abdominal infection. Frequently involved in NI due to antibiotic resistance.	Antibodies against surface polysaccharides or teichoic acid capsule appear to be protective. Good target for passive immunotherapy. Target molecules include the AS virulence factor, adhesins (Ace, Efa A, Esp) and an ABC transporter protein.	Koch *et al.* (2004)
Legionella pneumophila	Pontiac (flu-like) fever, Legionnaire's disease	A prophylactic vaccine would be useful in oatients with severe immunosuppression and the elderly. Fifteen per cent of cases of Legionella infection are nosocomial. A protective antibody response is induced in animal models against the MSP, MCMP, AmpS and type IV pili proteins.	Blander *et al.* (1993), Stone *et al.* (1998)
Klebsiella (K. pneumoniae, K. oxytoca)	Ventilator-associated pneumonia	Capsule (K antigen)-specific antibodies are opsonic and protect against disseminated disease. O antigen elicits opsonizing antibodies against non-encapsulated strains. Target for passive immunotherapy. In humans, passive immunotherapy with anti K and O immunoglobulins prevents acquired infections in intensive care units	Trautmann *et al.* (2004)
Candida albicans and other opportunistic fungal pathogens (e.g. *Aspergillus fumigatus*)	Tissue candidiosis, most particularly vulvovaginal candidiosis	Effective antimycotics are available (e.g. amphotericin B), but a high rate of infection recurrence justifies the development of a vaccine. Candidate target antigens include HSP 90, ashesins. The commensal nature of *C. albicans* could represent an obstacle for a classical prophylactic vaccine. Vaccines should be developed against the mycelial rather than the yeast form. In animal models, protection is partial. In humans, there is a close correlation between recovery from infection and the development of an antibody response to HSP90. Ongoing clinical study with amphotericin B and a human recombinant antibody to HSP90. Attempts, at preclinical stage, to develop vaccines based on dendritic cells (transfected with RNA from *C albicans*, or *A fumigatus*) to elicit protective cellular immune responses, as well as a conjugate vaccine targeting surface mannans	Matthews *et al.* (2004), Bozza *et al.* (2004), Magliani *et al.* (2002)

frequent serotypes covalently coupled to exotoxin A has been tested in CF patients. In a 10-year open-label phase II longitudinal study in 25 previously non-colonized CF patients compared with a non-immunized matched control group, the vaccine led to a statistically significantly lower rate of infection in the vaccinated group compared with the control group ($P < 0.001$). Furthermore, time to colonization was longer in the vaccination group than in the control group, and vaccination led to preservation of lung function (assessed by FEV measurement). Altogether, vaccination proved to be useful in preventing and/or delaying colonization of CF patients with *Pseudomonas aeruginosa* (Lang, 2003).

In most cases however, active immunoprophylaxis is not applicable for the treatment of immunocompromised patients, and passive immunotherapy is the preferred treatment option (Holder *et al.*, 2004). Fully human monoclonal antibodies (MAbs) reactive with *Pseudomonas aeruginosa* O-polysaccharides are being developed (Lang, 2003). Such MAbs exhibit excellent efficacy in relevant models *in vitro* (opsonophagocytosis) and *in vivo* (murine burn wound sepsis).

Clostridium difficile

Clostridium difficile is a spore-forming anaerobic bacterium, commonly associated with infectious diarrhea in hospitalized patients (with about 300,000 cases annually in the US alone). Infection may be asymptomatic, moderate or result in fulminant pseudomembranous colitis. Disruption of normal colonic bacterial flora by broad-spectrum antibiotics appears to be the major risk factor of colonization (Warny, 2003). Other host factors include advanced age, pre-existing severe illness and impaired immune defenses (Giannasca *et al.*, 2004). Pathogenic strains of *Clostridium difficile* cause colitis and intestinal mucosal injury by releasing two protein exotoxins, toxin A and toxin B exhibiting a 49% identity at amino-acid level. Although administration of metronidazole or vancomycin is effective in most patients, a fraction (10 to 20%) of such patients relapse when these agents are discontinued. As a consequence, in the last two decades *Clostridium difficile* has become one of the most common nosocomial pathogens worldwide.

Several studies in animal models indicate that the host antibody response to toxins plays a key role in controlling *Clostridium difficile* infection. For example, following colonization, an early increase in serum IgG against toxin A leads to asymptomatic carriage of *Clostridium difficile*. Moreover, relapsing infection is associated with low serum IgG levels to toxin A. Hamsters vaccinated with formalin-inactivated toxins A and B are protected against challenge (Giannasca *et al.*, 2004). In humans, intravenous passive immunization with pooled human immunoglobulin has been successful in treating severe and recurrent *Clostridium difficile* colitis (Kyne *et al.*, 1998). Also, following symptomatic infection, many patients develop antitoxin A and B antibodies in serum, and are protected against subsequent infection. This explains why only a small proportion of high-risk hospitalized patients develop symptomatic infection while up to 31% are colonized with *Clostridium difficile*. These results suggest that passive or active immunization strategies eliciting anti toxin antibodies may be effective in severe, prolonged or recurrent *Clostridium difficile* diarrhea.

A vaccine based on formalin-inactivated toxin A and toxin B is being developed. In phase I studies, this vaccine was shown to elicit serum antitoxin A and B IgG levels that were 50-fold higher than the threshold associated with protection against relapses (Kyne *et al.*, 1998; Giannasca *et al.*, 2004). A trial was also conducted in chronically infected patients receiving vancomycin: patients remained symptom-free during the two-month follow-up period after antibiotic cessation. This vaccine can also be used to produce human antitoxin immunoglobulins for passive immunization trials. Intraveinous immunoglobulins (IVIG) containing antitoxins antibodies have improved symptoms in adults and children. Also human trials of oral passive immunotherapy have been conducted, using bovine IgG administered within enteric capsules. Efficacy was limited due to rapid degradation of IgGs by intestinal proteases. Monoclonal antibodies against the toxins are being developed for passive immunotherapy.

Uropathogenic *Escherichia coli*

Urinary tract infections (UTIs), commonly affect the bladder (cystitis) and kidney (pyelonephritis), and as such are amongst the most common bacterial infections, most particularly in women (Consensus Conference, 2002). Females of all ages as well as elderly men are mostly susceptible to UTIs caused by the Gram-negative bacterium *Escherichia coli*. Uropathogenic *E. coli* (UPEC) is thought to originate in the intestine. This infectious disease is characterized by a high rate of recurrence. A woman treated for an uncomplicated UTI has a 25–50% chance of developing a recurrent infection. Uropathogenic *E. coli* represent a heterogeneous collection of strains expressing various O: K: H serotypes. Serogroups 01, 02, 04, 06, 075 are the most frequent (collectively accouting for 40% of bacteriemic *E. coli* UTI) (Barnett *et al.*, 1997). Vaccines developed against recurrent *E. coli* (UTI) are based on inactivated bacteria or subunit proteins. In animal models, partial protection is obtained with the P fimbriae, type I fimbriae, hemolysin, and the K antigen. Ongoing clinical studies are conducted with P fimbriae and Fim H. Other candidates tested in humans include a mixture of *E. coli* membrane glycoproteins (Uro-Vaxom) as well as whole cell heat killed bacteria (Schmidhammer *et al.*, 2002). Protection conferred by these two vaccines appears to be short lived.

Enterococci

Enterococci are currently the third most common pathogen(s) isolated from bloodstream infections (Jones *et al.*, 1997). Enterococci are physiologic commensals of the gastrointestinal, and also female genital tracts in humans. These bacteria are responsible for up to four cases of nosocomial bloodstream infection per 10,000 hospital discharges in the US. Enterococci can cause bacteremia, meningitis, endocarditis or intraabdominal infections. Since the development of resistance to glycopeptides, crude mortality rates of up to 100% have been reported among certain patient populations infected with vancomycin-resistant enterococci (Huebner, 2003). Enterococci are increasingly acquiring resistance mechanisms to multiple antibiotics, allowing them to prevail in hospital and nursing home settings. Also they can transfer resistance determinants to other more virulent Gram-positive bacteria (e.g. *Staphylococcus aureus*).

E. faecalis* and *E. faecium* are the most frequently involved species. A limited number of clinically relevant serotypes has been isolated thus far. Fifty-seven percent of pathogenic enterococci express an extracellular teichoic acid capsule, which is a target for opsonic antibodies. Mice immunized with purified capsular polysaccharide have reduced bacterial counts in their kidneys, livers and spleens as compared with those in control animals following intravenous challenge with live enterococci (Huebner, 2003). Rabbit antibodies raised to the purified polysaccharide used as passive immunotherapy were effective even when the sera were administered up to 48 hours after challenge. A serotyping system based on capsular polysaccharides establishes four major serogroups.

Enterococcal capsular polysaccharide antigens could be used to develop active or passive immunotherapy regimens for the treatment and prevention of enterococcal infections in immunocompromised patients. For example, the ENT-1 polysaccharide expressed by 80% of *E. faecalis* clinical isolates, conjugated to a carrier protein was found to elicit a protective antibody response in mice. Other potential target antigens for vaccination purposes or for passive immunotherapy include ABC transporter proteins as well as the 'aggregation substance' (AS). The latter is a glycoprotein acting as a virulence factor expressed at the surface of the bacterium (Koch *et al.*, 2004). Also adhesins (e.g. Ace, EfaA, Esp) acting as colonization factors represent interesting vaccine targets. Regarding enterococci, prevention of infections by prophylactic vaccination would reduce mortality as well as hospital stay in high-risk patients. Passive immunotherapy might represent a more cost-effective approach, since most patients likely require protection only during hospitalization (Koch *et al.*, 2004).

CONCLUSIONS

Nosocomial infections represent a growing concern, most particularly in the context of a serious threat posed by antibiotic resistance. Numerous therapeutic strategies based on vaccines and passive immunotherapy are in relatively early stages of development, and for most of these vaccines, their utility remains to be established. Promising results in efficacy studies have been obtained in large-scale human studies with candidate vaccines against *Staphylococcus aureus* and *Pseudomonas aeruginosa*. Many of the organisms involved in nosocomial infections are able to colonize mucosal surfaces. In this context, a better understanding of the role of neutralizing antibodies and mucosal immunity in protection has to be developed.

If proven successful, vaccines against nosocomial infections could be used before admission at the hospital, i.e. before colonization. Thus, when an effective vaccine is available, a recommendation would be to vaccinate all patients going for elective surgical or immunosuppressive therapy. Patients who are detected as carriers of a nosocomial pathogen could be vaccinated before discharge from the hospital. Alternatively, some of these vaccines could be associated with antibiotic therapy, in order to prevent recurrence following antibiotic cessation. For some targets (e.g. enterococci), passive immunotherapy with appropriate poly-, or better, monoclonal antibodies might be preferred, in terms of cost effectiveness, to ensure immediate and short term protection during hospitalization.

References

Archer, G.L. 1998. Staphylococcus aureus: a well-armed pathogen. Clin. Infect. Dis. 26: 1179–1181.

Balaban, N., Goldkorn, T., Nhan, R.T., Dang, L.B., Scott, S., Ridgley, R.M., Rasooly, A., Wright, S.C., Larrick, J.W., Rasooly, R., and Carlson, J.R. 1998) Autoinducer of virulence as a target for vaccine and therapy against *Staphylococcus aureus*. Science 280: 438–440.

Barnett, B.J., and Stephens, D.S. 1997. Urinary tract infection: an overview. Am. J. Med. Sci. 314: 245–249.

Bauer, H.W., Rahlfs, V.W., Lauener, P.A., and Bleßmann, G.S.S. 2002. Prevention of recurrent urinary tract infections with immuno-active *E. coli* fractions: a meta-analysis of five-placebo-controlled double-blind studies. Int. J. Antimicrob. Agents 19: 451–456.

Blander, S.J., and Horwitz, M.A. 1993. Major cytoplasmic membrane protein of Legionella pneumophila, a genus common antigen and member of the hsp 60 family of heat shock proteins, induces protective immunity in a ginea pig model of Legionnaire's disease. J. Clin. Invest. 91: 717–723.

Bozza, S., Montagnoli, C., Gaziano, R., Rossi, G., Nkwanyuo, G., Bellocchio, S., and Romani, L. 2004) Dendritic cell-based vaccination against opportunistic fungi. Vaccine 22: 857–864.

Brandt, E., Currie, B., Marrnmo, L. Pruksakorn, S., and Good, M.F. 1998. Can class I epitope of M protein be a diagnostic marker for rheumatic fever in populations endemic for group A streptococci? Lancet 351: 1860.

Brandt, E., Sriprakash, K.S., Hobb, R.I., Hayman, W.A., Zeng, W., Batzloff, M.R., Jackson, D.C., and Good, M.F. 2000. New multi-determinant strategy for a group A streptococcal vaccine designed for the Australian Aboriginal population. Nature Med. 6: 455–461.

Brouillette, E., Lacasse, P., Shkreta, L., Belanger, J., Grondin, G., Diarra, M., Fournier, S., and Talbot, B. 2002. DNA immunisation against the clumping factor A (Elf A) of Staphylococcus aureus. Vaccine 20: 2348–2357.

Consensus conference. 2003. Nosocomial urinary tract infections (NUTI) in adult patients. Med. Mal. Infect. 33: 218–222.

Fattom, A.I., Horwith, G., Fuller, S., Propst, M., and Naso, R. 2003. Development of StaphVAX™, a polysaccharide conjugate vaccine against S. aureus infection: from the lab bench to phase III clinical trials. Vaccine 22: 880–887.

Fischer, G. 2003. Passive imunoprophylaxis of Staphylococcus aureus and S epidermidis. 'Immunological approaches against nosocomial infections'. Mérieux Foundation Ed. p. 49.

Foster, T.J., and Hook, M. 1998. Surface protein of Staphylococcus aureus. Trends Microbiol. 6: 484–488.

Genestier, A.L. 2003. Panton-Valentine leukocidin-producing methicillin-resistant Staphylococcus aureus: a potential threat to both hospital and community patients. 'Immunological approaches against nosocomial infections'. Mérieux Foundation Ed. pp. 25–26.

Ghigo, J.M. 2001. Natural conjugative plasmids induce bacterial biofilm development. Nature 412: 442–444.

Giannasca, P.J., and Warny, M. 2004. Active and passive immunization against Clostridium difficile diarrhea and colitis. Vaccine, 22: 848–856.

Giraudo, J.A., Calzolari, A., Rampone, H., Giraudo, A.T., Bogni, C., Larriestra, A., and Nagel, R. 1997. Field trials of a vaccine against bovine mastitis. 1. Evaluation in heifers. J. Dairy Sci. 80: 845–853.

Goldman, D.A. 2003. The burden of nosocomial infection in the context of antimicrobial resistance, in 'Immunological approaches against nosocomial infections'. Mérieux Foundation Ed. p. 19.

Götz, F. 2002. Staphylococcus and biofilms. Mol. Microbiol. 43: 1367–1378.

Hiramatsu, K. 2003. Genetic characterization of meticillin-resistant Staphylococcus aureus. 'Immunological approaches against nosocomial infections'. Mérieux Foundation Ed. p. 23.

Holder, I.A. 2004. Pseudomonas immunotherapy: a historical overview. Vaccine 22: 831–839.

Huebner, J. 2003. Immunotherapy of enterococcal infections. 'Immunological approaches against nosocomial infections'. Mérieux Foundation Ed. p. 57.

Iglewski, B. 2003. Pseudomonas aeruginosa virulence factors. 'Immunological approaches against nosocomial infections'. Mérieux Foundation Ed. p 31.

Jones, R.N., Marshall S.A., Pfaller M.A., Wilke W.W., Hollis R.J., Erwin M.E., and SCOPE Hospital Study Group. 1997. Nosocomial enterococcal blood stream infections in the SCOPE program: antimicrobial resistance, species occurrence, Molecular testing results, and laboratory testing accurancy. Diag. Microbiol. Infect. Dis. 29: 95–102.

Kluytmans, J., Van Belkum, A., and Verbrugh, H. 1997. Nasal carriage of Staphylococcus aureus: epidemiology, underlying mechanisms, and associated risks. Clin. Microbiol. Rev. 10: 505–520.

Kmietowicz, Z. 2000. Hospital infection rates in England out of control. Br. Med. J. 320: 534–535.

Koch, S., Hufnagel M., Theilacker C., and Huebner J. 2004) Enterococcal infections: host response, therapeutic, and prophylactic possibilities. Vaccine 22: 822–830.

Kyne, L., and Kelly, C.P. 1998. Prospects for a vaccine for Clostridium dfficile. Biodrugs 3: 173–181.

Lang, A. 2003. Prophylaxis and therapy of Pseudomonas aeruginosa infection in cystic fibrosis and immunocompromised patients. 'Immunological approaches against nosocomial infections'. Mérieux foundation Ed. p. 61.

Lee, J.C. 2003. Limitations of current approaches towards Staphylococcus aureus vaccines development. 'Immunological approaches against nosocomial infections'. Mérieux Foundation Ed. p. 53.

Lindahl, G. 2003. Host-pathogen interactions in Streptococcus pyogenes infections, with special reference to puerperal fever. 'Immunological approaches against nosocomial infections'. Mérieux Foundation Ed. p. 37.

Lowy, F.D. 1998. Staphylococcus aureus infections. N. Engl. J. Med. 339: 520–532.

Magliani, W., Conti, S., Cassone, A., De Bernardis, F., and Polonelli, L. 2002. New immunotherapeutic strategies to control vaginal candidiasis. Trends Mol. Med. 8: 121–126.

Maira-Litran, T., Kropec, A., Goldmann, D., and Pier, G.B. 2004. Biologic properties and vaccine potential of the staphylococcal poly-N-acetyl glucosamine surface polysaccharide. Vaccine 22: 872–879.

Matthews, R.C., and Burnie, J. 2004. Recombinant antibodies: a natural partner in combinatorial antifungal therapy. Vaccine 22: 865–871.

McKenney, D., Pouliot, K.L., Wang, Y., Murthy, V., Ulrich, M., Doring, G., Lee, J.C., Goldmann, D.A., and Pier, G.B. 1999. Broadly protective vaccine for Staphylococcus aureus based on an in vivo-expressed antigen. Science 284: 1523–1527.

NNIS. 2003) National nosocomial infections surveillance (NNIS) system report, data summary from January 1992 through June 2003. Am J. Infect Control 31: 481–498.

Orsi, G.B., Di Stefano, L., and Noah, N. 2002. Hospital-acquired, laboratory-confirmed bloodstream infection: increased hospital stay and direct costs. Infect. Control. Hosp. Epidemiol. 23: 190–197.

Patti, J. 2003. Aurexis, a humanized monoclonal antibody targeting *Staphylococcus aureus*. 'Immunological approaches against nosocomial infections'. Mérieux Foundation Ed. p. 51.

Pier, G.B. 2003. Promises and pitfalls of *Pseudomonas aeruginosa* lipopolysaccharide as a vaccine antigen. Carbohydrate Res. 338: 2549–2556.

Plowman, R., Graves, N., Griffin, M.A.S., Roberts, J.A., Swan A.V., Cookson B., and Taylor, L. 2001. The rate and cost of hospital-acquired infections occurring in patients admitted to selected specialties of a district general hospital in England and the national burden imposed. J. Hosp. Infect. 47: 198–290.

Polonelli, L., Gerloni, M., Conti, S., Fisicaro, P., Cantelli, C., Portincasa, P., Alomondo, F., Barea, P.L., Hernando, F.L., and Ponton, J. 1994. Heat-shock mannoproteins as targets of secretory IgA in *Candida albicans*. J. Infect. Dis. 169: 1401–1405.

Prince, A. 2002. Biofilms, antimicrobial resistance, and airways infection. N. Engl. J. Med. 14: 1110–1111.

Roberts, R.R., Scott, R.D., Cordell, R., Solomon, S.L., Steel, L., Kampe, L.M., Trick, W.E., and Weinstein, R.A. 2003. The use of economic modelling to determine the hospital costs associated with nosocomial infections. Clin. Infect. Dis., 36: 1424–32.

Schmidhammer, S., Ramoner, R., Höltl, L., Bartsch, G., Thurnher, M., and Zelle-Rieser, C. 2002. An *Escherichia coli*-based oral vaccine against urinary tract infections potently activates human dendritic cells. Urology 60: 521–526.

Shinefield, H., Black, S., Fattom, A., Horwith, G., Rasgon, S., Ordonez, J., Yeoh, H., Law, D., Robbins, J.B., Scheerson, R., Muenz, L., and Naso, R. 2002. Use of a *Staphylococcus aureus* conjugate vaccine in patients receiving hemodialysis. N. Engl. J. Med. 346: 491–496.

Spencer, RC. 1998) Predominant pathogens found in the European prevalence of infection in intensive care study. Eur. J. Clin. Microbiol. Infect Dis. 15: 281–285.

Stone, B.J., and Kwaik, A.Y. 1998. Expression of multiple pili by Legionella pneumophila: identification and characterization of a type IV pilin gene and its role in adherence to mammalian and protozoan cells. Infect. Immun. 66: 1768–1775.

Sturtevant J., and Calderone R. 1997. *Candida albicans* adhesions: biochemical aspects and virulence. Rev. Iberoam. Micol. 14: 90–97.

Suei, Hung C. 2003. From bug to pod: the journey of uropathogenic *E. coli*. 'Immunological approaches against nosocomial infections'. Mérieux Foundation Ed. p. 59.

Trautmann, M., Held, T.K., and Cross, A.S. 2004. O antigen seroepidemiology of *Klebsiella* clinical isolates and implications for immunoprophylaxis of Klebsiella infections. Vaccine 818–821.

Vegni, F.E., Panceri, M.L., Biffi, M., Banfi, E., Porretta, A.D., and Privitera, G. 2004. Three scenarios of clinical claim reimbursement for nosocomial infection: the good, the bad, and the ugly. J. Hosp. Infect., 56: 150–155.

Vincent, J.L. 2003. Nosocomial infections in adult intensive-care units. Lancet 361: 2068–77.

Walker, R.I., Blanchard, T., Braun, J.M., Cebra, J.J., Cross, A.S., Fattom, A., Giannasca, P.J., Holder, I.A., Huebner, J., Matthews, R., Pier, G.B., Romani, L., von Specht, B.U., and Trautmann, M. 2004. Meeting summary possibilities for active and passive vaccination against opportunistic infections. Vaccine 22: 801–804.

Warny, M. 2003. Prospects for a vaccine against Clostridium difficile. Immunological approaches against nosocomial infections. Mérieux Foundation Ed. p. 63.

Weidenmaier, C., Kokai-Kun, J.F., Kristian, S.A., Chanturiya, T., Kalbacher, H., Gross, M., Nicholson, G., Neumeister, B., Mond, J.J., and Peschel, A. 2004. Role of teichoic acids in *Staphylococcus aureus* nasal colonization, a major risk factor in nosocomial infections. Nature Med. 10: 243–248.

Wenzel, R.P. 1995. The economics of nosocomial infections. J. Hosp. Infect. 31: 79–87.

Yokoyama, K., Doi, Y., Yamane, K., Kurokawa, H., Shibata, N., Shibayama, K., Yagi, T., Kato, H., and Arakawa, Y. 2003. Acquisition of 16S rRNA methylase gene in *Pseudomonas aeruginosa*. Lancet 362: 1888–1893.

Chapter 10

TB Vaccine Development: Opportunity and Imperative

Anne S. De Groot and Julie A. McMurry

Abstract

On the short list of the following health threats – HIV, tuberculosis, and bioterror pathogens – tuberculosis (TB) should be considered the most significant threat to global health. One form of tuberculosis, latent TB infection (LTBI), affects one-third of the world's population or nearly 2 billion individuals, most of whom live in the developing world. These individuals are at very high risk of developing active TB from latent infection, especially if they become co-infected with the HIV virus. Therefore, the development of a TB vaccine to prevent disease or to curb the development of active TB disease from the latent state of infection would have an enormous impact on developing world economies. Despite the global importance of TB disease, no new TB vaccine has been licenced for human use since the late 1800s. One reason for the lack of new TB vaccine candidates may be that the correlates of TB immunity remain poorly defined. Furthermore, any new TB vaccine must be developed for use in a population that has already been immunized against TB with BCG. This chapter frames the opportunity for developing a new TB vaccine and describes several recent TB vaccine development efforts.

TB VACCINE DEVELOPMENT: OPPORTUNITY AND IMPERATIVE

Framing the opportunity

Given the wide distribution of tuberculosis (TB) in the world and its adverse impact on the health of adults, any intervention that reduces the prevalence of *Mycobacterium tuberculosis* (Mtb) infection and TB disease presents an opportunity to improve global health. Due to the sheer number of economically active adults who are at risk of TB disease, the development of a TB vaccine would also have important economic implications. Yet no new TB vaccine has been developed since that late 1800s when bacille Calmette–Guerin (BCG), a live attenuated vaccine against TB, was first discovered. TB represents a significant challenge for vaccine developers as the correlates of TB immunity remain poorly defined and any new vaccine must be developed for use in a population that has already been immunized against TB with BCG. Fortunately, an infusion of funding from the Bill and Melinda Gates Foundation recently regenerated interest in the development of TB vaccines. As a result, large numbers of TB vaccine candidates are entering preclinical studies and several phase I trials are expected to take place in the next few years.

Epidemiology

There can be no doubt that developing an effective TB vaccine would have a positive impact on world health. TB claims more human life at present than any other infectious disease. According to the World Bank, the disease accounts for more than 25% of avoidable adult deaths in developing countries with an estimated 8.7 million new cases of active TB and 3 million deaths annually (World Bank, 1993). Latent TB infection (LTBI) affects one third of the world population – nearly 2 billion individuals (Raviglione *et al.*, 1997). TB is accelerated and exacerbated in the context of HIV infection. As the global epidemic of HIV continues to expand into countries with high rates of TB, more active TB cases can be expected. TB has already become the most common cause of death in AIDS patients (Sepkowitz, 2001) (Figure 10.1).

TB is also expanding because latent TB infection usually goes untreated. As a rule, physicians in developing countries wait until TB develops (from latent infection) and then identify and treat TB cases (or not, depending on access to care). WHO has supported this approach to TB case identification and use of directly observed short course therapy, or DOTS. With DOTS, TB is curable (95% cure rates) and affordable (a six month supply costs $11–37). Unfortunately, despite the low cost and high cure rate associated with DOTS, treatment remains inaccessible for many individuals who are affected by the disease. As of 2000, only 12% of all TB patients were receiving DOTS, and only 95 out of 212 countries in the world had implemented DOTS in their national TB programs (Dye *et al.*, 1999). Due to concerns about possible failure of the DOTS strategy, the World Health Organization (WHO) recently re-emphasized the development of TB vaccines (WHO, 2000).

WHO is now reporting that resistance to first line antituberculous medications (such as those included in the DOTS treatment) is as high as 40% in some countries (Mendez *et al.*, 1998) and that associated mortality due to multidrug resistant strains (MDR TB) is now 40–60%, i.e. as high as it was in the pre-chemotherapy era. In the USA, MDR TB has

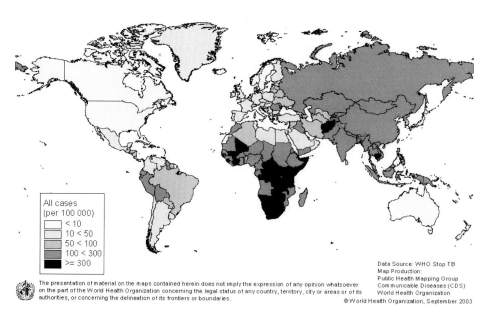

Figure 10.1 Global estimates of TB disease (WHO, 2001). This figure is also reproduced in colour in the colour section at the end of the book.

been detected in 43 states in the US and the District of Columbia. Even more worrisome, infection by MDR TB strains exceeds 10% of all new cases in parts of the former Soviet Union and is on the rise in regions of Eastern Europe, Africa and Asia, and resistance to INH, the first line drug against Mtb, is nearly 100% in parts of Russia and Eastern Europe (Andersen, 2001). These observations attest to the urgency of developing a vaccine against tuberculosis, latent tuberculosis in particular.

Existing vaccines and treatments

BCG, the live attenuated vaccine for tuberculosis developed by Koch in the late 1800s, remains the most widely distributed vaccine in use in the world today. More than 90% of the world's children are vaccinated with BCG; that is to say, vaccination against TB is very well accepted by the public. Any vaccine that does as well or better than BCG, even if it is simply formulated in a consistent manner (BCG is highly variable), stands to be a tremendous commercial success.

Latent tuberculosis infection (LTBI), the form of TB that affects 10 to 15 million individuals in the US, has a 10% chance of progressing to full-blown tuberculosis disease. LTBI is currently managed with a medication called isoniazid (INH), a medication that must be taken once daily over the course of nine months (or 270 individual doses) for full eradication. Many individuals do not complete this course of therapy, while some (about 1 in 300) develop INH-related side-effects. When LTBI prophylaxis fails, active TB disease can develop.

INH treatment for LTBI provides a useful yardstick against which the potential commercial success of an effective TB vaccine can be measured. In the United States alone, between 1954 and 1997, the use of anti-TB treatment reduced the number of newly diagnosed cases of active TB by 32%, the number of mortalities by 81%, the number of life-years lost by 87%, and the cost of medical treatment by 76%. The total financial burden of illness over this time period (including the value of lost life-years) was reduced from $894 billion (in 1997 dollars) to $128 billion (Javitz and Ward, 2002). Thus, a TB vaccine that would prevent the progression of LTBI to active disease would reduce medical expenditures in the United States by approximately $250 million per year.

An effective TB vaccine will also have a significant economic benefit in terms of global health. Experts estimate that such a vaccine would be worth at least $25 billion in terms of avoided medical spending, worldwide. More specifically, the 1 billion people who are currently at risk of developing TB following exposure could expect to save $25.00 in medical costs if they had received a 75% effective vaccine of 10 years' duration (Weis et al., 1999; Bishai and Mercer, 2001). An effective LTBI vaccine could easily be priced in the same range as the hepatitis vaccine ($50 per dose or $150 per three dose regimen) in the developed world. Pricing in that range would generate more than $500 million in revenue in the US market and as much or more in developed countries overseas where the LTBI rate is as much as 50 times higher than the rate in the US. In the developing world, the current intervention for active TB costs $5 per DALY. An effective vaccine priced at $1 per dose would be equivalent to the cost per DALY of directly observed short course therapy for LTBI, or DOTS. According to the WHO, an acceptable price for an effective TB vaccine might be as high as $10 per dose, in developing countries, given the urgency of the TB epidemic.

Why not BCG?

Why develop a new vaccine against TB? A vaccine against TB already exists. The reason that a new TB vaccine is desperately needed is that BCG only provides partial protection against TB. Bacille Calmette–Guerin vaccine (BCG) is derived from a number of different live attenuated strains of *Mycobacterium bovis* (BCG 'Pasteur', BCG 'Copenhagen', etc.). BCG is primarily used in developing countries to vaccinate children. Despite the fact that BCG is one the most widely implemented vaccines, people vaccinated with BCG still go on to develop TB as adults, and the contribution of BCG to TB control worldwide is limited (Styblo, 1976). The mechanism of action of this vaccine is not well understood, and different strains of BCG have demonstrated wide-ranging degrees of efficacy in studies carried out in different regions of the world (from 0% protective efficacy to greater than 80%).

Some studies suggest that the efficacy of BCG is inversely related to levels of exposure to environmental mycobacteria. Areas in which environmental mycobacteria are prevalent tend to be those in which TB is endemic, thereby making BCG often least effective against pulmonary TB in the areas it is most desperately needed. Researchers attempting to explain BCG's variable efficacy (80% to 0% depending on the trial site and the strain of BCG; Colditz *et al.*, 1994) have also performed molecular sequence and proteome comparisons. Behr and Small (1999) suggested that the progressive loss of genetic material over the years might reflect a progressive adaptation of BCG strains to laboratory conditions that has compromised their capacity to survive in the host, impairing their ability to stimulate a durable immune response. Thus, even though BCG is widely accepted, there is room for improvement and a great need for a more effective TB vaccine (Table 10.1).

Organizations such as the 'Stop TB' program at WHO, the Global Fund, and the Sequella TB Foundation have been working hard to raise awareness about the prevalence of TB, the need for directly observed therapy (DOTS) and the need for a new TB vaccine. No fewer than 20 research teams are currently hard at work on novel approaches to TB vaccine development, due in part to these efforts and to the Bill and Melinda Gates Foundation's $25 million gift to the Sequella Global TB Foundation.

Immune responses in TB infection and disease

TB immunopathogenesis

Tuberculosis infection only rarely results in the immediate development of TB disease. More often, infection is followed by latency, during which time Mtb remains dormant in the body, inside macrophages and within the extra cellular matrix of granulomas. Unknown

Table 10.1 Pros and cons of existing TB vaccine (BCG)

Pro	Cons
Reliable protection of children against TB meningitis and miliary TB and against leprosy	Primary (neonatal) immunization is probably not protective beyond late childhood/early adolescence
Advantages related to long and extensive use, e.g. price, logistics, public awareness, etc.	Typical drawbacks of live vaccines, e.g. side-effects, vaccine stability, genetic variability, etc.
Significant and boostable protection	Non-boostable immunity
Immunotherapy, e.g. bladder cancer	Highly geographically variable protection against adult pulmonary TB

Adapted from table compiled by Uli Fruth, WHO (2003).

factors influence the progression of Mtb infection to TB disease. Stress, immunodeficiency, and malnutrition can each play a role. TB disease primarily affects the lungs, although other organs (bone marrow, spleen, intestine, blood, meninges) can also be involved.

Correlates of immunity

While the full correlates of protection from TB disease and Mtb infection still remain to be clearly defined, antigen dependent cell-mediated immunity to Mtb protein antigens nevertheless appears to be one of the critical components of effective host defense against the development of TB disease (Kaufmann et al., 1992; Kaufmann, 2001).

The importance of CD4+ helper T cells in the response to TB is perhaps best illustrated by patients who also have human immunodeficiency virus (HIV) infection. These individuals are not necessarily more susceptible to Mtb infection, but HIV results in progressive loss of CD4+ T cell clones that has been associated with accelerated progression to active TB (Rieder et al., 1989; Brandt et al., 2000). CD4+ T cells appear to orchestrate the activation of Mtb-infected macrophages, and marshal other components of cellular immune defense to the locus of Mtb infection; interferon-gamma (IFN-γ) release by these T cells induces Mtb-infected macrophages to engage intracellular immune defenses (Kampmann et al., 2000; Pearl et al., 2001). Additionally, while IFN-γ is not the sole correlate, and its role in human immunity to TB is still under study, IFN-γ responses have been shown to be strong in PPD-positive healthy subjects and patients with minimal TB (Barnes et al., 1993; Huygen et al., 1988; Torres et al., 1998; Wilkinson et al., 1998; Ravn et al., 1999) and weaker in TB patients with advanced disease (Huygen et al., 1988; Torres et al., 1998; Fomsgaard et al., 1999) Thus, it is generally believed that ideal post-infection vaccine components should be those antigens that (a) are recognized by the CD4+ lymphocytes of Mtb-immune individuals, (b) stimulate Th1-type responses including IFN-γ secretion (Flynn et al., 1992) and (c) activate macrophages (Kampmann et al., 2000; Kaufmann, 2001). Although CD8+ CTL do play a role in murine models of tuberculosis, the role of CD8+ T cells in *human* immune response to Mtb is still under study (Flynn et al., 1992; Hussain et al., 2002).

Defining immune-competent responses in vitro

One method for empirically identifying protective Mtb antigens and/or peptides for vaccine development has been to use T cells derived from Mtb-exposed human subjects, to test for response to candidate proteins and peptide epitopes *in vitro*. This *ex vivo* method of screening has been utilized by several research groups (Vordemeier et al., 1992; De Groot et al., 1996). The rationale for this approach is that 90% of Mtb-infected individuals remain asymptomatic, containing their Mtb infection over the course of many years. Individuals who are exposed to Mtb but have not demonstrated clinical illness after two years following the date of exposure are generally presumed to be Mtb-immune. Identifying and characterizing the responses of these immune individuals may provide vital direction for vaccine development.

While researchers are in general agreement that T cell responses are important and that screening Mtb-infected individuals for response to antigens is an acceptable approach to identifying candidate antigens, criteria to be used for the selection of these antigens from the vast repertoire of TB proteins (there are approximately 4000 open reading frames in the Mtb genome) remain vague. Antigens that are secreted by Mtb have been the focus of several TB vaccine development efforts since these antigens have been shown to induce potent immune responses in humans (Andersen, 1994; Boesen *et al.*, 1995; Andersen, 1997; Horwitz *et al.*, 2000). Additionally, some studies have shown that responses to secreted TB antigens have been greater than to those antigens of cytosolic origin (Mustafa *et al.*, 1998). Secreted antigens have been shown to elicit significant protection (in animal models), equal in magnitude to BCG, while also priming responses to a wider range of the antigens than does BCG (Andersen, 1994; Boesen *et al.*, 1995; Demissie *et al.*, 1999) Accordingly, much research has been done to characterize the individual antigens and to evaluate their potential use in vaccines and diagnostics. Nevertheless, the full potential of the spectrum of secreted antigens has yet to be harnessed (Andersen, 1994; Boesen *et al.*, 1995; Sonnenberg *et al.*, 1997; Denis *et al.*, 1998; Demissie *et al.*, 1999).

TB vaccines: to prevent or to treat?

Vaccines against TB can be divided into two types: vaccines to prevent primary TB infection and vaccines to prevent reactivation of latent TB disease. Vaccination to prevent primary TB infection would eliminate mycobacteria before they are able to take up residence in host macrophages, thereby eliminating the potential for the development of latency, and eliminating the potential for later development of full-blown TB disease. Vaccination during latent TB infection (LTBI) would contain infection, preventing the multiplication of Mtb bacilli and the development of full-blown TB disease. The advantages and disadvantages of each approach are discussed here below.

Preventing TB infection

Researchers have traditionally approached the problem of TB vaccine development with the goal of prevention. In order to be implemented, a preventive vaccine would have to demonstrate clear superiority over BCG. For a number of reasons (such as efficacy against meningeal tuberculosis, protective effect against leprosy [Stern *et al.*, 1996]), efforts to remove BCG from the repertoire of childhood vaccinations in the developing world and to replace it with a new TB vaccine are unlikely to succeed. Demonstrating clear superiority would also be difficult, since a phase III study comparing BCG to a new vaccine would have to take place over at least 10, if not 20, years.

Preventing LTBI

In contrast, vaccines to prevent latent TB infection (LTBI) would significantly reduce the global burden of TB. Vaccines targeting latent TB infection would also reduce the global burden of TB since one third of the world's population has LTBI, and each of these individuals has 10% lifetime risk of developing TB disease. Furthermore, LTBI individuals who are also HIV-infected have a 7–10% risk of developing TB disease within 1 year (Selwyn *et al.*, 1989), Consequently, TB is currently the leading cause of death from AIDS, resulting in 30% of AIDS deaths world-wide (Raviglione *et al.*, 1997).

Which approach should be used when building a vaccine for TB? Clearly, the most relevant approach would be to stimulate immune responses that correlate with protective immune response in natural TB infection. Fortunately, a protective immune response to TB can indeed be generated (unlike the situation with HIV), since only 8–10% of Mtb-infected individuals go on to develop TB. Unfortunately, it is not perfectly clear what the critical components, or correlates, of immunity to TB might be.

TB vaccine concepts

New TB vaccines in development

A number of vaccines to prevent TB are under development although few of these vaccines are directed at the problem of LTBI. As no adequate animal model of TB exists, most TB vaccine research is performed in mice (who, unlike humans, do not develop cavitary TB lesions in their lungs) and guinea pigs (who do develop TB lesions that resemble human disease). Prophylactic TB vaccines under development include modified BCG overexpressing antigen 85a (Horwitz, 1995), a DNA prime/boost approach also targeting either hsp 65 (Lowrie *et al.*, 2003) or 85A (Tanghe *et al.*, 2000), a recombinant MVA vaccine encoding 85A (Goonetilleke *et al.*, 2003) and a vaccine based on Mtb auxotrophs (Pavelka *et al.*, 2003) (Table 10.2). Since animal models are poor predictors of TB vaccine efficacy, trial sites are being prepared in locations where TB is highly prevalent around the world (Figure 10.2).

Intramuscular injection of plasmid DNA expressing the single antigen, hsp 65, a mycobacterial protein, was one of the first approaches to be shown to be equivalent to bacillus Calmette–Guerin (BCG) (Lowrie *et al.*, 1997). Plasmids expressing some other mycobacterial antigens, hsp70, 36 kDa and 6 kDa, were also proven to be effective. However, mice immunized with the same constructs, in studies performed by another group (Orme and colleagues in Fort Collins, Colorado), did not appear to be effectively protected. Immunization with the Ag85 antigen of *M. tuberculosis* was equally disappointing (Taylor *et al.*, 2003).

Immunization studies performed with the live attenuated Mtb auxotroph vaccine (a lysine auxotrophic mutant of *Mycobacterium tuberculosis* strain H37Rv) has also been shown to be equivalent to that of the *Mycobacterium bovis* BCG vaccine (Pavelka *et al.*, 2003). Again, these studies were performed in a mouse model with an aerosol challenge. More recently, a team of researchers reported that the Rpf protein of the tuberculosis organism itself and four out of five of its mycobacterial homologues, administered as subunit vaccines, are highly immunogenic. Vaccination of mice with Rpf-like proteins resulted in a significant level of protection against a subsequent high-dose challenge with virulent *M. tuberculosis* H37Rv, both in terms of survival times and mycobacterial multiplication in lungs and spleens (Yeremeev *et al.*, 2003).

Table 10.2 Candidate TB vaccines in preclinical development

Candidate	Vaccine type	Stage	Reference
M. vaccae	Killed mycobacteria	Phase II, 2002	von Reyn *et al.* (2002)
Ag 85	Virus-vectored	Phase I, 4/2001	McShane *et al.* (2001
Ag 85	Recombinant BCG	Phase I, 2/2004	Horwitz *et al.* (2000
5 Mtb epitopes	Peptides + adjuvant	Phase I, (2004?)	Meister *et al.* (1995)
72f fusion protein	Subunit + adjuvant	Phase I, 1/2004	Reed (personal communication)
ESAT6/85A	Subunit + adjuvant	Phase I, 1/2004	Weinrich *et al.* (2001)
Ag85	DNA vaccine	Phase I ,*UD	Ulmer *et al.* (1997)
HSP70	DNA vaccine	Phase I, *UD	Tascon *et al.* (1996)
Listeriolysin	Recombinant BCG	Phase I, *UD	Conradt *et al.* (1999)
Attenuated Mtb	Albert Einstein, NY	Phase I, *UD	Chambers *et al.* (2000)
Attenuated Mtb	Pasteur, Paris	Phase I, *UD	Jackson *et al.* (1999)

*UD = date undetermined at this time. Adapted from table compiled by Uli Fruth, WHO (2003).

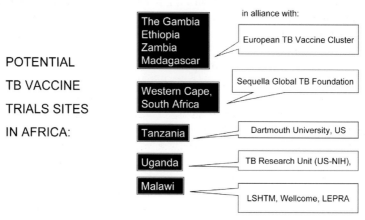

POTENTIAL

TB VACCINE

TRIALS SITES

IN AFRICA:

The Gambia
Ethiopia
Zambia
Madagascar

in alliance with:

European TB Vaccine Cluster

Western Cape,
South Africa

Sequella Global TB Foundation

Tanzania — Dartmouth University, US

Uganda — TB Research Unit (US-NIH),

Malawi

LSHTM, Wellcome, LEPRA

Figure 10.2 Proposed TB vaccine trial sites, 2003 (adapted from Uli Fruth, WHO, 2003).

Another approach under development is based on combining a number of Mtb antigens in one vaccine. This DNA-based TB gene 'cocktail' is delivered in conjunction with intracellular targeting sequences (TPA and ubiquitin). Protection of mice against primary Mtb infection using this approach was successful. Histopathological studies of mice vaccinated with the constructs and then challenged with live Mtb displayed less histopathology than naïve controls; accordingly, specific cellular immune responses and interferon gamma secretion were detected. Finally, in three different long-term experiments, survival periods following challenge were shown to increase by sevenfold for vaccinated mice compared with naïve controls, although mean times to death for mice immunized with the vaccine were unchanged, relative to BCG-immunized controls (Delogu *et al.*, 2002).

And finally, newer approaches to prevention of TB disease may involve 'boosting' BCG with improved vaccines. Boosting BCG-immunized guinea pigs with a fusion protein '72f' was recently shown to be more effective than immunization with BCG alone in challenges studies (Reed *et al.*, 2003). Another research group (Huygen *et al.*, 1988) is also using this approach in combination with a DNA vaccine encoding 85A and the 40KD antigen of Mtb.

Vaccines to prevent Mtb disease in the LTBI host

Re-vaccinating subjects who have LTBI with BCG has never been considered to be a very effective means for preventing TB disease – indeed, the first trial of BCG for this indication failed more than 80 years ago. One reason this approach may have failed is that exposure to Mtb antigens could exacerbate latent disease. This effect was recently demonstrated in the context of live or heat treated BCG, with or without lipid adjuvants, on the recurrence of Mtb in latently infected mice (Moreira *et al.*, 2002). In these experiments, increased antigen-specific T-cell proliferation was observed but there was no reduction in bacterial load in the lungs of BCG vaccinated mice re-challenged with Mtb and, perhaps more worrisome, larger lung granulomas were discovered. This effect seemed to be due to increased expression of tumor necrosis factor alpha (TNF-α) and interleukin 6 (IL-6). The studies appeared to demonstrate that providing Mtb antigens in the context of prior *M. tuberculosis* infection leads to immune activation, exacerbating lung pathology. The exacerbation may be due to TNF alpha-induced inflammation. It is however possible that the effect of immunizing with whole BCG including bacterial cell membranes, lipids, and other components shifted the immune response to Th-2 type responses, which would be associated with TNF secretion.

In contrast, immunization of mice with pure (recombinant) antigen, as in experiments performed with DNA in the experiments of Morris *et al.*, did not appear to exacerbate LTBI or increase disease pathology following re-challenge. Yet, using the same vaccine 'cocktail' combination described earlier in mice that had LTBI, Morris reported no protection against latent TB infection (Repique *et al.*, 2002). A number of other researchers have also failed to demonstrate that post-exposure vaccination prevents relapse in mice with latent tuberculosis. For example, Turner *et al.* (2000) showed that a DNA vaccine that was effective against a primary infection did not protect when administered immunotherapeutically in a post-exposure model. In addition, immunization with either BCG or a heat-killed *Mycobacterium vaccae* vaccine did not alter the relapse rate in a murine model of dormant tuberculosis (Collins and Mackaness, 1970).

A DNA vaccine expressing hsp 65 vaccine has been the subject of a great deal of controversy over the last two years. This vaccine was first shown to be successful in the prevention of TB recurrence in the Cornell model of MDRTB by Lowrie and associates (Tascon *et al.*, 1996). Only a few years later, another group of researchers claimed that the hsp 65 vaccine might exacerbate TB in mice (Orme *et al.*, 2001). In the latter studies, mice appeared to develop discrete regions of cellular necrosis throughout the lung. Similar reactions were seen in mice given a vaccine with DNA coding for the Ag85 antigen of *M. tuberculosis* (Taylor *et al.*, 2003). The relevance of this study to DNA immunization in humans has yet to be determined.

Thus, at least four recent attempts at developing LTBI vaccines have failed in murine models or have had equivocal results. Morris and others have postulated that this failure may be due to the effect of latent TB infection itself on immune cells. While competent immune response against latent TB appears to be maintained in most hosts because the bacteria are contained inside the granulomas, the type of response that is required to clear infection may be qualitatively different. To reduce or eliminate *latent* TB infection, a vaccine may need to promote greater macrophage (or dendritic cell) activation. For example, Britton *et al.* have shown that DNA immunization in conjunction with plasmids expressing IL-12 are effective means of inducing TB immunity. IL-12 can also be given as a recombinant protein (which avoids the problem of prolonged IL-12 exposure due to DNA delivery). Alternatively, coadministration with adjuvants that increase Th-1 response such as CPG motif-containing plasmids may overcome the refractory nature of local immune response.

New approach to TB vaccine development: epitope-driven vaccines

Taking the Lowrie, Morris and Kaplan studies in context, 'whole' TB vaccines (based on BCG, or attenuated Mtb) for LTBI may have an adverse effect on the immune response due to the priming of the immune system for Th-2 type responses. As neither Lowrie nor Morris observed exacerbation in LTBI mice vaccinated with DNA vaccines, removing the protein antigens from the context of the whole or killed bacteria appears to reduce the Th2 effect associated with mycobacterial cell wall components, which may in turn be responsible for the increased pathology. This suggests that it is worth pursuing a vaccine based on the delivery of multiple antigens – or epitopes derived from these antigens – in an immunostimulatory adjuvant or perhaps in conjunction with the TB vaccine developed by Lowrie. Thus, as an alternative to replacing BCG, it may be possible to develop such a genome-derived multi epitope/multiantigen vaccine as would afford additional protection from TB disease in individuals already either vaccinated with BCG or latently infected with Tuberculosis.

A new paradigm of TB vaccine development is therefore emerging, based on the concept that an *ensemble of epitopes* could stimulate protective Th1 immune responses, while whole antigen and/or the whole organism might suppress immune response. This new paradigm is based on the following observations. Following exposure to a pathogen, epitope-specific memory T cell clones are established (Blattman *et al.*, 2000). These clones respond rapidly and efficiently upon any subsequent infection, elaborating cytokines, killing infected host cells, and marshalling other cellular defenses against the pathogen.

It is now known that protective immune response requires the development of broad T cell response to an ensemble of different epitopes (Harrer *et al.*, 1996; Gillespie *et al.*, 2000; Gianfrani *et al.*, 2000). The link between broad epitope response and protection from disease has been confirmed for HIV, hepatitis B (HBV), hepatitis C (HCV), LCMV, and malaria (Rowland-Jones, 1999; Cooper *et al.*, 1999; Propato *et al.*, 2001). Many of the constituents of the protective epitope ensemble may be subdominant epitopes (van der Most *et al.*, 1998; Geginat *et al.*, 2001; Yamada *et al.*, 2001). Using computer-driven epitope mapping tools it is now possible to map entire genome sequences for that ensemble of epitopes that may induce a protective immune response (De Groot *et al.*, 2001). This approach has been used to define epitopes for one peptide-in-adjuvant TB vaccine currently under investigation in HLA-transgenic mice (Meister *et al.*, 1995).

Researchers carrying out a variety of epitope-based (epitope-driven) vaccination studies in a range of animal models have obtained proof that vaccines composed of epitopes, not whole proteins, can stimulate protective immune responses. For example, CTLs elicited by peptide immunization have been shown to afford protection against RSV challenge (Simmons *et al.*, 2001), malaria (Franke *et al.*, 2000), measles virus (Schadeck *et al.*, 1999), and HSV challenge (Rosenthal *et al.*, 1999) in mice and in larger mammals such as sheep (Hislop *et al.*, 1998). These studies of epitope-driven vaccines have also confirmed the need to combine T helper epitopes with CTL epitopes (Fomsgaard *et al.*, 1999; Hsu *et al.*, 1999).

Epitope-driven vaccines may offer a safety advantage over attenuated, live vaccines, which have the potential to cause disease in pediatric, elderly, or immune-compromised populations. Epitope-driven vaccines could also be found to be safer than whole protein vaccines if any parts of the whole protein are cross-reactive with self-proteins. In addition, multiple epitopes derived from more than one antigen (and representative of many genes in a genome) can be packaged into a relatively small delivery vehicle. Furthermore, in some studies, epitope-based vaccines have induced more potent responses than whole protein vaccines (Ishioka *et al.*, 1999). By simultaneously targeting multiple dominant and subdominant epitopes, epitope-based vaccines appear to side step the propensity for the immune system to focus on a single immunodominant epitope (Oukka *et al.*, 1996; Tourdot *et al.*, 1997). It should be noted that the field of epitope-driven vaccines is relatively new. For this reason, few epitope-driven vaccine constructs have reached the stage of efficacy trials in humans, although several have been shown to be effective in animal models.

Why would vaccination with TB epitopes, presumably the same epitopes being expressed by the Mtb infected cells present in LTBI patients, enhance the effectiveness of immune response to Mtb? In LTBI patients, Mtb replication is limited and effectively isolated within granulomata. The ability of Mtb to overcome these defenses probably depends on local conditions – such as the presence of Th-1-directed T cell clones that can activate host macrophages and recruit additional T cells to the area of Mtb reactivation (Kaufmann and Hess, 1999).

An examination of the reactivation of TB in HIV infected individuals clearly reveals that an ongoing T cell immune response is critical for the containment of LTBI; however, there is much yet to be studied about the escape of LTBI from immune containment. A number of questions remain unanswered. For example, is there too little diversity in the memory T cell repertoire initially established during primary infection. Or perhaps the repertoire is even focused on T cell epitopes that are no longer present when LTBI reactivates? In the course of HIV infection, there appears to be a shift in the T cell epitopes which are recognized (Harrer et al., 1996). Alternatively, if reactivation of LTBI occurs in the context of limited T cell response, are enough T-memory cells present in the region surrounding the granuloma, when Mtb infection is reactivated? Even if the right memory T cell repertoire is present during reactivation, is the response of these cells robust enough or are there enough of them to contain the infection? Should Mtb succeed in replicating – either within the infected macrophage or the surrounding matrix of the granuloma – can sufficient additional T-memory clones be recruited? And furthermore, should Mtb disseminate either locally or distantly through the migration of infected macrophages, can the disseminated infection be contained? If local defenses can be overcome, the circulating T memory cells created following an initial Mtb infection may be insufficient to counter dissemination of the Mtb bacillus. Moreover, relevant memory T cell clones may be lost either gradually over time (immunosenesence) or by active depletion by HIV. While epitope-driven vaccines remain untested in the context of TB, there is sufficient indirect proof to support the evaluation of an epitope-based, T cell directed vaccine. Indeed, as there is no effective vaccine against latent TB, and development of an effective vaccine is critically important in terms of global health, this hypothesis deserves further investigation.

Mapping the TB immunome

The availability of two *Mycobacterium tuberculosis* genomes has provided a unique opportunity for directly deriving vaccine candidates using bioinformatics. In a collaboration directed at rapid development of a novel genome-derived TB vaccine, McMurry et al. used EpiMatrix, a computer-driven pattern-matching algorithm that predicts T cell epitopes, to analyze the sequences of putative secreted proteins derived from the *M. tuberculosis* 1551 and H37Rv genomes for vaccine candidates.

First, putative secreted proteins were identified by bioinformatics analysis of the aligned genomes using algorithms that identify transmembrane domains and cell membrane attachment sites (SignalP and SPScan, TMpred and Prosite Scan). A set of 73 proteins was identified in this manner. The protein sequences were scanned for epitopes using EpiMatrix, an epitope-mapping algorithm. Ninety-seven putative T cell epitopes were selected for *in vitro* screening. Using this approach, the number of potential *M. tuberculosis* epitopes for preliminary evaluation was narrowed to just a few candidates from more than 1.3 million overlapping peptide candidates.

T cell responses to the selected peptides were then evaluated in interferon-gamma release ELIspot assays and in T cell proliferation assays, using peripheral blood mononuclear cells (PBMC) obtained from healthy, asymptomatic tuberculin skin test positive (*M. tuberculosis* immune) donors. Thirteen of 17 genome-derived peptides stimulated an IFN-γ response *in vitro*. One highly promiscuous epitope induced IFN-γ secretion in PBMCs from more than 60% of the *M. tuberculosis* immune subjects tested. Twelve genome-derived epitopes were selected for inclusion in a multiepitope TB vaccine.

An immunome-derived TB vaccine
The importance of bioinformatics in the evaluation of the proteomes of pathogenic organisms is underscored by this approach to *M. tuberculosis* vaccine development. Whereas a function has been assigned to 2220 of the 4203 proteins in the CDC-1551 genome, the remaining 1983 are TB unique hypothetical proteins with no known function. None of these hypothetical proteins has been cloned, and their structures are, as yet, unknown. While the exact identities, structure, and functions of the proteins from which most of these epitopes are derived remains unknown, this lack of knowledge has not impeded the selection of TB vaccine candidates.

CONCLUSION
TB remains endemic in most countries in the world despite more than 30 years of DOT campaigns by the WHO and other world health agencies. TB afflicts adults in these countries even though most have received BCG (Styblo and Meiger, 1976). For a number of reasons (efficacy against meningeal tuberculosis, protective effect against leprosy), efforts to remove BCG from the repertoire of childhood vaccinations in the developing world and to replace it with a new TB vaccine are unlikely to succeed. In a TB endemic country, a vaccine trial in children would have to take place against the background of BCG and would have to span 10 to 20 years. Likewise, though perhaps faster, an adult vaccine trial in a TB endemic country must take place against the background of not just BCG immunization but also perhaps prior TB infection. Development of a post-infection vaccine that can be administered against a background of BCG immunization *and/or* pre-existing Mtb infection is one path to TB control that deserves further investigation.

BCG, the existing vaccine, is unlikely to be replaced by a new, prophylactic TB vaccine. There are a number of reasons why replacement is not possible (Table 10.2). However, the most important is that it provides protection against TB disease in infancy and also appears to protect against other infections, an effect that may prove difficult to evaluate in a clinical trial. Fortunately, a number of different TB vaccine candidates are now undergoing preclinical testing, some of which appear to have potential for use following BCG immunization.

The number of candidates under evaluation represents a relative flurry of activity in the field of TB vaccines, which is due in part to increased funding at the foundation level (specifically due to Bill and Melinda Gates Foundation funding of the Sequella Global TB Foundation in 2001). New approaches to TB vaccine development deserve even greater support, since none of the 'tried and true' methods of vaccine development have been successful to date. Lack of knowledge about the correlates of protection in particular and TB immunopathogenesis in general need not impair our ability to build, and test, new vaccines for TB. The development of an entirely novel, TB vaccine composed of an ensemble of genome-derived epitopes which may promote a broad T cell-mediated protective immune response against LTBI is one approach that may prove successful. Indeed, the development of a novel TB vaccine is both an opportunity for exploring new vaccine approaches and a global health imperative.

Disclosure

One of the contributing authors, Anne S. De Groot, is a senior officer and majority shareholder at EpiVax, a privately owned vaccine design company located in Providence, RI. Dr De Groot acknowledges that there is a potential conflict of interest related to her relationship with EpiVax and attests that the statements contained in this review are free of any bias that might be associated with the commercial goals of the company.

References

Andersen, P. 1994. Effective vaccination of mice against *Mycobacterium tuberculosis* infection with a soluble mixture of secreted mycobacterial proteins. Infect. Immun. 62: 2536–2544.

Andersen, P. 1997. Host responses and antigens involved in protective immunity to *Mycobacterium tuberculosis*. Scand. J. Immunol. 452: 115–1131.

Andersen, P. 2001. TB vaccines: progress and problems [Review]. Trends Immunol. 22: 160–168.

Barnes, P.F., Lu, S., Abrams, J.S., Wang, E., Yamamura, M.and Modlin, R.L. 1993. Cytokine production at the site of disease in human tuberculosis. Infect. Immun. 61: 3482–3489.

Behr, M.A., Wilson, M.A., Gill, W.P., Salamon, H., Schoolnik, G.K., Rane, S. and Small, P.M. 1999. Comparative genomics of BCG vaccines by whole-genome DNA microarray. Science 284: 1520–1523.

Bishai, D.M. and Mercer, D. 2001. Modeling the economic benefits of better TB vaccines. Int. J. Tuberc. Lung Dis. 5: 984–993.

Blattman, J.N., Sourdive, D.J., Murali-Krishna, K., Ahmed, R. and Altman, J.D. 2000. Evolution of the T cell repertoire during primary, memory, and recall responses to viral infection. J. Immunol. 165: 6081–6090.

Boesen, H., Jensen, B.N., Wilcke, T. and Andersen, P. 1995. Human T-cell responses to secreted antigen fractions of *Mycobacterium tuberculosis*. Infect. Immun. 63: 1491–1497.

Bonner, J. Report: Leading Immunologist questions TB vaccine safety. Biomednet News (Jul 26th, 2001).

Brandt, L., Elhay, M., Rosenkrands, I., Lindblad, E.B., and Andersen, P. 2000. ESAT-6 subunit vaccination against *Mycobacterium tuberculosis*. Infect. Immun. 68: 791–795.

Chambers, M.A., Williams, A., Gavier-Widen, D., Whelan, A., Hall, G., Marsh, P.D., Bloom, B.R., Jacobs, W.R. and Hewinson, R.G. 2000. Identification of a *Mycobacterium bovis* BCG auxotrophic mutant that protects guinea pigs against *M. bovis* and hematogenous spread of *Mycobacterium tuberculosis* without sensitization to tuberculin. Infect. Immun. 68: 7094–7099.

Colditz, G.A., Brewer, T.F., Berkey, C.S., Wilson, M.E., Burdick, E., Fineberg, H.V.and Mosteller, F. 1994. Efficacy of BCG vaccine in the prevention of tuberculosis. Meta-analysis of the published literature. JAMA 271: 698–702.

Collins, F.M. and Mackaness, G.B. 1970. The relationship of delayed hypersensitivity to acquired antituberculous immunity. I. Tuberculin sensitivity and resistance to reinfection in BCG-vaccinated mice. Cell. Immunol. 1: 253–265.

Conradt, P., Hess, J. and Kaufmann, S.H. 1999. Cytolytic T-cell responses to human dendritic cells and macrophages infected with *Mycobacterium bovis* BCG and recombinant BCG secreting listeriolysin. Microbes Infect. 1: 753–764.

Cooper, S., Erickson, A.L., Adams, E.J., Kansopon, J., Weiner, A.J., Chien, D.Y., Houghton, M., Parham, P. and Walker, C.M. 1999. Analysis of a successful immune response against hepatitis C virus. Immunity. 10: 439–449.

De Groot, A.S., Carter, E.J., Roberts, C.G.P., Edelson, B.T., Jesdale, B.M., Meister, G.E., Houghten, R.A., Montoya, J., Romulo, R.C., Berzofsky, J.A. and B.D.L.L. Ramirez. 1996. A novel algorithm for the efficient identification of T cell epitopes: prediction and testing of candidate TB vaccine peptides in genetically diverse populations, Vaccines 96, Cold Spring Harbor Laboratory, Cold Spring Harbor, NY, pp. 127–134.

De Groot, A.S., Bosma, A., Chinai, N.S., Frost, J., Jesdale, B.M., Gonzalez, M.A., Martin W. and Saint-Aubin, C. 2001. From genome to vaccine: In silico predictions, ex vivo verification. Vaccine 19: 4385–4395.

Delogu, G., Li, A., Repique, C., Collins, F. and Morris, S.L. 2002. DNA Vaccine combinations expressing either tissue plasminogen activator signal sequence fusion proteins or ubiquitin-conjugated antigens induce sustained protective immunity in a mouse model of pulmonary tuberculosis. Infect. Immun. 70: 292–302.

Demissie, A., Ravn, P., Olobo, J., Doherty, T.M., Eguale, T., Geletu, M., Hailu, W., Andersen, P. and Britton, S. 1999. T-cell recognition of *Mycobacterium tuberculosis* culture filtrate fractions in tuberculosis patients and their household contacts. Infect. Immun. 67: 5967–5971.

Denis, O., Tanghe, A., Palfliet, K., Jurion, F., van den Berg, T.P., Vanonckelen, A., Ooms, J. Saman, E., Ulmer, J.B., Content, J. and Huygen, K. 1998. Vaccination with plasmid DNA encoding mycobacterial antigen

85A stimulates a CD4[+] and CD8[+] T-cell epitopic repertoire broader than that stimulated by *Mycobacterium tuberculosis* H37Rv infection. Infect. Immun. 66: 1527–1533.

Dye, C., Scheele S., Dolin P., Pathania V. and Raviglione, M.C. 1999. Global burden of tuberculosis: estimated incidence, prevalence, and mortality by country. JAMA 282: 677–686.

Flynn, J.L., Goldsein, M.M., Triebold, K.H., Koller, B. and Bloom, B.R. 1992. Major histocompatability complex class I-restricted T cells are required for resistance to Mycobacterium TB infection. Proc. Natl. Acad. Sci. USA 89: 12013–12017.

Fomsgaard, A., Nielsen, H.V., Kirkby, N., Bryder, K., Corbet, S., Nielsen, C., Hinkula, J. and Buus, S. 1999. Induction of cytotoxic T cell responses by gene gun DNA vaccination with minigenes encoding influenza A virus HA and NP CTL-epitopes. Vaccine 18: 681–691.

Franke, E.D., Sette, A., Sacci, J. Jr., Southwood, S., Corradin, G. and Hoffman, S.L. 2000. A subdominant CD8(+) cytotoxic T lymphocyte (CTL) epitope from the Plasmodium yoelii circumsporozoite protein induces CTLs that eliminate infected hepatocytes from culture. Infect. Immun. 68: 3403–3411.

Gallimore, A., Hengartner, H. and Zinkernagel, R. 1998. Hierarchies of antigen-specific cytotoxic T cell responses. Immunol. Rev. 164: 29–36.

Geginat, G., Schenk, S., Skoberne, M., Goebel, W. and Hof, H. 2001. A novel approach of direct ex vivo epitope mapping identifies dominant and subdominant CD4 and CD8 T cellepitopes from *Listeria monocytogenes*. J. Immunol. 166: 1877–1884.

Gianfrani, C., Oseroff, C., Sidney, J., Chesnut, R.W. and Sette, A. 2000. Human memory CTL response specific for influenza A virus is broad and multispecific. Hum. Immunol. 61: 438–452.

Gillespie, G.M., Wills, M.R., Appay, V., O'Callaghan, C., Murphy, M., Smith, N., Sissons, P., Rowland-Jones, S., Bell, J. I. and Moss, P.A. 2000. Functional heterogeneity and high frequencies of cytomegalovirus-specific CD8(+) T lymphocytes in healthy seropositive donors. J. Virol. 74: 8140–8150.

Goonetilleke, N.P., McShane, H., Hannan, C.M., Anderson, R.J. and Brookes, R.H. 2003. Hill AV 8: Enhanced immunogenicity and protective efficacy against *Mycobacterium tuberculosis* of bacille Calmette–Guerin vaccine using mucosal administration and boosting with a recombinant modified vaccinia virus Ankara. J. Immunol. 171: 1602–1609.

Harrer, T., Harrer, E., Kalams, S.A., Barbosa, P., Trocha, A., Johnson, R.P., Elbeik, T., Feinberg, M.B., Buchbinder, S.P. and Walker, B.D. 1996. Cytotoxic T lymphocytes in asymptomatic long-term nonprogressing HIV-1 infection. Breadth and specificity of the response and relation to in vivo viral quasispecies in a person with prolonged infection and low viral load. J. Immunol. 156: 2616–2623.

Hislop, A.D., Good, M.F., Mateo, L., Gardner, J., Gatei, M.H., Daniel, R.C., Meyers, B.V., Lavin, M.F. and Suhrbier, A. 1998. Vaccine-induced cytotoxic T lymphocytes protect against retroviral challenge. Nature Med. 4: 1193–1196.

Horwitz, M.A., Lee, B.W.E., Dillon, B.J. and Harth, G. 1995. Protective immunity against tuberculosis induced by vaccination with major extracellular proteins of myocbacterium tuberculosis. Proc. Natl. Acad. Sci. USA 92: 1530–1534.

Horwitz, M.A., Harth, G., Dillon, B.J., and Maslesa-Galic, S. 2000. Recombinant bacillus Calmette–Guerin (BCG) vaccines expressing the *Mycobacterium tuberculosis* 30-kDa major secretory proteine induce greater protective immunity against tuberculosis than conventional BCG vaccines in a highly susceptible animal model. Proc. Natl. Acad. Sci. USA. 97: 13853–13858.

Hsu, S.C., Chargelegue, D., Obeid, O.E. and Steward, M.W. 1999. Synergistic effect of immunization with a peptide cocktail inducing antibody, helper and cytotoxic T cell responses on protection against RSV. J. Gen. Virol. 80: 1401–1405.

Hussain, R., Kaleem, A., Shahid, F., Dojki, M., Jamil, B., Mehmood, H., Dawood, G. and Dockrell, H.M. 2002. Cytokine profiles using whole-blood assays can discriminate between tuberculosis patients and healthy endemic controls in a BCG-vaccinated population. J. Immunol. Meth. 264: 95–108.

Huygen, K., Van-Vooren, J.P., Turneer, M., Bosmans, R., Diercks, P. and De Bruyn, J. 1988. Specific lymphoproliferation, gamma interferon production and serum immunoglobulin G directed against a purified 32kDa mycobacterial protein antigen (P32) in patients with active tuberculosis. Scand. J. Immunol. 27: 187–194.

Ishioka, G.Y., Fikes, J., Hermanson, G., Livingston, B., Crimi, C., Qin, M.S., del Guercio, M.F., Oseroff, C., Dahlberg, C., Alexander, J. *et al.* 1999. Utilization of MHC class I transgenic mice for development of minigene DNA vaccines encoding multiple HLA-restricted CTL epitopes. J. Immunol. 162: 3915–3925.

Jackson, M., Phalen, S.W., Lagranderie, M., Ensergueix, D., Chavarot, P., Marchal, G., McMurray, D.N., Gicquel, B. and Guilhot, C. 1999. Persistence and protective efficacy of a *Mycobacterium tuberculosis* auxotroph Vaccine Infect. Immun. 67: 2867–2873.

Javitz, H.S., and Ward, M. 2002. Value of antimicrobials in the prevention and treatment of tuberculosis in the United States. Int. J. Tuberc. Lung Dis. 6: 275–288.

Kampmann, B., O'Gaora, P. Snewin, V.S., Gares, M.P., Young, D.B. and Levin, M. 2000. Evaluation of human anti-mycobacterial immunity using recombinant reporter mycobacteria. J. Infect. Dis. 182: 895–901.

Kaufmann, S.H., Gulle H., Daugelat, S. and Schoel, B. 1992. Tuberculosis and leprosy: attempts to identify T-cell antigens of potential value for vaccine design. Scand. J. Immunol. Suppl. 11: 85–90.

Kaufmann, S.H.E. 2001. How can immunology contribute to the control of tuberculosis? Nature Rev. Immunol. 1: 20–30.

Kaufmann, S.H.E., and Hess, J. 1999. Impact of intracellular location of and antigen display by intracellular bacteria: implications for vaccine development. Immunol. Lett. 65: 81–84.

Lowrie, D.B., Silva, C.L., Colston, M.J., Ragno, S. and Tascon, R.E. 1997. Protection against tuberculosis by a plasmid DNA vaccine. Vaccine 15: 834–838.

McShane, H., Brookes, R., Gilbert, S.C. and Hill, A.V. 2001. Enhanced immunogenicity of CD4(+) T-cell responses and protective efficacy of a DNA-modified vaccinia virus Ankara prime-boost vaccination regimen for murine tuberculosis. Infect. Immun. 69: 681–686.

Mendez, et al. 1998. Global Surveillance for antiTB drug resistance, 1994–1997. New Engl. J. Med. 338: 1641–1649.

Moreira, A.L., Tsenova, L., Melles Haile Amancheck name, Bekker, L.G., Freeman, S., Mangaliso, B., Schröder, U., Jagirdar, J., Rom, W.N., Tovey, M.G., Freedman, V.H., and Kaplan, G. 2002. Mycobacterial antigens exacerbate disease manifestations in Mycobacterium tuberculosis-infected mice. Infect. Immun. 70: 2100–2107.

Mustafa, A.S., Amoudy, H.A., Wiker, H.G., Abal, A.T., Ravn, P., Oftung, F. and Andersen, P., 1998. Comparison of antigen-specific T-cell responses of tuberculosis patients using complex or single antigens of Mycobacterium tuberculosis. Scand. J. Immunol. 48: 535–543.

Oukka, M., Manuguerra, J.C, Livaditis, N., Tourdot, S., Riche, N., Vergnon, I., Cordopatis, P. and Kosmatopoulos, K. 1996. Protection against lethal viral infection by vaccination with nonimmunodominant peptides. J. Immunol. 157: 3039–3045.

Palendira, U., Kamath, A.T., Feng, C.G., Martin, E., Chaplin, P.J., Triccas, J.A. and Britton, W.J. 2002. Coexpression of interleukin-12 chains by a self-splicing vector increases the protective cellular immune response of DNA and Mycobacterium bovis BCG vaccines against Mycobacterium tuberculosis. Infect. Immun. 70: 1949–1956.

Pavelka, M.S., Chen, B. Jr., Kelley, C.L., Collins and F.M., Jacobs, W.R Jr. 2003. Vaccine efficacy of a lysine auxotroph of Mycobacterium tuberculosis. Infect. Immun. 71: 4190–4192.

Pearl, J.E., Saunders, B., Ehlers, S., Orme, I.M. and Cooper, A.M. 2001. Inflammation and lymphocyte activation during mycobacterial infection in the interferon-deficient mouse. Cell. Immunol. 211: 43–50.

Propato, A., Schiaffella, E., Vicenzi, E., Francavilla, V., Baloni, L., Paroli, M., Finocchi, L., Tanigaki, N., Ghezzi, S., Ferrara, R., Chesnut, R., Livingston, B., Sette, A., Paganelli, R., Aiuti, F., Poli, G., and Barnaba, V. 2001. Spreading of HIV-specific CD8$^+$ T-cell repertoire in long-term nonprogressors and its role in the control of viral load and disease activity. Hum. Immunol. 62: 561–576.

Raviglione, M.C., Dye, C., Schmidt, S., and Kochi, A. 1997. Assessment of world wide TB control. Lancet 350: 624–627.

Ravn, P., Demissie, A., Eguale, T., Wondwosson, H., Lein, D., Amoudy, H.A., Mustafa, A.S., Jensen, A.K., Holm, A., Rosenkrands, I., Oftung, F., Olobo, F., von Reyn, F., and Andersen, P. 1999. Human T cell responses to ESAT-6 antigen from Mycobacterium tuberculosis. J. Infect. Dis. 179: 637–645.

Reed, S.G., Alderson,M.R., Dalemans, W., Lobet, Y., and Skeiky, Y.A.2003. Prospects for a better vaccine against tuberculosis. Tuberculosis (Edinb.) 83: 213–219.

Repique, C.R., Li, A., Collins, F.M., and Morris S.L. 2002. DNA immunization in a mouse model of latent tuberculosis: Effect of DNA vaccination on reactivation of disease and on reinfection with a secondary challenge. Infect. Immun. 70: 3318–3323.

Rieder, H.L., Cauthen, G.M., Comstock, G.W., and Snider, D.E. 1989. Epidemiology of tuberculosis in the United States. Epidemiol. Rev. 11: 79–98.

Rosenthal, K.S., Mao, H., Horne, W.I., Wright, C., and Zimmerman, D. 1999. Immunization with a LEAPS heteroconjugate containing a CTL epitope and a peptide from beta-2-microglobulin elicits a protective and DTH response to herpes simplex virus type 1. Vaccine 17: 535–542.

Rowland-Jones, S. 1999. Long-term non-progression in HIV infection: clinico pathological issues. J. Infect. Dis. 38: 67–70.

Schadeck, E.B., Partidos, C.D., Fooks, A.R., Obeid, O.E., Wilkinson, G.W., Stephenson, J.R., and Steward, M.W. 1999. CTL epitopes identified with a defective recombinant adenovirus expressing measles virus nucleoprotein and evaluation of their protective capacity in mice. Virus Res. 65: 75–86.

Selwyn, P.A., Hartel, D., Lewis, V.A., Schoenbaum, E.E., Vermund, S.H., Klein, S., Walker, A.T., and Friedland, G.H. 1989. A prospective study of the risk of tuberculosis among intravenous drug users with human immunodeficiency virus infection. N. Engl. J. Med. 320: 545–550.

Sepkowitz, K.A. 2001. Tuberculosis control in the 21st century. Emerg. Infect. Dis. 7: 259–262.

Simmons, C.P., Hussell, T., Sparer, T., Walzl, G., Openshaw, P., and Dougan, G. 2001. Mucosal delivery of a respiratorysyncytial virus CTL peptide with enterotoxin-based adjuvants elicits protective, immuno-pathogenic, and immunoregulatory antiviral CD8+ T cell responses. J. Immunol. 166: 1106–1113.

Sonnenberg, M.G. and Belisle, J.T. 1997. Definition of Mycobacterium tuberculosis culture filtrate proteins by two-dimensional polyacrylamide gel electrophoresis, N-terminal amino acid sequencing, and electrospray mass spectrometry. Infect. Immun. 65: 4515–4524.

Sterne, J.A., Fine, P.E., Ponnighaus, J.M., Sibanda, F., Munthali, M. and Glynn, J.R. 1996. Does bacille Calmette–Guerin scar size have implications for protection against tuberculosis or leprosy? Tuber. Lung Dis. 77: 117–23.

Styblo, K. and Meiger J. 1976. Impact of BCG vaccination programmes in children and young adults on the tuberculolosis problem. Tubercle 57: 17–43.

Tanghe, A., Denis, O., Lambrecht, B., Motte, V., van den Berg, T., and Huygen, K. 2000. Tuberculosis DNA vaccine encoding Ag85A is immunogenic and protective when administered by intramuscular needle injection but not by epidermal gene gun bombardment. Infect. Immun. 68: 3854–3860.

Tascon, R.E., Colston, M.J., Ragno, S., Stavropoulos, E., Gregory, D. and Lowrie, D.B. 1996. Vaccination against tuberculosis by DNA injection. Nature Med. 2: 888–892.

Taylor, J.L., Turner, O.C., Basaraba, R.J., Belisle, J.T., Huygen, K., and Orme, I.M. 2003. Pulmonary necrosis resulting from DNA vaccination against tuberculosis. Infect. Immun. 71: 2192–8.

Torres, M., Herrera, T., Villareal, H., Rich, E.A., and Sada, E. 1998. Cytokine profiles for peripheral blood lymphocytes from patients with active pulmonary tuberculosis and healthy household contacts in response to the 30-kilodalton antigen of Mycobacterium tuberculosis. Infect. Immun. 66: 176–180.

Tourdot, S., Oukka, M., Manuguerra, J.C., Magafa, V., Vergnon, I., Riche, N., Bruley-Rosset, M., Cordopatis, P., and Kosmatopoulos, K. 1997. Chimeric peptides: a new approach to enhancing the immunogenicity of peptides with low MHC class I affinity: application in antiviral vaccination. J. Immunol. 159: 2391–2398.

Turner, J., Rhoades, E.R, Keen, M., Belisle, J.T., Frank, A.A., and Orme, I.M. 2000. Effective preexposure tuberculosis vaccines fail to protect when they are given in an immunotherapeutic mode. Infect. Immun. 68: 1706–1709.

Ulmer J.B., Liu, M.A., Montgomery, D.L., Yawman, A.M., Deck, R.R., DeWitt, C.M., Content, J., and Huygen, K. 1997. Expression and immunogenicity of Mycobacterium tuberculosis antigen 85 by DNA vaccination. Vaccine 15: 792–794.

van der Most, R.G., Murali-Krishna, K., Whitton, J.L., Oseroff, C., Alexander, J., Southwood, S., Sidney, J., Chesnut, R.W., Sette, A., and Ahmed, R. 1998. Identification of Db- and Kb-restricted subdominant cytotoxic T-cell responses in lymphocytic choriomeningitis virus-infected mice. Virology 240: 158–167.

von Reyn, C.F., and Vuola, J.M. 2002. New vaccines for the prevention of tuberculosis. Clin. Infect. Dis. 35: 465–474.

Vordermeier, H.M., Harris, D.P., Friscia, G. et al. 1992. T cell repertoire in TB: selective anergy to an immunodominant epitope of the 38Kda antigen in patients with active disease. Eur. J. Immun. 22: 2631–7.

Weinrich OA, van Pinxteren LA, Meng OL et al. 2001. Protection of mice with a tuberculosis subunit vaccine based on a fusion protein of antigen 85b and esat-6. Infect. Immun. 69: 2773–2778.

Weis, S.E, Foresman, B, Matty, K.J., Brown, A., Blais, F.X. et al. 1999. Treatment costs of directly observed therapy and traditional therapy for mycobacterium tuberculosis: a comparative analysis. Int. J. Tuberc. Lung Dis. 3: 976–984.

Wilkinson, R.J., Zhu, X., Wilkinson, K.A., Lalvani, A., Ivanyi, J., Pasvol, G., and Vordermeir, H.M. 1998. 3800 MW antigen-specific major histocompatibility complex class I restricted interferon-gamma-secreting CD8+ T cells in healthy contacts of tuberculosis. Immunology 95: 585–590.

World Bank. World development report. 1993. Investing in Health. New York: Oxford University Press, p. 116.

World Health Organization Scientific Working Group on Tuberculosis. Recommendations. (February 2000. UNDP/World Bank/WHO Special Programme for Research and Training in Tropical Diseases (TDR) 9–11, Geneva, Switzerland.

Yamada, T., Uchiyama, H., Nagata, T., Uchijima, M., Suda, T., Chida, K., Nakamura, H., and Koide, Y. 2001. Protective cytotoxic T lymphocyte responses induced by DNA immunization against immunodominant and subdominant epitopes of Listeria monocytogenes are noncompetitive. Infect. Immun. 69: 3427–3430.

Yeremeev, V.V., Kondratieva, T.K., Rubakova, E.I., Petrovskaya, S.N., Kazarian, K.A., Telkov, M.V., Biketov, S.F., Kaprelyants, A.S., and Apt, A.S. 2003. Proteins of the Rpf family: immune cell reactivity and vaccination efficacy against tuberculosis in mice. Infect. Immun. 71: 4789–94.

Chapter 11

Development of a Vaccine Against Rotaviruses: Current Status

Duncan Steele, Roger Glass and Joseph Bresee

Abstract

Rotaviruses remain a major cause of morbidity and mortality in young children in developing countries and the development of a rotavirus vaccine is a high priority for the international community. Despite a setback for the reassortant rhesus rotavirus vaccine because of possible links to intussusception, the oral live, attenuated vaccine approach remains the strategy of choice and two candidates are in late-stage development and clinical evaluation. These vaccine candidates, which employ a different concept for protection against severe rotavirus disease, are being tested in large safety and efficacy trials designed to measure safety from an association with intussusception. The aim is to have a vaccine licensed within the next 12 to 24 months. Despite these advancements, challenges to the design of rotavirus vaccines and to the future usefulness and introduction of these vaccines remain. Several alternative live, attenuated vaccine candidates are in early-stage development and are building a partnership model with national vaccine manufacturers in emerging nations.

INTRODUCTION

Diarrheal diseases remain an important cause of morbidity in young children in developed countries and a major cause of morbidity and mortality in infants and young children in developing countries. The most recent review of diarrheal mortality indicates that although global mortality due to diarrheal disease has declined dramatically over the two past decades, the annual incidence of diarrheal episodes per child has remained high (Kosek *et al.*, 2003). In addition, in developing countries, diarrhea-related illnesses are associated with a median of 21% of all deaths in children less than 5 years of age, thus remaining a leading cause of death in this age group (Kosek *et al.*, 2003), and accounting for an estimated 2.5 million deaths annually.

Rotavirus is the major enteric pathogen associated with this high diarrhea-related mortality in infants and young children in developing countries, and worldwide it is associated with an estimated 440,000 to 600,000 deaths annually (Bresee *et al.*, 1999; Parashar *et al.*, 2003). The incidence rates of rotavirus infection do not vary significantly between industrialized countries and the developing countries of Africa and Asia, indicating that socio-economic improvements in water and sanitation may not reduce rotavirus diarrhea (Bresee *et al.*, 1999). Nevertheless, inequities in healthcare mean that the vast majority of deaths are in children in the poorest countries. This has prompted the international prioritization of rotavirus vaccines as a primary strategy for the reduction of the mortality associated with this infection.

Since the hallmark publication by de Zoysa and Feachem (1985), which noted that rotavirus resulted in 20% of all diarrheal deaths in young children, the international community has given the development of a rotavirus vaccine a high priority. Despite improvements in the overall management and outcome of diarrheal diseases, resulting in part from interventions such as oral rehydration therapy (ORT) and the Integrated Management of Childhood Illnesses, the proportion of diarrheal illnesses attributable to rotavirus has not declined. In a recent review, rotavirus remained associated with over 25 million clinic or emergency room visits, 2 million hospitalizations, and a median of 440,000 deaths annually in children under 5 years of age (Parashar *et al.*, 2003). This tremendous burden of disease, of which over 82% occurs in developing countries, has driven the urgency of developing a rotavirus vaccine.

The recognition of the association between RotaShield®, a previously licensed reassortant rhesus rotavirus vaccine, and intussusception was a major setback in the development of an efficacious rotavirus vaccine for infants and young children (Centers for Disease Control and Prevention (CDC), 1999b). Nevertheless, the current status of rotavirus vaccine development has never been more promising, with two candidates in late-stage development by multinational pharmaceutical companies and several other candidates under clinical development.

Classification

Rotaviruses were first identified by Ruth Bishop (1973). These viruses display a distinctive wheel-like morphology by electron microscopy (Figure 11.1), leading to the name *Rotavirus*. The viral particles are approximately 75 nm in diameter and have spikes that protrude from the surface, extending the diameter to approximately 100 nm (Prasad and

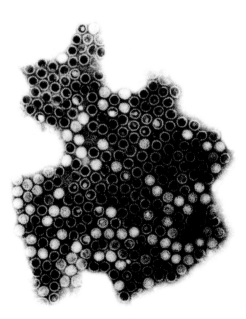

Figure 11.1 Rotavirus particles observed by direct negative staining electron microscopy in the stool from a child with acute rotavirus diarrhea (courtesy of Nicola Page).

Ckiu., 1994). Rotaviruses are classified in the family *Reoviridae* because of the presence of a segmented, double-stranded RNA viral genome (Estes, 2001).

The 11 segments of the double-stranded RNA genome can be easily separated by polyacrylamide gel electrophoresis (PAGE), the standard method of differentiating viral strains and monitoring the molecular epidemiology of the virus (reviewed in Estes *et al.*, 1984; Desselberger *et al.*, 2001). The migration profiles of the RNA segments by polyacrylamide gel electrophoresis (PAGE) are called RNA electropherotypes and indicate considerable strain diversity amongst circulating strains in nature. Human rotaviruses have two predominant RNA electropherotypes exist that are distinguishable by the migration of the 11th gene segment to yield either a 'short' or a 'long' electropherotype (Estes *et al.*, 1984).

The triple-layered virus particle consists of an inner core that surrounds the segments of double-stranded RNA. This layer comprises proteins VP1, VP2, and VP3 (Estes, 2001) (Figure 11.2). The inner capsid, which is made up of the major structural protein VP6, is the major antigenic mass of the virion and constitutes the group-specific antigen of the virus. The outer capsid consists of two proteins, VP7 and VP4, which are important viral antigens for vaccine development because both elicit neutralizing antibodies in the host (Estes, 2001).

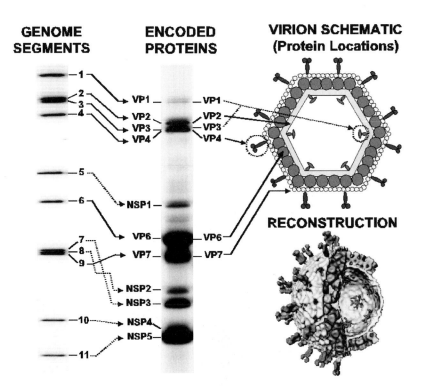

Figure 11.2 Rotavirus particle showing the important antigens required for vaccine development. Reproduced from http://www.iah.bbsrc.ac.uk/dsRNA_virus_proteins/rotavirus%20figure.htm with permission from Frank Ramig.

Ten of the 11 distinct segments of double-stranded RNA each encode a single gene product except for gene 11 segments encodes two. Thus, six structural and six non-structural proteins are produced, of which several are important for viral pathogenesis and vaccine development as described below.

The VP6 inner capsid constitutes approximately 55% of the antigenic mass of the viral particle. This protein is associated with antigenic specificity but is not involved in neutralization specificity (Estes and Cohen; 1989; Kapikian *et al.*, 2001). The VP6 protein is highly antigenic and immunogenic and it is the most frequently targeted protein in diagnostic assays for the detection of rotavirus particles in stool samples (Estes and Cohen, 1989). VP6 contains common epitopes shared by other group A rotaviruses as well as subgroup antigens (Svensson *et al.*, 1988). The VP6 protein contains two distinct domains. The first domain is made up of a common group-specific epitope shared by all rotaviruses of a given group. This site is located between amino acid residues 48 and 75 (Kohli *et al.*, 1992). The second domain, which has been defined serologically by ELISA, complement fixation, immune adherence haemagglutination assay, and immune electron microscopy (Taniguchi *et al.*, 1984), is antigenically polymorphic and called the subgroup antigens. These epitopes are the targets for antigenic classification of rotavirus strain subgroups.

Monoclonal antibodies to the VP6 antigen have been generated (Greenberg *et al.*, 1983; Taniguchi *et al.*, 1984) and extensively used in molecular epidemiologic studies of human and animal rotaviruses. Urasawa *et al.*, 1990, speculated that both epitopes exist on all rotavirus strains and that the monoclonal antibodies used to differentiate subgroup specificity react with overlapping conformational determinants formed by interaction with other viral proteins. Monoclonal antibodies specific for the VP6 epitopes shared by all rotaviruses react with monomeric and trimeric forms of VP6, while monoclonal antibodies specific for subgroup I or II epitopes react only with the trimeric form of VP6, suggesting that the subgroup antigenic specificity is determined by conformational epitopes produced by the folding of VP6 or the interaction between VP6 monomers (Gorziglia *et al.*, 1988). The common epitopes are continuous determinants while subgroup specific antigenic sites are dependent upon interaction between VP6 monomers for their mature configuration (Gorziglia *et al.*, 1988).

Currently, four rotavirus VP6 subgroup specificities have been recognized by how they react with the monoclonal antibodies: VP6 subgroup I is found in some human and most animal rotaviruses. Subgroup II is found most often in human rotaviruses and more rarely among animals strains. Combinations of subgroups I and II are rare in human strains, and non-subgroups I and II are even rarer among rotaviruses from mammals.

These subgroup antigens have been used for rotavirus molecular epidemiological studies of rotavirus and constitute one of four important antigenic and molecular markers that are used to describe rotaviruses in nature (Kapikian *et al.*, 2001; Desselberger *et al.*, 2001).

Characteristics of rotavirus important for vaccine development

The outer capsid structural proteins of the virion, VP7 and VP4, determine the serotype of the virus strain by the specificity of the neutralizing antibody response and therefore are considered important for vaccine development. The relevance of the neutralizing antibody response in vaccine development is less clear and the two late stage vaccine candidates employ different approaches (see below). It is assumed that the neutralizing antibody response in serum reflects the 'vaccine take' and the magnitude of the response and the specificity of the immune response to the virus (Ward *et al.*, in press).

Both of the rotavirus surface proteins, VP4 and VP7, elicit the production of distinct neutralizing antibodies and thus are considered important in vaccine development. The genes encoding these two proteins segregate separately, which has led to a binomial system of classification for the VP7 glycoprotein (*G* types) and the protease-sensitive VP4 (*P* types) (Estes, 2001).

The outer capsid layer, VP7, is a glycoprotein and constitutes the major neutralization antigen of the particle. Early studies showed that VP7 elicits an immune response in the host (Hoshino *et al.*, 1985) and that use of hyper-immune sera could distinguish rotavirus serotypes (Hoshino *et al.*, 1984). At least 14 serotypes are recognized (reviewed in Estes, 2001; Desselberger *et al.*, 2001) and a 15th has been proposed (Rao *et al.*, 2001). Nucleic acid sequence analysis of VP7 genes has revealed regions of the gene that are distinct between serotypes. Monoclonal antibody studies indicate that these are antigenic domains, which may be important for evoking neutralizing antibody. The major antigenic domains are labelled A (lying between amino acids 87 and101), B (amino acids 145–150) and C (amino acids 211–223) (Kapikian *et al.*, 2001).

VP7 is encoded by gene segment 7, 8 or 9, depending on the rotavirus strain (Estes and Cohen; 1989; Estes, 2001). Genotyping methods that utilize the VP7 gene in a multiplex, nested polymerase chain reaction assay have become popular for determining the VP7 type of a strain (Gentsch *et al.*, 1996; Desselberger *et al.*, 2001). The VP7 based genotype and the neutralizing antibody-based serotype systems of analysis and characterization have been compared and correlate completely.

Five VP7 serotypes are identified commonly amongst human rotaviruses (G1 – G4 and G9) although some other serotypes are regionally important (Gentsch *et al.*, 1996). For instance, G5 strains were detected in Brazil (Santos *et al.*, 1998), G8 strains in Africa (Cunliffe *et al.*, 1999; Armah *et al.*, 2001), and G10 strains in India (Das *et al.*, 1994). Because serotype distribution is believed to be important epidemiologically and possibly to affect vaccine-related efficacy, strain diversity and surveillance studies are a prime research tool for ongoing studies (Desselberger *et al.*, 2001).

VP4 is a non-glycosylated outer capsid protein with several important functions. It acts as the viral receptor, and has haemagglutinin, neutralization and virulence characteristics (Estes, 2001). VP4 forms 60 short spikes that protrude through the surface, is encoded by gene segment 4. Both VP4 and VP7 proteins act as antigens in neutralizing immune responses and contribute to the diverse antigenic complexities of rotaviruses (Hoshino, *et al.*, 1985; Offit, *et al.*, 1986). The diversity and distribution of VP4 has also been investigated widely in molecular epidemiology studies, but most have centered on genotyping of the VP4 gene due to difficulties in generating immunological reagents for VP4 serotyping.

The VP4 gene product is cleaved by trypsin to produce VP8*, which carries the type-specific epitopes and VP5*, which carries more cross-reactive epitopes (Gorziglia *et al.*, 1986; Estes, 2001). The cross-reactivity makes it difficult to generate a panel of serotype-specific monoclonal antibodies to the VP4. VP4 types are shown as a serotype (indicated by an open number when known) and a genotype that is indicated in square brackets, e.g. P1A[8] (Estes, 2001).

To date, studies have identified more than 20 rotavirus serotypes in nature (Estes, 2001; Kapikian *et al.*, 2001; Rao *et al.*, 2001), although relatively few are common in human rotaviruses worldwide (Gentsch *et al.*, 1996; Desselberger *et al.*, 2001). The most common types are designated as P1A[8], P1B[4] and P2[6], although some VP4 types occur sporadically, e.g. P[9] and P[14] (Desselberger *et al.*, 2001). Some other VP4 types are common in limited geographic areas [e.g. P[11] in India (Das *et al.*, 1994)].

Among human rotaviruses, there is usually an association between the VP7 serotype and the VP4 type. Thus P1A[8] strains tend to be associated with strains bearing a G1, G3 or G4 VP7 serotype, while P1B[2] strains are associated with the G2 serotype system. P1A[8] strains, regardless of G serotype, tend to be of the VP6 subgroup II and to have a long RNA electropherotype, while strains with a P1B[4]G2 type tend to be VP6 subgroup I with a short RNA electropherotype [reviewed in Estes and Cohen, 1989; Desselberger *et al.*, 2001]. The P2[6] and the G9 strains seem to be more promiscuous and have been identified in strains with multiple configurations (Iturriza-Gomara *et al.*, 2002). This is likely to be a factor of viral strain evolution as these strains were described more recently in the literature.

Epidemiology of rotavirus

The epidemiology and pathogenesis of rotavirus infection is well defined and provide important clues for the development of rotavirus vaccine strategies. Rotaviruses are ubiquitous in nature, infecting virtually all young children by the second or third year of life (Kapikian *et al.*, 2001), although in developing countries rotavirus tends to infect almost 75% of infants before their first birthday (Bresee *et al.*, 1999; Steele *et al.*, 2003). Typically, symptomatic rotavirus infection occurs most frequently in children between the ages of 3 and about 18 months, resulting in mild-to-severe acute watery diarrhea with a subsequent loss of fluids and electrolytes (Kapikian *et al.*, 2001). Infections in infants less than 3 months of age are more likely to be associated with mild or subclinical infection (Bresee *et al.*, 2003). Finally, neonatal infections are in general asymptomatic, perhaps due to protection conferred by passively acquired maternal antibodies or an immature intestinal epithelial system (Bishop *et al.*, 1983; Dearlove *et al.*, 1983) or by viral characteristics (Hoshino *et al.*, 1984). Re-infections in older children are common but tend to be subclinical and probably reflect the natural immunity offered by the primary infection.

Natural rotavirus infection protects against severe diarrhea in subsequent reinfections as shown by an early study in which neonatal rotavirus infection, which were asymptomatic, conferred protection against subsequent severe rotavirus diarrhea, although reinfection was common (Bishop *et al.*, 1983). Furthermore, two longitudinal natural history studies that followed birth cohorts in Mexico and Guinea Bissau, have confirmed that a primary rotavirus infection, whether associated with symptomatic or asymptomatic infection, confers significant protection against disease associated with subsequent reinfection (Velazquez *et al.*, 1996; Fischer *et al.*, 2002). This phenomenon was seen in other studies and led to the hypothesis that a live, orally administered rotavirus vaccine would confer protective efficacy against severe rotavirus disease.

Rotavirus infections exhibit a seasonal pattern in temperate countries, where most rotavirus infections occur during the winter (Kapikian *et al.*, 2001). In tropical areas and in some developing countries, rotavirus infection tends to occur with some increased activity during cooler months of the year (Cunliffe *et al.*, 1998; Kapikian *et al.*, 2001).

Infections in infants less than 3 months of age are more likely to be associated with mild or subclinical infection (Bresee *et al.*, 2003). Finally, neonatal infections are in general asymptomatic, perhaps due to protection conferred by passively acquired maternal antibodies or an immature intestinal epithelial system (Bishop *et al.*, 1983; Dearlove *et al.*,

1983) or by viral characteristics (Hoshino *et al.*, 1984). Re-infections in older children are common but tend to be subclinical and probably reflect the natural immunity offered by the primary infection.

Pathogenesis

Rotavirus particles were first visualized in humans by thin-section electron microscopy of the duodenal mucosa of an infant with acute watery diarrheal illness (Bishop *et al.*, 1973). The distinctive viral particles (Figure 11.1) were soon identified worldwide in the faeces of infants and young children with gastroenteritis (Flewett *et al.*, 1974; Schoub *et al.*, 1975). Rotaviruses were found to be an important aetiological agent of acute infantile diarrhea, and were soon recognized as the most important of the known agents of severe diarrheal illness in infants and young children (Kapikian *et al.*, 2001).

Rotavirus particles are shed in large numbers in faeces ($>10^{11}$/g) during the acute infection and are transmitted by the faecal–oral route. The virus is stable in the environment (Ansari *et al.*, 1991), which facilitates the rapid and efficient transmission of the infection. Speculation on the respiratory transmission of rotaviruses, due to the seasonality and rapid transmission of the infection (Cook *et al.*, 1990), has not been substantiated by clinical or laboratory studies, although rotavirus is occasionally recovered from the respiratory tract (Santosham *et al.*, 1983; Zheng *et al.*, 1991). Nevertheless, aerosol droplet and person-to-person spread does seem to be a primary mode of transmission.

Rotavirus infection has a short incubation period (1–3 days). The disease is characterized by the sudden onset of acute watery diarrhea, often accompanied by fever and vomiting (Staat *et al.*, 2002). Although most rotavirus infections are relatively mild, approximately 1 in every 5 children will develop symptoms and dehydration severe enough to warrant a visit to a medical facility, and as many as 1 in 65 will be admitted to hospital and about 1 in every 293 children will die of rotavirus infection (Parashar *et al.*, 2003). Typically, the acute infection which is accompanied by diarrhea and fever for 3 to 5 days. Vomiting is a

Table 11.1 Implications for rotavirus vaccine defined by the differences in the epidemiology of rotavirus infection between developing countries and developed countries (adapted from Bresee *et al.*, 2003)

Epidemiology	Developed country	Developing country	Implications for vaccine trials
Percent infected by age 12 months	40%	75%	Vaccine must be given earlier. Potential interference of maternal antibody with vaccine 'take'
Median age (months) of first infection	12–18	6–12	
Seasonality	Winter peak	Year round	Year-round exposure to infants, earlier age of acquisition. Need for earlier vaccination
Case fatality rate	Low	High	Outcomes and measurements in vaccine trial design
Mixed infection with other enteropathogens	Uncommon	Common	May limit vaccine take, and affect diarrhea outcomes of trial design. Necessitate additional vaccine doses
Multiple virus serotypes	One major type circulating	More than one type circulating	Vaccine efficacy may be challenged in trial design. Vaccine candidates may need different formulations

predominant early symptom of rotavirus infection, which may undermine the effectiveness of ORT. Furthermore, in the animal model, full recovery of the absorptive function of the enterocytes of the villa may take up to 6 weeks.

The virus infects and replicates almost exclusively in the mature enterocytes at the tips of the intestinal villi (Mebus *et al.*, 1974; Pearson and McNulty, 1977). Following infection in calves or piglets, the cells at the tips of the villus become denuded and blunted, resulting in the loss of absorptive capacity of sodium, glucose, and water. This is consistent with the migration of undifferentiated, immature enterocytes towards the villous tip (Clark *et al.*, 2003). Rotaviruses do not seem to replicate in the immature epithelial cells of the villous crypt, nor in the M cells covering the Peyer's patches (Greenberg *et al.*, 1994). Rotavirus infection is often accompanied by serious fluid and electrolyte loss with dehydration, especially in small infants, which is related to similar damage of the intestinal epithelial cells (Holmes *et al.*, 1975).

At least four rotavirus proteins are associated with virulence in the gnotobiotic piglet model (Hoshino *et al.*, 1993). Reassortant virus studies in this model indicate that VP3, VP4, VP7 and NSP4 are all necessary for virulence.

The rotavirus non-structural NSP4 protein acts as a viral enterotoxin and induces diarrhea in the mouse model in an age-dependent and dose-dependent manner (Ball *et al.*, 1996). It is believed that NSP4 is thought to selectively regulates extracellular Ca^{2+} entry into the infected cells (Ball *et al.*, 1996). Intracellular calcium concentration ($[Ca^{2+}]_i$) increases in virus-infected cells and accumulation of NSP4 and its concomitant effect on $[Ca^{2+}]_i$ mobilization may be responsible for cytotoxicity and cell death during the later stages of viral infection (Michelangeli *et al.*, 1995). NSP4 may stimulate a Ca^{2+}-dependent signal transduction pathway that alters epithelial transport and that NSP4-specific receptors may decrease in number as mice age (Ball *et al.*, 1996). If so, this would explain the preferential infection of children versus adults but would not explain adult rotavirus infections.

Finally, rotavirus infections evoke intestinal fluid and electrolyte secretion by activation of the enteric nervous system (ENS) in the intestinal wall. Although, the involvement of the ENS in rotavirus diarrhea may provide potential sites of action for drugs in the treatment of this disease (Lundgren *et al.*, 2000) and provide an alternative intervention to vaccination. However, it is unlikely to be a potential strategy to protect children in developing countries against severe rotavirus disease.

Immunity against rotavirus infection

The immunological mechanism that confers protection against rotavirus disease is unknown for both natural infection (Velazquez *et al.*, 1996) and immunization (Midthun and Kapikian, 1996). Rotavirus infection does result in both serum and intestinal antibodies responses and in general does protect against severe diarrheal illness upon subsequent infection (Bishop *et al.*, 1983; Velazquez *et al.*, 1996; Fischer *et al.*, 2002). Although the role of intestinal neutralizing antibodies is usually accepted as playing an important role in protection against disease, results have been inconsistent, possibly due to variations in experimental design. Three questions remain:

1 Is serum antibody indicative of protection of rotavirus disease?
2 Is neutralizing antibody the most important mechanism of protective immunity?
3 What other immune mechanisms may play a role?

The role of serum antibodies in protection

The role of serum antibodies remains elusive as shown by studies the examined the natural history of rotavirus infection (Ward and Bernstein, 1994; Velazquez *et al.*, 1996; Gorrell *et al.*, 1999), vaccine trials (Clark *et al.*, 1996; Midthun and Kapikian, 1996) and adult challenge studies (summarized in Jiang *et al.*, 2002). In brief, most studies have indicated that the presence of serum antibodies was a good surrogate marker for protection (Jiang *et al.*, 2002), although it is believed that other effector mechanisms of the immune response were important (Ward and Bernstein, 1994; Jiang *et al.*, 2002). Thus, from these studies, it is difficult to assess whether serum antibodies are active components of the protective immune response or just a correlate of protection.

In two studies of adult volunteers (Kapikian *et al.*, 1983; Ward *et al.*, 1989), serum antibodies in both studies correlated with protection against disease but intestinal neutralizing antibodies did not. Natural rotavirus infection in young children also differed. In Danish children, IgA correlated with protection but IgG did not (Hjelt *et al.*, 1987), whereas in Bangladeshi infants, IgG correlated with protection (Clemens *et al.*, 1992) but another study reported a correlation for both immunoglobulins (O'Ryan *et al.*, 1994). Finally, in vaccine trials in children, some degree of protection was usually observed, although this correlated better with overall immune response and not with serotype-specific neutralizing antibody (Bernstein *et al.*, 1990; Clark *et al.*, 1996; Kapikian *et al.*, 1996; Jiang *et al.*, 2002).

Serotype-specific neutralizing antibody

A major debate concerns the need for serotype-specific neutralizing antibody and whether other immune effector mechanisms play a role. Although serotype specific epitopes have been described for the rotavirus strains, it must be borne in mind, that cross-reactive epitopes exist on both the VP7 and the VP4 serotypes, which means that protection against multiple rotavirus strains may be affected through these cross-reactive domains.

Two philosophical approaches exist as to the putative role of serum neutralizing antibody in the protection and the two rotavirus vaccine candidates in late stage development utilize these different approaches. On the one hand, the belief that serotype-specific neutralizing antibody is necessary for protection has driven the approach of reassortant rotavirus vaccines, such as the rhesus quadrivalent (Kapikian *et al.*, 1996) or the bovine reassortant strains (Clark *et al.*, 1996). Thus, although monovalent rhesus (G3) and bovine strains (RIT, WC3 and UK, which are G6) have been tested in clinical settings with different results, reassortant vaccines covering the four common human rotavirus VP7 serotypes (Gentsch *et al.*, 1996) were developed as discussed below. An alternative approach utilises the idea that natural rotavirus infection generates a broad protective response against reinfection and that protective efficacy is generated by alternative immune responses in addition to the neutralizing antibody response (Ward, 2003).

Results of several studies in human populations have indicated that neutralizing antibodies are not the major mechanism in protection. For instance, in separate neonatal studies, the serotype of the endemic neonatal strain that infected newborns conferred protection against other circulating serotypes in those same infants (Bishop *et al.*, 1983; Aijaz *et al.*, 1996). Also, in older children a severe primary rotavirus infection usually confers protection against subsequent severe rotavirus disease upon reinfection even with different serotypes (Velazquez *et al.*, 1996; Fischer *et al.*, 2002). When the reinfection is associated with symptomatic disease, the infecting strain is usually of a different VP7 serotype, indicating that serotype-specific neutralizing antibody does have a role to play.

In clinical trials utilizing monovalent rotavirus vaccine strains (described below) indicated that serotype-specific neutralizing antibody responses against the circulating rotavirus strains appear to be important in protection (reviewed in Midthun and Kapikian, 1996). Thus evidence that neutralizing antibody be important for protection is based on empirical data from early vaccine clinical trials. Nevertheless, in other vaccine trials in children, protection did not always correlate with neutralizing antibody (Bernstein *et al.*, 1990; Clark *et al.*, 1996; Kapikian *et al.*, 1996). The difficulty in understanding the mechanism of protection has made interpretation of various clinical trials difficult – especially if they produced different efficacy results (Jiang *et al.*, 2002).

The role of other immune effector mechanisms

Although few studies have investigated T cell responses in humans, lympho-proliferative assays indicate that children did develop measurable levels of circulating rotavirus-specific T cells after a primary infection (Offit *et al.*, 1993). Furthermore, Jaimes *et al.* (2002) found elevated levels of virus-specific CD4$^+$ and CD8$^+$ T cells secreting gamma-interferon, after rotavirus infection.

Animal models have demonstrated the interplay of humoral and cell-mediated immunity. Studies in the adult mouse model show that the B, CD8$^+$ and CD4$^+$ T cells all play a role in the protection of rotavirus shedding in the mouse (Ward, 2003). For instance, in B-cell-deficient mice, which are unable to produce any antibody, long-term protection against rotavirus was essentially lost, demonstrating the importance of antibody in clearance of the infection (Franco and Greenberg, 1995). Cytotoxic T cells were observed to be necessary for the initial resolution of the infection and where B-cell-deficient mice were depleted of their CD8 cells, resolution of the initial shedding was lost (Franco and Greenberg, 1993). Finally, CD4 cells were shown to confer protection against challenge in B-cell deficient, CD8 depleted mice, whereas if the CD4 cells were depleted, the protection against challenge was lost (McNeal *et al.*, 2002; Ward *et al.*, 2003).

Rotavirus vaccines

The global burden of rotavirus disease and the high mortality associated with rotavirus infection in children in the developing world has prompted international prioritization of the development of a rotavirus vaccine (Bresee *et al.*, 1999). The fact that rotaviruses occur with equal frequency in children in developing and developed countries indicates that improvements in water supply, sewage disposal and sanitation are not sufficient to stop the spread of the disease. Thus, a rotavirus vaccine would have universal applicability for children (Bresee *et al.*, 1999).

Rotavirus vaccine development was initiated soon after the discovery of the virus for several reasons. Among these were the universal burden of disease and mortality in infants and young children (de Zoysa and Feachem, 1985); the observation that primary natural infection led to protection against severe disease upon reinfection (Bishop *et al.*, 1983; Bernstein *et al.*, 1991; Velazquez *et al.*, 1996); the antigenic relatedness of animal and human rotaviruses (Hoshino *et al.*, 1984; Estes and Graham, 1985); the restricted interspecies transmission of rotaviruses, and the fact that human strains were attenuated when administered to the young of animal species (Wyatt *et al.*, 1983).

The major effort towards the development of rotavirus vaccines has utilized human or animal rotavirus strains in a live, attenuated oral approach. Early animal studies indicated that protection against rotavirus disease was mediated primarily by intestinal immunity (see below).

JENNERIAN APPROACH TO ROTAVIRUS VACCINES

The protection offered by primary rotavirus infection and the antigenic relatedness of animal and human rotaviruses stimulated a 'Jennerian' approach to rotavirus vaccination which relied on immunization with animal rotavirus or animal-human reassortant rotavirus strains (Midthun and Kapikian, 1996). Thus, the use of attenuated animal rotavirus strains produced the first rotavirus vaccine candidates (Table 11.2), and these continue to be a major focus of vaccine.

Monovalent animal rotavirus candidates

The early rotavirus vaccine candidates included bovine strains (RIT4237 and WC3) and the monovalent parent rhesus rotavirus (MMU18006). After variable results with the bovine strains, which both carried a G6 serotype specificity that is not found in human strains, the RIT4237 candidate was dropped from clinical development and WC3 was developed into a multivalent candidate as described below.

The monovalent G3 rhesus rotavirus candidate was also developed and early results seemed promising with the strain showing a good immune response, although it was slightly reactogenic (Christy et al., 1986). However, clinical studies investigating the protective efficacy of the vaccine yielded highly variable results. In some studies in which the circulating rotavirus was serotype G3 (similar to the vaccine), protective efficacy was demonstrated (Flores et al., 1987). However, in other studies in which the circulating strains were predominantly G1, the vaccine failed to offer heterotypic protection against rotavirus diarrhea (Santosham et al., 1991). The early animal rotavirus vaccine candidates have been reviewed (Midthun and Kapikian, 1996 and Bresee et al., 2003) and will not be discussed further here.

Failure of the monovalent strains to offer heterotypic cross-protection against rotaviruses resulted in the hypothesis that serotype-specific immunity was important for vaccine efficacy and protection (Midthun and Kapikian, 1996) and led to the development of reassortant rotavirus vaccine candidates.

Table 11.2 Early rotavirus vaccine candidates that have been discontinued from development

Vaccine strain	Type of vaccine	Company/developer (year)	Reason for discontinuation
RIT 4237	Bovine monovalent G6P6[1]	SmithKline (1983)	Poor protective efficacy in developing country infants
RIT4256	Bovine monovalent G6P7[5]	SmithKline (1986)	Lower passage than RIT4237 but immunogenicity similar
WC3	Bovine monovalent G6P7[5]	Wistar Institute (1984)	Variable efficacy in developing countries[1]
RRV	Rhesus monovalent G3P5B[3]	NIH (1985)	Variable efficacy in developing countries[2]
M37	Neonatal mono-valent G1P2[6]	NIH (1989)	Poor efficacy in trial with low titre in Finland

[1]Parent strain of the reassortant bovine rotavirus strain developed by Merck Research Laboratories.
[2]Parent strain of the reassortant rhesus rotavirus strain developed by Wyeth Ayerst .

Lamb rotavirus (LLR)

A monovalent lamb rotavirus strain (G10P[12]) that was isolated in primary calf kidney cells in China in 1985 has been developed as a vaccine after multiple passage (World Health Organization, WHO, 2000; Bresee *et al.*, 2003). The strain, called LLR (Lanzhou Lamb Rotavirus), does not contain the antigenic determinants commonly found in human rotavirus strains. In clinical trials in China, the vaccine exhibited a serum neutralizing response in 61% of vaccinees (WHO, 2000). However, the trials were in older children and the immune response resembled a 'booster' response with a similar elevation in titre to neutralizing antibody to G1–G4 strains. LLR was licensed for use in China in 2000 and remains in use locally.

Modified Jennerian approach to vaccine development

The concept of the Jennerian approach animal rotaviruses that are attenuated for human disease was modified to generate reassortant vaccines carrying the four common human rotavirus VP7 genes (G1–G4) on the genetic background of the early animal rotavirus strains. These reassortant vaccine candidates were developed to yield strains that would offer a multivalent serotype exposure upon immunization, while retaining the attenuated nature of the parent strain.

Rhesus-human reassortant rotavirus vaccine

The quadrivalent rhesus-human reassortant rotavirus vaccine is based on the rhesus rotavirus (RRV) strain, which shares G3 specificity with human rotaviruses. Three reassortant rhesus strains with the VP7 gene from human rotaviruses for G1 (human strain D), G2 (strain DS-1) and G4 (strain ST3) respectively were created (Midthun *et al.*, 1985). The vaccine candidate consisted of a pool of these reassortant strains with the parent RRV strain, and early studies showed each reassortant strain to be similar to the parent RRV strain in infants with regard to safety, reactogenicity, shedding and immunogenicity (Halsey *et al.*, 1988; Midthun and Kapikian, 1996). These studies also showed that protective efficacy was associated with the serologic response as measured by the serum IgA response (Vesikari *et al.*, 1992; Midthun and Kapikian, 1996).

A series of efficacy trials were conducted in different populations and at different vaccine concentrations (10^4 pfu and 10^5 pfu per dose) and in general showed consistent protective efficacy against all types of rotavirus diarrhea (50–60%) and against severe rotavirus disease (70–100%) (reviewed in Midthun and Kapikian, 1996). More vaccine than placebo recipients experienced a mild (38.0 – 38.9°C) short-lived fever 3–5 days after vaccination 21–25% and 4 respectively. Higher fevers, >39°C, were also observed to be more common in vaccine recipients than in the placebo group (approximately 2% versus 1%) (Vesikari *et al.*, 1992; Midthun and Kapikian, 1996).

The pivotal phase III efficacy trials, which used three doses of the vaccine at 4×10^5 pfu per dose, showed 50–60% protection against any rotavirus diarrhea and 70–100% protection against severe rotavirus diarrhea (that requiring hospitalizations or rehydration (Rennels *et al.*, 1996; Joensuu *et al.*, 1997; Perez-Schael *et al.*, 1997; Santoshan *et al.*, 1997). The protective efficacy was exhibited against different circulating VP7 serotypes and was evident over two to three rotavirus seasons.

On the basis of these results, RotaShield® was licensed in the United States in 1998 and quickly added to the routine immunization schedule for USA infants (CDC, 1999). However, within 9 months more than 500,000 infants had received the vaccine, there was a reported association between the vaccine and intussusception (CDC, 1999). Although the debate about the true attributable risk of intussusception continues today, (Murphy B et al., 2003; Murphy T et al., 2003), the vaccine was withdrawn by the manufacturer in October 1999, and the recommendation for its use was withdrawn by the Advisory Committee for Immunization Practices.

Although RotaShield® remains licensed in the USA, the vaccine is no longer produced and has not been evaluated in clinical trials in children in developing countries. Questions remain as to whether the vaccine should have had more clinical evaluation in the developing world due to the high risk–benefit of a rotavirus vaccine where rotavirus disease-associated mortality is high (Bresee et al., 2000; Weijer, 2000).

Reassortant WC3 bovine–human rotavirus vaccine

WC3 is a bovine rotavirus, bearing a G6P7[5] serotype that is not found among human rotaviruses. It was developed as an early monovalent vaccine candidate and adapted after efficacy clinical trials yielded variable results (reviewed in Midthun and Kapikian, 1996; Clark et al., 1996).

The parent WC3 strain was consistently found to be safe and immunogenic in early studies, with neutralizing antibody responses in 71–97% of recipients, although the immune response was specific to bovine rotavirus (Clark et al., 1986; Clark et al., 1996). However, the vaccine was not consistent in protective efficacy (Clark et al., 1986; Bernstein et al., 1990) and no clear correlate of protection could be discerned.

Nevertheless, due to the good safety profile and the high immunogenicity demonstrated, WC3 was developed as a reassortant vaccine candidate. Various reassortant combinations with human rotavirus genes for serotypes G1–G4 and/or P1A[8] on the bovine WC3 background have been generated (Clark et al., 1996). A series of clinical trials utilizing the monovalent WC3 reassortant strains with human rotavirus G1 or G2 specificity illustrated the safety and immunogenicity of the vaccine components and that the immune response to the bovine rotavirus VP4 was significant (Clark et al., 1990). These study results suggested that WC3 components should be included in future vaccine candidates. The reassortant rhesus rotavirus trials showed similar results (Bernstein et al., 1995).

Clark et al. (1996) have described the vaccine development, its safety and immunogenicity (similar to a quadrivalent candidate) (Clark et al., 1995; Clark et al., 2004) and the final combination, a pentavalent reassortant strain with the G1–G4 and P1A human rotavirus genes (Table 11.3).

A clinical trial examining the efficacy of three doses of a quadrivalent WC3 candidate (containing human rotavirus genes for VP7 G1–G3 and VP4 P1A[8]) showed immunogenicity of 88%, as measured by serum IgA antibody response to rotavirus (Clark et al., 1995). The proportion of children who developed neutralizing antibodies to G1, G3 and P1A was ~57%, although that to G2 was slightly lower (Clark et al., 1995). During the trial both G1 and G3 wild type strains were circulating, and the vaccine provided 68% protection against rotavirus disease and against severe rotavirus infection.

In a more recent report, the quadrivalent WC3 vaccine was shown to be safe and well tolerated with 75% efficacy against rotavirus diarrhea of any severity and 100% efficacy against severe rotavirus infection through one season (Clark et al., 2004). A three-fold or greater serum anti-rotavirus IgA response was noted in 88% of the vaccinees.

The pentavalent WC3 reassortant rotavirus vaccine candidate (human rotavirus genes G1–G4 and P1A[8]) was recently evaluated in an immunogenicity and efficacy trial in

Table 11.3 Live rotavirus vaccine candidates that are currently licensed or under clinical development

Vaccine strain	Type of vaccine	Company/developer	Status	Inventor
Licensed vaccines				
RotaShield®	Quadrivalent reassortant rhesus rotavirus strain with human rotavirus genes	Wyeth Ayerst (USA)	License remains in USA (1998)	AZ Kapikian, NIH
LLR	Monovalent lamb rotavirus	Lanzhou Institute (China)	Licensed in China (2000)	ZS Bai, Lanzhou Institute
RotaRix	Monovalent human rotavirus strain	GlaxoSmithKline (Belgium)	Phase III safety and efficacy trial	R Ward, Gamble Institute
Late stage clinical development				
RotaTeq	Multivalent reassortant bovine strain with human rotavirus genes	Merck Research (USA)	Phase III safety and efficacy trial	HF Clark, Wistar Institute
Early clinical development				
UK	Multivalent reassortant bovine strain with human rotavirus genes	Wyeth Ayerst/NIH	Phase II trial	AZ Kapikian, NIH
RV3	Monovalent human neonatal rotavirus strain	University of Melbourne	Phase II trial	RF Bishop, Melbourne University
116E and I321	Monovalent human–bovine reassortant strains	Indian/USA consortium	Phase I trial	RI Glass, MK Bhan, HB Greenberg, CD Rao *et al.*
Preclinical development				
VLPs	Virus-like particles	Baylor College of Medicine	Preclinical	MK Estes, M Conner
DNA	DNA vaccines	Massachusetts School of Medicine	Preclinical	JE Herrman

Adapted from Bresee *et al.* (2003).

1,946 Finnish infants aged 2–8 months. All received three doses of different vaccine concentrations (Vesikari *et al.*, 2002). The vaccine showed 81–97% immunogenicity and gave protection against any rotavirus disease of 59–77%. On the basis of this successful clinical trial, the pentavalent vaccine candidate is currently undergoing a phase III safety and efficacy trial in Europe and the USA.

The pentavalent candidate is constituted as a liquid in a sodium citrate buffer to improve stability at refrigerator temperature (Clark *et al.*, 2003). The vaccine will be given orally in three doses at 10^5 ffu doses to infants approximately 6–8 weeks apart, when infants will also be receiving routine childhood immunization. The large safety and efficacy trial has not administering the vaccine with the concomitant childhood vaccines, and thus the potential of this vaccine in young infants in developing countries where infants also receive oral poliomyelitis vaccine (OPV), remains to be elucidated.

Reassortant UK bovine–human vaccine

A second bovine-human reassortant vaccine is based on the bovine strain UK (also G6P7), and contains the human rotavirus genes for serotype G1–G4 and P1A[8] reassorted onto the bovine rotavirus UK background (Hoshino *et al.*, 1997). The individual components of the vaccine were shown to be safe and immunogenic after two doses, as indicated by the presence of serum IgA (Clements-Mann *et al.*, 1999). Subsequently the quadrivalent VP7-specific vaccine was administered in three doses at 10^5 ffu to infants with concomitant childhood immunizations (Clements-Mann *et al.*, 2001). There was no adverse reaction with the other concomitant vaccines and 95% of the infants developed neutralizing antibody responses to the vaccine strain. Efficacy trials with the vaccine candidate are planned.

Attenuated human rotavirus strains

Rotavirus vaccine candidates have been generated from either putatively naturally attenuated neonatal strains and from strains that were associated with symptomatic infection in older children. Of note, the natural human rotavirus infection induced a broad serum of immune responses across the rotavirus serotypes, although it was not clear how this occurred (Gorrell and Bishop, 1999). Therefore, the process of attenuation should not restrict this broad immune response, while sufficiently attenuating the strain for safe use in infants.

Neonatal human rotavirus strain (M37)

M37, a serotype G1 strain, was recovered from stools of an asymptomatic neonate in Venezuela. Early studies investigating rotavirus strains from neonates showed that neonatal infection was often asymptomatic and that the strains may be naturally attenuated. VP4 was apparently distinct as it was P2[6], and this was thought to explain the attenuation (Flores *et al.*, 1986; Gorziglia *et al.*, 1986). This concept has since been challenged by the finding of P2[6] VP4 rotavirus strains in symptomatically infected older children (Steele *et al.*, 1993; Cunliffe *et al.*, 1999; Armah *et al.*, 2002). Furthermore, neonatal infection is now known to confer protection against symptomatic rotavirus diarrhea (Bishop *et al.*, 1983). Nevertheless, M37 has been evaluated as a vaccine candidate.

Phase I studies in which doses of 10^4 and 10^5 pfu were administered showed that the vaccine was safe and well tolerated, but only moderately immunogenic (Flores *et al.*, 1990; Vesikari *et al.*, 1991). In a small phase II immunogenicity and efficacy trial in

Finnish infants aged 2–6 months a single dose of M37 vaccine at either 10^4 or 10^5 pfu was administered. The lower dose of vaccine showed no clinical efficacy against circulating G1 strains, and an IgA immune response of only 47% (Vesikari *et al.*, 1991). However, the higher dose gave a better immune response (76%), but the study lacked sufficient statistical power to ascertain clinical efficacy. The vaccine candidate was not evaluated further.

Neonatal human rotavirus strain (RV3)

Neonatal rotavirus infection in Melbourne, Australia conferred clinical protection against subsequent rotavirus disease in infants (Bishop *et al.*, 1983). This study and other longitudinal surveillance studies (Bernstein *et al.*, 1991; Ward and Bernstein, 1994; Velazquez *et al.*, 1996) indicated that natural infection with a single wildtype rotavirus invariably conferred protection against moderate-to-severe rotavirus disease upon reinfection. The naturally attenuated neonatal rotavirus strain identified in this study (RV3) was developed as a vaccine candidate due to these observations (Barnes *et al.*, 1997).

The vaccine candidate was safe and well tolerated in phase I trials in adults, children, and infants (Barnes *et al.*, 1997). In a phase II trial in which three doses of vaccine (10^5ffu) were administered at ages 3, 5 and 7 months, only 46% of vaccinees showed an immune response (Barnes *et al.*, 2002); however, the infants with an immune response were partially protected against rotavirus disease in the second year, supporting the observation that this strain offered protection after natural infection.

Further clinical trials are planned with the RV3 strain at a higher vaccine titre to determine if a higher immune response is generated and will be efficacious. This neonatal candidate is of special interest because of the good natural protection seen and because of the other neonatal strain (M37) was discontinued at a higher titre.

Naturally occurring neonatal bovine–human reassortant strains

Neonatal rotavirus strains identified in India also conferred protection against subsequent rotavirus disease (Bhan *et al.*, 1993). Strain 116E is a naturally occurring reassortant strain (G8P8[11]), between bovine and human rotaviruses with only the VP4 gene derived from a bovine rotavirus (Das *et al.*, 1993). A second naturally occurring bovine human rotavirus strain in neonates was detected in Bangalore (Aijaz *et al.*, 1996). Strain I321 carries G10P8[11] specificity and is predominantly a bovine strain, with only two human rotavirus non-structural proteins present. These strains are being developed further as vaccine candidates by an international consortium consisting of Indian and US collaborators.

Monovalent human rotavirus strain (89-12)

A naturally circulating human rotavirus strain associated with diarrheal disease was found to confer natural immunity to subsequent rotavirus infection in infants and young children (Ward and Bernstein, 1994). The strain, 89-12 (G1P1A[8]), was recovered from stools of a 15-month-old toddler with rotavirus diarrhea and was shown to be protective against rotavirus disease in the following season. Strain 89-12 was adapted to tissue culture and serially passaged to attenuate the strain as a vaccine candidate (Bernstein *et al.*, 1990; Bernstein *et al.*, 1998). A clinical trial of the attenuated 89-12 vaccine strain offered 89% protective efficacy against any rotavirus disease and 100% against protection against severe rotavirus infection in the subsequent season (Bernstein *et al.*, 1999), and this protection extended over at least two years (Bernstein *et al.*, 2002). Initial trials demonstrated that the vaccine strain was safe and immunogenic and that after two doses nearly every child (94%) developed an immune response.

The parent strain, 89-12, which was further attenuated passaged in tissue culture, and cloned and purified (now designated Rix4414), is being developed as a vaccine by GlaxoSmithKline Biologicals. The vaccine was evaluated in immunogenicity and efficacy trials in Finland (Vesikari et al., 2002) and Latin America (Perez-Schael et al., 2002), where it is now in phase III safety and efficacy trials. In the Finnish trial, 405 infants were vaccinated with two doses of vaccine (10^5 ffu) at ages 2 and 4 months; 80% immunogenicity was demonstrated and the vaccine gave protective efficacy of 69% against any rotavirus disease and 90% against severe rotavirus disease (Vesikari et al., 2002; De Vos et al., 2004).

The phase III efficacy trial was undertaken in Brazil, Mexico and Venezuela. In all, 1,986 infants were vaccinated at ages 2 and 4 months with different vaccine concentrations ($\approx 10^4$, 10^5 and 10^6 ffu) (Perez-Schael et al., 2002). Immunogenicity was detected in 60–65% of infants and the vaccine conferred protection of 68–87% against severe rotavirus infection and 61–92% against rotavirus hospitalizations.

The philosophy behind the concept of a monovalent vaccine strain relies on the idea that neutralizing antibody is not the only immune effector of protection and that other immune factors play a role (Ward, 2003). In this latter trial, rotavirus-associated diarrheal episodes during the efficacy phase of follow-up were almost evenly distributed between the G1 and non-G1 circulating strains. Protection against severe rotavirus diarrhea was observed to be comparable between G1 and non-G1 strains (76.5% versus 76.7%) (Perez-Schael et al., 2002; Ruiz-Palacios et al., 2002).

The vaccine is being further evaluated in phase III safety and efficacy trials in Latin America and Asia, which are also designed to separate the rotavirus vaccine administration with the routine childhood vaccines. In addition, specific trials examining specific issues for infants in developing countries (such as the potential interaction with OPV and dose ranging) are ongoing in South Africa and Bangladesh.

The vaccine is intended as a two-dose vaccine. It is currently prepared in a lyophilized formulation, which is not optimal for the Expanded Programme of Immunization (EPI) schedule in developing countries due to problems related to storage capacity, vaccine or buffer wastage, and vaccine re-constitution at the field clinic. The vaccine Rotarix™, was licensed in Mexico in July 2004.

CHALLENGES TO ROTAVIRUS VACCINE DEVELOPMENT

Rotavirus vaccine development faces several challenges, the greatest of which may well be the safety of new vaccine candidates in regard to intussusception and recent reports of rotavirus antigenaemia after natural infection in the animal model.

Association with intussusception

The reported association of the RotaShield® vaccine with intussusception – a rare but serious type of bowel obstruction found in infants worldwide – has had a lasting effect on rotavirus vaccine development (CDC, 1999; B. Murphy et al., 2003). The continuing debate about the association of the rhesus-specific rotavirus vaccine, RotaShield® with intussusception (B. Murphy et al., 2003; T. Murphy et al., 2003) does not alter the fact that both candidate vaccines in late stage development (Merck Research Laboratories and GlaxoSmithKline Biologicals) are enrolling between 60,000–70,000 infants in safety trials designed primarily to prove safety against an association with intussusception. Nevertheless, with the rarity of intussusception and the relatively small elevated risk of the rhesus rotavirus vaccine (estimated to be approximately 1 additional case in every 10,000 infants vaccinated (Peters and Myers, 2002), these two large safety trials may be underpowered to detect a real risk. Therefore, it is likely that post-licensure surveillance will be the final harbinger of the long-term safety of the new generation rotavirus vaccines.

Rotavirus antigenaemia

A transient rotavirus antigenaemia has been reported in an animal model and in children (Blutt *et al.*, 2003). Rotavirus antigen was detected in sera of 22 of 33 children with acute rotavirus infection but in none of 35 controls. The antigen in the serum was transient, disappeared quickly and seemed to be directly related to the concentration of the rotavirus antigen in stool (Blutt *et al.*, 2003). Further studies are warranted to elucidate our understanding of the pathogenesis and clinical manifestations of rotavirus infection. It may also be important to examine the role of antigenaemia in vaccine trial, although it seems likely that the transient nature of the event and the attenuated nature of the vaccine candidates will not affect the safety profile of the vaccines.

References

Aijaz, S., Gowda, K., Jagannath, H.V., Reddy, R.R., Maiya, P.P.,Ward, R.L., Greenberg, H.B., Raju, M., Babu, A., and Rao, C.D. 1996. Epidemiology of symptomatic human rotaviruses in Bangalore and Mysore, India from 1988 to 1994 as determined by electropherotype, subgroup and serotype analysis. Arch. Virol. 141: 715–726.

Ansari, S.A., Springthorpe, V.S., and Sattar, S.A. 1991. Survival and vehicular spread of human rotaviruses. Possible relation to seasonality of outbreaks. Rev. Infect. Dis. 13: 488–491.

Armah, G.E., Pager, C.T., Asmah, R.H., Anto, F.R., Oduro, A.R., Binka, F.N., and Steele, A.D. 2001. Prevalence of unusual human rotavirus strains in Ghanaian children. J. Med. Virol. 63: 67–71.

Ball, J.M., Tian, P., Zeng, C.Q., Morris, A.P., and Estes, M.K. 1996. Age-dependent diarrhea induced by a rotaviral non-structural glycoprotein. Science 272: 101–104.

Barnes, G.L., Lund, J.S., Adams, L., Mora, A., Mitchell, S.V., Caples, A., and Bishop, R.F. 1997. Phase I trial of a candidate rotavirus vaccine (RV3) derived from a human neonate. J. Paediatr. Child Health 33: 300–304.

Barnes, G.L., Lund, J.S., Mitchell, S.V., de Bruyn, L., Piggford, L., Smith, A.L., Furmedge, J., Masendycz, P.J., Bugg, H.C., Bogdanovic-Sakran, N., Carlin, J.B., and Bishop, R.F. 2002. Early phase II trial of human rotavirus vaccine candidate RV3. Vaccine 20: 2950–2956.

Bernstein, D.I., Glass, R.I., Rodgers, G., Davidson, B.L., and Sack, D.A. 1995. Evaluation of rhesus rotavirus monovalent and tetravalent reassortant vaccines in US children. US Rotavirus Vaccine Efficacy Group. JAMA 273: 1191–1196.

Bernstein, D.I., Sack, D.A., Rothstein, E. Reisinger, K., Smith, V.E., O'Sullivan, D. Spriggs, D.R., and Ward, R.L. 1999. Efficacy of live, attenuated human rotavirus vaccine 89-12 in infants: A randomised placebo-controlled trial. Lancet 354: 287–290.

Bernstein, D.I., Sack, D.A., Reisinger, K., Rothstien, E., and Ward, R.L. 2002. Second year follow-up evaluation of live, attenuated human rotavirus 89-12 vaccine in healthy infants. J. Infect. Dis. 186: 1487–1489.

Bernstein, D.I., Sander, D.S., Smith, V.E., Schiff, G.M., and Ward, R.L. 1991. Protection from rotavirus reinfection. Two year prospective study. J. Infect. Dis. 164: 277–283.

Bernstein, D.I., Smith, V.E., Sander, D.S., Pax, K.A., Schiff, G.M., and Ward, R.L. 1990. Evaluation of WC3 rotavirus vaccine and correlates of protection in healthy infants. J. Infect. Dis. 162: 1055–1062.

Bernstein, D.I., Smith, V.E., Sherwood, J.R., Schiff, G.M., Sander, D.S., deFeudis, D., Spriggs, D.R., and Ward, R.L. 1998. Safety and immunogenicity of live, attenuated human rotavirus vaccine 89-12. Vaccine 16: 381–387.

Bhan, M.K., Lew, J.F., Sazawal, S., Das, B.K., Gentsch, J.R., and Glass, R. 1993. Protection conferred by neonatal rotavirus infection against subsequent diarrhea. J. Infect. Dis. 168: 282–287.

Bishop, R.F., Davidson, G.P., Holmes, I.H., and Ruck, B.J. 1973. Virus particles in epithelial cells of duodenal mucosa of children with gastroenteritis. Lancet 2: 1281–1283.

Bishop, R.F., Barnes, G.L., Cipriani, E., and Lund, J.S. 1983. Clinical immunity after neonatal rotavirus infection: A prospective longitudinal study in young children. N. Engl. J. Med. 309: 72–76.

Blutt, S.E., Kirkwood, C.D., Parreno, V., Warfield, K.L., Ciarlet, M., Estes, M.K., Bok, K., and Bishop, R.F. 2003. Rotavirus antigenaemia and viraemia: A common event? Lancet 362: 1445–1449.

Bresee, J.S., Glass, R.I., Ivanoff, B., and Gentsch, J. 1999. Current status and future priorities for rotavirus vaccine development, evaluation and implementation in developing countries. Vaccine 17: 2207–2222.

Bresee, J.S., El Arifeen, S., Azim, T., Chakraborty, J., Mounts, A.W., Podde, G., Gentsch, J.R., Ward, R.L., Black, R., Glass, R.I., and Yunus, M. 2001. Safety and immunogenicity of tetravalent rhesus based rotavirus vaccine in Bangladesh. Pediatric Infect. Dis. J. 20: 1136–1143.

Bresee, J.S., Glass, R.I., Parashar, U.D., and Gentsch, J.R. 2003. Rotavirus. In: B.S. Bloom and P.H. Lambert eds. The Vaccine Book. Academic Press, London, pp. 225–243.

Centers for Disease Control and Prevention. 1999. Rotavirus Vaccines for the prevention of rotavirus gastroenteritis among children – Recommendations of the Advisory Committee on Immunization Practices. MMWR 48: 1–23.

Centers for Disease Control and Prevention. 1999. Intussusception among recipients of rotavirus vaccine – United States 1998–1999. MMWR 48: 577–581.

Christy, C., Madore, H.P., Treanor, J.J., Pray, K., Kapikian, A.Z., Chanock, R.M,. and Dolin, R. 1986. Safety and reactogenicity of the live attenuated rhesus monkey rotavirus vaccine. J. Infect. Dis. 154: 1045–1047.

Clark, H.F., Bernstein, D.I., Dennehy, P.H., Offit, P., Pichichero, M., Treanor, J., Ward, R.L., Krah, D.L., Shaw, A., Dallas, M., Laura, D., Eiden, J.J., Ivanoff, N., Kaplan, K.M., and Heaton, P. 2004. Safety, efficacy and immunogenicity of a live quadrivalent human-bovine reassortant rotavirus vaccine in healthy infants. J. Pediatr. 144: 184–190.

Clark, H.F., Borian, F.E., and Plotkin, S.A. 1990. Immune protection of infants against rotavirus gastroenteritis by a serotype 1 reassortant of bovine rotavirus WC3. J. Infect. Dis. 161: 1099–1104.

Clark, H.F., Burke, C.J., Volkin, D.B., Offit, P.A., Ward, R.L., Bresee, J.S., Dennehy, P., Gooch, W.M., Malacaman, E., Matson, D., Walter, E., Watson, B., Krah, D.L., Dallas, M.J., Schodel, F., Kaplan, M., and Heaton, P. 2003. Safety, immunogenicity and efficacy in healthy infants of G1 and G2 human reassortant rotavirus vaccine in a new stabiliser/buffer liquid formulation. Pediatr. Infect. Dis. J. 22: 914–920.

Clark, H.F., Furukawa, F., Bell, L.M., Offit, P.A., Perella, P.A., and Plotkin, S.A. 1986. Immune response of infants and children to low passage bovine rotavirus (strain WC3). Am. J. Dis. Child. 140: 350–355.

Clark, H.F., Offit, P.A., Ellis, R.W., Eiden, J.J., Krah, D., Shaw, A.R., Pichichero, M., Treanor, J.J., Borian, F.E., Bell, L.M., and Plotkin, S.A. 1996. The development of multivalent bovine rotavirus (strain WC3) reassortant vaccine for infants. J. Infect. Dis. 174S: s73–80.

Clark, H.F., Offit, P.A., Glass, R.I., and Ward, R.L. 2003. Rotavirus Vaccines. In: S.A. Plotkin and Orenstein W.A. Vaccines, 4th Ed. Saunders, pp. 1327–1345.

Clark, H.F., White, C.J., Offit, P.A., et al. 1995. Preliminary evaluation of safety and efficacy of quadrivalent human-bovine reassortant rotavirus vaccine. Pediatr. Res. 37: 172.

Clemens, J.D., Ward, R.L., Rao, M.R., Sack D.A., Knowlton, D.R., van Loon, F.P., Huda, S., McNeal, M., Ahmed, F., and Schiff G. 1992. Sero-epidemiologic evaluation of antibodies to rotavirus as correlates of the risk of clinically significant rotavirus diarrhea in rural Bangladesh. J. Infect. Dis. 165: 161–165.

Clements-Mann, M.L., Makhene, M.K., Mrukowicz, J., Wright, P.F., Hoshino, Y., Midthun, K., Sperber, E., Karron, R., and Kapikian. A.Z. 1999. Safety and immunogenicity of live attenuated human-bovine (UK) reassortant rotavirus vaccines with VP7-specificity for serotypes 1, 2, 3, or 4 in adults, children and infants. Vaccine 17: 2715–2725.

Clements-Mann, M.L., Dudas, R., Hoshino, Y., Nehring, P., Sperber, E., Wagner, M., Stephens, I., Karron, R., Deforest, A., and Kapikian, A.Z. 2001. Safety and immunogenicity of live attenuated quadrivalent human-bovine (UK) reassortant rotavirus vaccine administered with childhood vaccines to infants. Vaccine 19: 4676–4684.

Cunliffe, N.A., Gondwe, J.S., Broadhead, R.L., Mol.yneaux, M.E., Woods, P.A., Bresee, J.S., Glass, R.I., Gentsch, J.E., and Hart, C.A. 1999. Rotavirus G and P types in children with acute diarrhea in Blantyre, Malawi from 1997 to 1998. Predominance of novel P[6]G8 strains. J. Med. Virol. 57: 308–312.

Cunliffe, N.A., Kilgore, P.E., Bresee, J.S., Steele, A.D., Luo, N., Hart, C.A., and Glass, R.I. 1998. Epidemiology of rotavirus diarrhea in Africa: A review to assess the need for rotavirus immunization. Bull. W.H.O. 76: 525–537.

Das, B.K., Gentsch, J.R., Hoshino, Y., Ishida, S.I., Nakagomi, O., Bhan, M.K., Kumar, O., and Glass, R. 1993. Characterisation of the G serotype and genogroup of New Delhi newborn rotavirus strain 116E. Virology 197: 99–107.

Das, S., Genstch, J.R., Cicirello, H.G., Woods, P.A., Gupta A., Ramachandran, M., Kumar, R., Bhan, M.K., and Glass, R.I. 1994. Characterisation of rotavirus strains from newborns in New Delhi, India. J. Clin. Microbiol. 32: 1820–1822.

De Vos, B., Vesikari, T., Linhores, A.C., Salinas, B., Perez-Schael, I., Ruiz-Palacios, G.M., Guerrero Mde, L., Phua, K.B., Delem, A., and Hardt, K. 2004. A rotavirus vaccine for prophylaxis of infants against rotavirus gastroenteritis. Pediatr. Infect. Dis. J. 23: S179–S182.

De Zoysa, I., and Feachem, R.G. 1985. Interventions for the control of diarrheal disease among young children: Rotavirus and cholera immunization. Bull. WHO 63: 569–583.

Dearlove, J., Latham, P., Dearlove, B., Pearl, K., Thomson, A., and Lewis, I.G. 1983. Clinical range of neonatal rotavirus infection. BMJ 286: 1473–1475.

Desselberger, U., Iturriza-Gomara, M., and Gray, J.J. 2001. Rotavirus epidemiology and surveillance. In: Gastroenteritis Viruses. Novartis Foundation Symposium 238. John Wiley and Sons, Lrd, London. pp. 125–152.

Estes, M.K. 2001. Rotaviruses and their replication. In: Fields Virology, fourth edition. D.M. Knipe, P.M. Howley, D.E. Griffin, R.A. Lamb, M.A. Martin, B. Roizman, S.E. Strauss, eds. Lippincott, Williams & Wilkins, Philadelphia, pp. 1747–1785.

Estes, M.K., and Graham, D.Y. 1985. Rotavirus antigens. Adv. Exp. Med. Biol. 185: 201–214.

Estes, M.K., Graham, D.Y., and Dimitrov, D.H. 1984. The Molecular epidemiology of rotavirus gastroenteritis. Prog. Med. Virol. 29: 1–22.

Fischer, T.H., Valentiner-Branth, P., Steinsland, H., Perch, M., Santos, G., Aaby, P., Mol.bak, K., and Sommerfelt, H. 2002. Protective immunity after natural rotavirus infection: A community cohort study of newborn children in Guinea Bissau, West Africa. J. Infect. Dis. 186: 593–597.

Flores, J., Midthun, K., Hoshino, Y., Green, K.Y., Gorziglia, M., Kapkian, A.Z., and Chanock, R.M. 1986. Conservation of the fourth gene among rotaviruses recovered from asymptomatic newborn infants and its possible role in attenuation. J. Virol. 60: 972–979.

Flores, J., Perrez-Schael, I., Blanco, M., White, L., Garcia, D., Vilar, M., Cunto, W., Gonzalez, R., Urbina, C., Boher, J., Mendez, M., and Kapikian, A.Z. 1990. Comparison of the reactogenicity and antigenicity of M37 rotavirus vaccine and rhesus rotavirus based quadrivalent vaccine. Lancet 336: 330–334.

Flores, J., Perez-Schael, I., Gonzalez, M., Garcia, D., Perez, M., Daoud, N., Cunot, W., and Kapikian, A.Z. 1987. Protection against severe rotavirus diarrhea by rhesus rotavirus vaccine in Venezuelan infants. Lancet i: 882–884.

Franco, M.A., and Greenberg, H.B. 1995. Role of B cells and cytotoxic T lymphocytes in clearance of and immunity to rotavirus infection in mice. J. Virol. 69: 7800–7806.

Gentsch, J.,R,, Woods, P,A,, Ramachandran, M., Das, B.K., Leite, J.P., Alfieri, A., Kumar, R., Bhan, M.K., and Glass, R.I. 1996. Review of G and P typing results from a global collection of rotavirus strains: Implications for vaccine development. J. Infect. Dis. 174: 530–536.

Gorrell, R.J., and Bishop, R.F. 1999. Homotypic and heterotypic serum neutralising antibody response to rotavirus proteins following natural primary infection and reinfection in children. J. Med. Virol. 59: 204–211.

Gorziglia, M., Hoshino, Y., Buckler-White, A., Blumentals, I., Glass, R., Flores, J., Kapikian, A.Z., and Chanock, R.M. 1986. Conservation of amino acid sequence of VP8 and the cleavage region of 84kDa outer capsid protein among rotaviruses recovered from asymptomatic neonatal infection. Proc. Natl. Acad. Sci. USA 83: 7039–7043.

Gorziglia, M., Hoshino, Y., Nishikawa, K., Maby, W.L., Jones, R., Kapikian, A.Z., and Chanock, R.M. 1988. Comparative sequence analysis of the genomic segment 6 of four rotaviruses each with different subgroup specificity. J. Gen. Virol. 69: 1659–1669.

Gorziglia, M., Larralde, G., Kapikian, A.Z., and Chanock, R.M. 1990. Antigenic relationships among human rotaviruses as determined by outer capsid protein VP4. Proc. Natl. Acad. Sci. USA 87: 7155–7159.

Greenberg, H.B., McAuliffe, A., Valdesuso, J., Wyatt, R.G., Flores, J., Kalica, A.R., Hoshino Y., and Singh, N.H. 1983. Serological analysis of the subgroup protein of rotavirus, using monoclonal antibodies. Infect. Immun. 39: 91–99.

Greenberg, H.B., Clark, H.F., and Offit, P.A. 1994. Rotavirus pathology and pathophysiology. Curr. Top. Microbiol. Immunol. 185: 255–283.

Halsey, N.A., Anderson, E.L., Sears, S.D., Steinhoff, M., Wilson, M., Belshe, R.B., Midthun, K., Kapikian, A.Z., Chanock, R.M., Samorodin, R., Burns, R., and Clemens, M. 1988. Human-rhesus reassortant rotavirus vaccines. Safety and immunogenicity in adults, children and infants. J. Infect. Dis. 158: 1261–1267.

Hjelt, K., Grauballe, P.C., Paerregaard, A., Nielsen, O.H., and Krasilnikoff, P.A. 1987. Protective efficacy of pre-existing rotavirus-specific immunoglobulin A against naturally acquired rotavirus infection in children. J. Med. Virol. 21: 39–47.

Holmes, I.H., Ruck, B.J., Bishop, R.F., and Davidson, G.P. 1975. Infantile enteritis viruses: Morphogenesis and morphology. J.Virol. 16: 937–943.

Hoshino, Y., Jones, R.W., Chanock, R.M., and Kapikian, A.Z. 1997. Construction of four double gene substitution human x bovine rotavirus reassortant vaccine candidates. J. Med. Virol. 51: 319–325.

Hoshino, Y., Sereno, M.M., Midthun, K., Flores, J., Kapikian, A.Z., and Chanock, R.M. 1985. Independent segregation of two antigenic specificities (VP3 and VP7) involved in neutralisation of the rotavirus infectivity. Proc. Natl. Acad. Sci. USA 82: 8701–8704.

Hoshino, Y., Wyatt, R.G., Greenberg, H.B., Flores, J., and Kapikian, A.Z. 1984. Serotypic similarity and diversity among rotaviruses of mammalian and avian origin as studied by plaque-reduction neutralization. J. Infect. Dis. 149: 694–702.

Hoshino, Y., Sereno, M.M., Kapikian, A.Z., and Chanock, R.M. 1993. Genetic determinants of rotavirus virulence studied in the gnotobiotic piglets. In: Vaccine 93. Cold Spring Harbor, N.Y., Cold Spring Harbor Laboratory Press, pp. 277–283.

Iturriza-Gomara, M., Isherwood, B., Desselberger, U., and Gray J.J. 2002. Reassortment in vivo. A driving force for diversity of human rotavirus strains isolated in the UK between 1995 and 1999. J. Virol. 8: 3696–3705.

Jaimes, M.C., Rojas, O.L., Gonzalez, A.M., Cajiao, I., Charpilienne, A., Pothier, P., Kohli, E., Greenberg, H.B., Franco, M.A., and Angel, J. 2002. Frequencies of virus-specific CD4 and CD8 T lymphocytes secreting gamma interferon after acute natural rotavirus infection in children and adults. J. Virol. 76: 4741–4749.

Jiang, B., Gentsch, J.R., and Glass, R.I. 2002. The role of serum antibodies in the protection against rotavirus disease: An overview. Clin. Infect. Dis. 34: 1351–1361.

Joensuu, J., Koskenniemi, E., Pang, X.L., and Vesikari, T. 1997. Randomised placebo controlled trial of the rhesus-human reassortant rotavirus vaccine for prevention of severe rotavirus gastroenteritis. Lancet 350: 1205–1209.

Kapikian, A.Z., Hoshino, Y., Chanock, R.M., and Perez-Schael, I. 1996. Efficacy of a quadrivalent rhesus rotavirus-based vaccine aimed at preventing severe rotavirus diarrhea in infants and young children. J. Infect. Dis. 174S: s65-s72.

Kapikian, A.Z., Hoshino, Y., and Chanock, R.M. 2001. Rotaviruses. In: Fields Virology, fourth edition. D.M. Knipe, P.M. Howley, D.E. Griffin, R.A. Lamb, M.A. Martin, B. Roizman, S.E. Strauss, eds. Lippincott, Williams, Wilkins & Philadelphi, pp. 1787–1833.

Kapikian, A.Z., Wyatt, R.G., Levine, M.M., Yolken, R.H., van Kirk, D.M., Dolin, R. Greenberg, H.B., and Chanock, R.M. 1983. Oral administration of human rotavirus to volunteers: Induction of illness and correlates of resistance. J. Infect. Dis. 147: 95–106.

Kohli, E., Maurice, L., Vautherot, J.F., Bourgeios, C., Bour, J.B., Cohen, J., and Pothier, P. 1992. Localisation of group-specific epitopes on the major capsid protein of group A rotavirus. J. Gen. Virol. 73: 907–914.

Kosek, M., Bern, C., and Guerrant, R.L. 2003. The global burden of diarrheal disease, as estimated from studies published between 1992 and 2000. Bull. WHO 81: 197–204.

Lundgren, O., Peregrin, A.T., Persson, K., Kordasti, S., Uhnoo, I., and Svensson, L. 2000. Role of the enteric nervous system in the fluid and electrolyte secretion of rotavirus diarrhea. Science 287: 409–411.

McNeal, M.M., rae, M.N., and Ward, R.L. 1997. Evidence that resolution of rotavirus infection in mice is due to both CD4 and CD8 cell-dependent activities. J. Virol. 71: 8735–8742.

Mebus, C.A., Stair, E.L., Underdahl, N.R., and Twiehaus, M.J. 1974. Pathology of neonatal calf diarrhea induced by a reo-like virus. Vet. Pathol. 8: 490–505.

Michelangeli, F., Lipriandi, F., Chemello, M.E., Ciarlet, M., and Ruiz, M.C. 1995. Selective depletion of stored calcium by thapsigargin blocks rotavirus maturation but not cytopathic effect. J. Virol. 69: 3838–3847.

Midthun, K., Greenberg, H.B., Hoshino, Y., Kapikian, A.Z., Wyatt, R.G., and Chanock, R.M. 1985. Reassortant rotaviruses as potential live rotavirus vaccine candidates. J. Virol. 53: 949–954.

Midthun, K., and Kapikian, A.Z. 1996. Rotavirus Vaccines: An overview. Clin. Microbiol. Rev. 9: 423–434.

Murphy, B.R., Morens, D.M., Simonsen, L., Chanock, R.M., La Montagne, J.R., and Kapikian, A.Z. 2003. Reappraisal of the association of intussusception with the licensed live rotavirus vaccine challenges initial conclusions. J. Infect. Dis. 187: 1301–1308.

Murphy, T.V., Smith, P.J., Gargiullo, P.M., and Schwartz, B. 2003. The first rotavirus vaccine and intussusception: Epidemiological studies and policy decisions. J. Infect. Dis. 187: 1309–1313.

Offit, P.A., and Blavat, G. 1986. Identification of the two rotavirus genes determining neutralisation specificities. J. Virol. 57: 376–378.

Offit, P.A., Hoffenberg, E.J., Santos, N., and Gouvea V. 1993. Rotavirus-specific humoral and cellular immune response after primary symptomatic infection. J. Infect. Dis. 167: 1436–1440.

O'Ryan, M.L., Matson, D.O., Estes, M.K., and Pickering, L.K. 1994. Anti-rotavirus G type specific antibodies in children with natural rotavirus infections. J. Infect. Dis. 169: 504–511.

Parashar, U.D., Hummelman, E.G., Bresee, J.S., Miller, M.A., and Glass, R.I. 2003. Global illness and deaths caused by rotavirus disease in children. Emerg. Infect. Dis. 9: 565–572.

Pearson, G.R., and McNulty, M.S. 1977. Pathological changes in the small intestine of neonatal pigs infected with a pig reo-like agent (rotavirus). J. Comp. Pathol. 87: 363–375.

Perez-Schael, I., Guntinas, M.J., Perez, M., Pagone, V., Rojas, A.M., Gonzalez, R. Cunto, W., and Kapikian, A.Z. 1997. Efficacy of the rhesus rotavirus based quadrivalent vaccine in infants and young children in Venezuela. N. Engl. J. Med. 337: 1181–1187.

Perez-Schael, I., Salinas, B., Linhares, A.C., Guerrero, M.L. Ruiz-Palacios, G., Clemens, S.A., Jacquet, J., and de Vos, B. 2002. Protective efficacy of an oral human rotavirus (HRV) vaccine in Latin American infants. Annual Meeting of the Interscience Conference on Anti-microbial Agents and Chemotyerapy. San Diego. Abstract.

Peters, G., and Myers, M.G. 2002. Intussusception, rotavirus and other oral vaccines: Summary of a Workshop. Pediatrics 110: e67.

Prasad, B.V.V., and Chiu, W. 1994. Structure of rotaviruses. Curr. Top. Microbiol. Immunol. 185: 9–29.

Rao, C.D., Gowda, K., and Reddy, B.S.Y. 2001. Sequence analysis of theVP4 and VP7 genes of nontypeable strains identifies a new pair of outer capsid proteins representing novel P and G genotypes in bovine rotaviruses. Virol. 276: 104–113.

Rennels, M.B., Glass, R.I., Dennehy, P.H., Bernstein, D.I. Pichichero, M.E., Zito, E.T., Mack, M.E., Davidson, B.L., and Kapikian, A.Z. 1996. Safety and efficacy of the high dose rhesus-human reassortant rotavirus vaccines: Report of the national multicentre trial. Pediatrics 97: 7–13.

Ruiz-Palacios, G.,. 2002. World Society for Paediatric Infectious Diseases Congress. Santiago, Chile. Abstract.

Santos, N., Lima, R.C.C., Pereira, C.F.A., and Gouvea, V. 1998. Detection of rotavirus types G8 and G10 among Brazilian children with diarrhea. J. Clin. Microbiol. 36: 2727–2729.

Santosham, M., Letson, G.W., Wolff, M., Reid, R., Gahagan, S., Adams, R., Callahan, C., Sack, R.B., and Kapikian, A.Z. 1991. A field study of the safety and efficacy of two candidate rotavirus vaccines in a Native American population. J. Infect. Dis. 163: 483–487.

Santosham, M., Yolken, R.H., Quiroz, E., Dillman, L., Oro, G., Reeves, W.C., and Sack, R.B. 1983. Detection of rotavirus in respiratory secretions of children with pneumonia. J. Pediatr. 103: 58.

Santosham, M., Moulton, L.H., Reid, R., Croll, J., Weatherholt, R., Ward, R., Forro, J., Zito, E., Mack, M., Brenneman, G., and Davidson, B.L. 1997. Efficacy and safety of high-dose rhesus-human reassortment rotavirus vaccine in Native American populations. J. Pediatr. 131: 632–638.

Schoub, B.D., Koornhof, H.J., Lecatsas, G., Prozesky, O.W., Freiman, I., Hartman, E., and Kassel, H. 1975. Viruses in acute summer gastroenteritis in black infants. Lancet ii: 1093–1094.

Staat, M.A., Azimi, P.H., Berke, T., Roberts, N., Bernstein, D.I., Ward, R.L., Pickering, L.K., and Matson, D.O. 2002. Clinical presentations of rotavirus infection among hospitalised children. Pediatr. Infect. Dis. J. 21: 221–227.

Steele, A.D., Garcia, D., Sears, J.F., Gerna, G., Nakagomi O., and Flores, J. 1993. Distribution of VP4 gene alleles in human rotaviruses using PCR-generated probes to the hyperdivergent region of the VP4 gene. J. Clin. Microbiol. 31: 1735–1740.

Steele, A.D., and Ivanoff, B. 2003. Rotavirus strains circulating in Africa. The emergence of G9 and P[6] strains. Vaccine 21: 361–367.

Svensson, L., Grhnquist, L., Pattersson, C.A., Grandien, M., Stintzing, G. and Greenberg, H.B. 1988. Detection of human rotaviruses which do not react with subgroup I and II specific monoclonal antibodies. J. Clin. Microbiol. 26: 1238–1240.

Taniguchi, K., Urasawa, T. Urasawa, S., and Yasuhara, T. 1984. Production of subgroup specific monoclonal antibodies against human rotaviruses and their application to an enzyme-linked immunosorbent assay for subgroup determination. J. Med. Virol. 14: 115–125.

Velazquez, F.R., Matson, D.O., Calva, J.J., Guerrero, M.L., Morrow, A.L., Carter- Campbell, S., Glass, R.I., Estes, M.K., Pickering, L.K., and Ruiz-Palacois, G.M. 1996. Rotavirus infection in infants as protection against subsequent infections. N. Engl. J. Med. 335: 1022–1028.

Vesikari, T., Clark, H.F., Offit, P.A. Schodel, F., Dallas, M., Heaton, P., Krah, D., Shaw, A., Garbarg-Chenon, A., Golm, G., Kaplan, K.M., and Sadoff, J. 2002. The effect of dose and composition of a pentavalent rotavirus reassortant vaccine (RotaTeq™) upon safety, efficacy and immunogenicity in healthy infants. Annual Meeting of the Infectious Diseases Society of America. Chicago, Abstract.

Vesikari, T., Green, K.Y., Flores, J., and Kapikian, A.Z. 1992. Protective efficacy against serotype 1 rotavirus diarrhea by live oral rhesus reassortant rotavirus vaccines with human rotavirus VP7 serotype specificity. Pediatr. Infect. Dis. J. 11: 535–542.

Vesikari, T., Karvonen, A., Espo, M. Korhonen, T., Bernstein, D.I., Delem, A., and de Vos, B. 2002. Evaluation of an oral human rotavirus (HRV) vaccine RIX4414 in Europe. Annual Meeting of the Interscience Conference on Anti-microbial Agents and Chemotherapy. San Diego, Abstract.

Vesikari, T., Ruuska, T., Koivu, H.P., Green, K.Y., Flores, J., and Kapikian, A.Z. 1991. Evaluation of the M37 human rotavirus vaccine in 2 to 6-month old infants. Pediatr. Infect. Dis. J. 10: 912–917.

Ward, R.L. 2003. Possible mechanisms of protection elicited by candidate rotavirus vaccines as determined with the adult mouse model. Viral Immunol. 6: 17–24.

Ward, R.L., and Bernstein, D.I. 1994. Protection against rotavirus disease after natural infection. J. Infect. Dis. 169: 900–904.

Ward, R.L., Bernstein, D.I., and Shukla, R. 1989. Effects of antibody to rotavirus on protection of adults challenged with human rotavirus. J. Infect. Dis. 159: 79–88.

Weijer, C. 2000. The future of research into rotavirus vaccines. Development, current issues and future prospects. BMJ 321: 525–526.

World Health Organisation. 2000. Report of the meeting on the Future Directions for Rotavirus Research in Developing Countries. Geneva, WHO/V&B/.00.23.

Zheng, B.J., Chang, R.X., Ma, G.Z., Xie, J.M., Liu, Q., Liu, X.R., and Ng, M.H. 1991. Rotavirus infection of the oropharynx and respiratory in young children. J. Med. Virol. 34: 29–37.

Chapter 12

Development of Vaccines Against Human Papillomavirus (HPV)

Russell L. Basser, Stirling Edwards and Ian H. Frazer

Abstract

Human papillomavirus (HPV) is associated with a common and usually asymptomatic infection, and occurs especially after commencement of sexual activity. Pathology related to persistent HPV infection is a major cause of mortality and morbidity worldwide. While it has long been accepted as a major etiological agent in the development of cervical cancer and anogenital warts, it is increasingly recognized as having a critical role in the development of cancers involving other anogenital sites and distant locations, such as the head and neck. The pivotal discovery of how to produce virus-like particles (VLPs) of HPV capsid in the early 1990s has resulted in the development of a prophylactic vaccine. Early clinical trials of VLPs have demonstrated remarkable efficacy in preventing persistent HPV infection, and results from phase III trials are expected in the next 2 to 3 years. A variety of approaches to therapy for established HPV infection and its consequences are currently being pursued, but progress has been slow and, as yet, no controlled clinical data have been published. Successful development of prophylactic and therapeutic vaccines for HPV infection will have a profound impact on healthcare in both developed and developing countries.

INTRODUCTION

Human papillomviruses (HPVs) are epitheliotropic viruses that infect cutaneous and mucosal tissue. Papillomaviruses are species-specific and while many animals harbor the virus, cross-infection does not occur. They are non-enveloped DNA viruses with a double stranded genome of approximately 8 kbp, and the virion is an icosahedral particle of around 55nm diameter. There are over 100 different HPV genotypes and these show a high degree of specificity for infection of particular tissues (McMurray *et al.*, 2001; Sisk *et al.*, 2002; Stanley, 2001), with approximately 30 types infecting only the anogenital region (Stubenrauch *et al.*, 1999). HPV is one of the most common sexually transmitted diseases and exposure to the virus generally occurs within a short time after the onset of sexual activity (Burk *et al.*, 1996; Ho *et al.*, 1998). It is estimated that at any one time there are 20 million people with anogenital HPV infection in the USA alone, and 5.5 million new infections every year (Tracking the Hidden Epidemics, 2001).

HPV genotypes are generally divided into two classes, depending on the pathology they cause. 'Low risk' types are aetiologically linked to benign lesions such as warts and low grade dysplasia, with HPV 6 and 11 causing most cases of anogenital warts. 'High-risk' types are associated with premalignant lesions and cancer of the cervix and a number of other sites (McMurray *et al.*, 2001).

The epidemiological and molecular evidence for the role of HPV infection in anogenital intraepithelial neoplasia and anogenital cancer is no longer controversial. Indeed, cervical cancer is the first malignancy to be causally linked to an infection by the World Health Organization (Bosch *et al.*, 2002). Using nucleic acid amplification techniques, HPV DNA is detected in 99% of cervical cancer specimens. Detailed investigations of the few cervical cancer specimens which appear to be HPV DNA negative strongly suggest that these are false negatives (Walboomers *et al.*, 1999). There are about 370,000 cases of cervical cancer worldwide each year, making it the third most common cancer in females. However it is the most common cancer in women living in developing countries. The lack of population-based screening and modern treatment techniques also results in substantial mortality and morbidity in these regions.

NATURAL HISTORY OF HUMAN PAPILLOMAVIRUS INFECTION

Most knowledge of the natural history of HPV infection comes from studies in women undergoing screening and treatment for cervical pathology. Genital HPV infections are predominantly transmitted though contact during sexual intercourse. In the majority of people, HPV infection remains asymptomatic and resolves spontaneously (Moscicki *et al.*, 1998), although many women are later reinfected with a new genotype or may experience reactivation of their initial infection (Ho *et al.*, 1998; Richardson *et al.*, 2003).

Persistent anogenital infection is associated with a range of benign and malignant epithelial lesions. The likelihood of persistent infection is related to HPV type, the number of sexual partners, sexual behaviour, age at acquisition and whether or not an individual is immunosuppressed (Schlecht *et al.*, 2001). The genotypes linked with different pathologies are shown in Table 12.1. The most common high-risk types are HPV16 and HPV18, which account for more than 70% of cervical pre-cancerous lesions and cancer (Munoz *et al.*, 2003). All HPV types may be associated with low-grade cytological abnormalities of the cervix, which are commonly found in response to recently acquired infection and generally spontaneously clear (Holowaty *et al.*, 1999). In contrast, one study

Table 12.1 Classification of papillomavirus

Group	Prototypes	Site of infection	Acute consequences	Chronic consequences	NB
Mucosal low risk	HPV6, 11, COPV, ROPV	Genital mucosa	Warts	Nil	Slow resolution in immunosuppressed subjects
Mucosal high risk	HPV16, 18, 31, 33, 35, 39, 45, 51, 52, 56, 58, 59, 68, 73, 82, BPV4	Anogenital mucosa (other mucosal surfaces)	Flat lesion (CIN)	~2% persist, ~1% progress to invasive cancer	Slow resolution in immunosuppressed subjects, variable malignant potential
Cutaneous low risk	HPV1, 2, BPV1	Skin	Warts	Nil	Synchronous regression, lasting immunity
Cutaneous high risk	HPV5, 8, CRPV	Skin	Flat lesion or nil	?Promotes squamous skin cancer (SqCC)	SqCC more common in immunosuppressed subjects

COPV, canine oral papillomavirus; ROPV, rabbit oral papillomavirus; BPV, bovine papillomavirus; CRPV, cottontail rabbit papillomavirus.

found that 28% of women with persistent high-risk HPV infection developed high-grade cervical intraepithelial neoplasia (CIN), the precursor lesion to cervical cancer, over a 2-year period (Koutsky et al., 1992). Although the majority of high-grade CIN lesions are found within 1 to 2 years of initial infection, there is usually an interval of many years to the development of cancer (Myers et al., 2000; Nobbenhuis et al., 2001; Wallin et al., 1999). High-grade CIN may regress spontaneously, but it is estimated that about 36% will progress to invasion if left untreated (McIndoe et al., 1984). There are currently no tools with which to identify those lesions that will progress, making it necessary to treat all women with high-grade CIN.

HPV infection is also associated with other anogenital malignancy, including vulvar (Hart, 2001), vagina (Sugase et al., 1997), penis (Dillner et al., 2000) and anal canal (Palefsky et al., 1991) cancers. Nonetheless, compared with cervical disease, HPV appears to be less commonly found in most of these cancers with the exception of anal cancer (Schiffman et al., 2003). HPV DNA is found in up to 94% of anal cancers and is often preceded by anal intraepithelial lesions (AIN) akin to those observed in the cervix (Holly et al., 2001; Palefsky et al., 1991; Palefsky et al., 1998). There are anatomical similarities between the cervix and anus in that both have a transformation zone which is especially susceptible to HPV infection with a high risk of neoplastic transformation. The risk of anal HPV infection and cancer is linked to the number of sexual partners, homosexual contact, other sexually transmitted diseases, and receptive anal intercourse. Patients with HIV infection have a particularly high incidence of anal HPV infection and pathology (Piketty et al., 2003), and the incidence of anal cancer in HIV infected people is about twice that of non-infected, matched controls (Palefsky et al., 2003). It should also be noted that cervical HPV infection and cancer are also more frequent in HIV-positive women (Palefsky, 2003). Furthermore, available data suggest that screening for abnormal anal cytology may well be cost-effective in people at risk for HIV infection (Goldie et al., 1999; Goldie et al., 2000).

Probably the most common anogenital pathology associated with HPV infection is genital warts, which are present in an estimated 1% of the population (Wiley et al., 2002), with an additional 500,000 to 1 million new cases per year in the USA (Gunter, 2003). Over 90% of warts result from infection with HPV type 6 or 11 (Beutner et al., 1999). Warts can spontaneously regress, remain unchanged over a long period of time, or increase in size and number. It should be noted that even if asymptomatic, they are often a source of anxiety for patients and may be cosmetically unsightly. There is no reliable way to determine in which patients lesions will resolve and when this might occur.

HPV infection is also thought to contribute to a number of non-genital benign lesions and cancers (Gillison et al., 2003). There is increasing evidence of a causal link to head and neck cancers, particularly of the oropharynx (Mork et al., 2001). Recurrent respiratory papillomatosis is a rare condition of infants related to HPV infection (nearly always HPV types 6 and 11) that is transferred from the mother at childbirth. It causes respiratory obstruction and may be life threatening (Wiatrak, 2003). Other less well-defined associations of disease and HPV infection include squamous cell carcinoma of the esophagus (Shen et al., 2002) and non-melanoma skin cancer (Harwood et al., 2000).

MANAGEMENT OF HPV-ASSOCIATED ANOGENITAL DISEASE

Management of HPV-associated anogenital disease varies with the site of the pathology and the risk carried for the sufferer. For instance, management of cervical HPV disease is based on identification and eradication of high-grade lesions to prevent the development of cancer. Decades of systematic cervical cytological screening programs in most developed countries have resulted in a drastic reduction in the incidence of and mortality from cervical cancer. Once detected, high-grade CIN is excised by removing the transformation zone of the cervix by one of several possible local surgical techniques. Such procedures carry little risk of acute problems such as bleeding or infection, and these usually resolve within four weeks if they occur. Long term damage to the cervix leading to cervical incompetence or stenosis is rare, and probably affects less than 0.1% of patients. Following local ablation of the cervical transformation zone, permanent clearance of the lesion can be achieved in more than 90% of women (Cox, 1999; Wright, Jr. *et al.*, 2003). Once cervical cancer is diagnosed, management is guided by the extent of cancer and general health of the patient (Cannistra *et al.*, 1996). In broad terms, treatment is multidisciplinary and involves appropriate combination of surgery, radiotherapy and chemotherapy.

The role of screening for anal HPV disease is much less well established. It is only recently that data relating to the benefit of screening in high-risk groups has been generated (Goldie *et al.*, 1999; Goldie *et al.*, 2000), and an understanding of which people are at risk is still evolving. Nevertheless, it is apparent that high-grade AIN is a premalignant condition and should be treated. In contrast to CIN, though, eradication of AIN is problematic. It tends to be multifocal, is often quite extensive in HIV-positive individuals, and removal of the transformation zone of the anus has obvious dramatic consequences. Most importantly, there has been little or no systematic, controlled evaluation of treatment for this disease, and most reports are anecdotal or, at best, retrospective reviews of practice. The common theme from such information is that relapse is common following local ablation of lesions, especially in immunocompromised patients (Chang *et al.*, 2002). Topical therapies, have been tried, but without much success (Chin-Hong *et al.*, 2002).

Anogenital condylomata (warts) are generally treated conservatively and may resolve without intervention. If required, a number of topical therapies (Gunter, 2003) are generally used, while surgical removal is usually only considered for more extensive and complicated lesions.

High-grade lesions at other sites are managed by attempting local removal, topical treatments, or a combination of both.

MOLECULAR BIOLOGY OF HUMAN PAPILLOMAVIRUS INFECTION

HPVs are exquisitely dependent upon epithelial cell differentiation for their replication. A general scheme of HPV replication begins with infection of the basal cells of the epithelium, the virus possibly gaining access through microlesions (Stubenrauch *et al.*, 1999). The viral DNA then undergoes amplification and remains in the basal cell in multiple episomal copies. When a basal cell divides one daughter progresses towards the top of the epithelial layer while differentiating. HPV manipulates this process of differentiation in a careful balancing act, forcing the cell to undergo DNA replication but not division. Under these conditions the virus is able to replicate its DNA into thousands of copies, which is then packaged into virions. Virion formation occurs only in the latter stages of differentiation as the cell approaches the top of the epithelium and becomes keratinized. The other daughter resulting from basal cell division retains HPV as multiple episomal copies until a further cell division repeats the process (McMurray *et al.*, 2001). In the absence of basal cell division HPV is able to remain in a quiescent state, which may explain why viral lesions can recur after long periods of apparent inactivity.

Given the dependence of viral replication upon cell differentiation, HPVs have proven to be virtually impossible to propagate in cell culture, except in conditions of low productivity such as the athymic mouse xenograft system and raft cultures (Kreider *et al.*, 1987; Meyers *et al.*, 1992). The inability to propagate HPV has hampered understanding of the biology of these viruses, in particular their ability to evade immune detection to avoid destruction. As well, the paucity of viral antigen material prevented definition of 'strains' based on serological comparisons, resulting in a classification of HPVs into 'genotypes' based on genomic DNA homology comparisons. It has only been since the availability of recombinant virus-like particles (VLPs) that the serological relationships of HPV genotypes have been determined (Kirnbauer *et al.*, 1992; Zhou *et al.*, 1991). In addition, the availability of pseudovirions (VLPs incorporating markers of cellular uptake) allowed the development of neutralization-like assays for a number of HPV genotypes (Unckell *et al.*, 1997; Yeager *et al.*, 2000; Zhou *et al.*, 1993). These studies suggested that genotypes essentially corresponded to serotypes and that neutralizing antibody responses were likely to be genotype specific (Cheng *et al.*, 1995; Giroglou *et al.*, 2001; Pastrana *et al.*, 2001). This has profound implications for design of prophylactic vaccines based on VLPs, as inclusion of a specific VLP for each genotype targeted by the vaccine will be required.

The genome of HPVs contains 8 to 9 open reading frames (ORFs) which code for proteins with a variety of functions and a large non-coding region, the long control region (LCR) or upstream regulatory region (URR). The LCR contains promoters for viral transcription and the origin of DNA replication. The ORFs are divided into two groups – the six to seven non-structural 'early' (E) proteins, which carry out a variety of functions related to viral replication and two 'late' (L) proteins, which form the coat of the virion. Currently identified functions of these proteins are outlined in Table 12.2, although fruitful research on discovering further functions and interactions of the E proteins is ongoing. Recent publications give a more complete analysis of E protein functions (Stanley, 2001; zur Hausen, 2000).

E6 and E7 play a central role in the oncogenicity of high risk HPVs. A clear role for E5 in oncogenesis has not been identified for HPVs, in contrast to that of bovine papillomavirus type 1 (BPV-1) (DiMaio *et al.*, 1986). Intracellular expression of E6 and E7 from HPV16 and other 'high' risk HPVs alters the growth characteristics of a variety of cell types *in vitro*, resulting in cell immortalization (E6 and E7) and transformation (E7). Significantly, E6 and E7 are the only HPV proteins consistently found to be expressed in cervical cancer tissue and in cell lines derived from the cancers (Schwarz *et al.*, 1985; Sherman *et al.*, 1992). The ongoing expression of these proteins is essential (but not sufficient) for the cellular events leading to the development and maintenance of malignancy (Alvarez-Salas *et al.*, 1999; von Knebel *et al.*, 1992; zur Hausen, 2000). As described below, E6 and E7 exert multiple effects upon cells (McMurray *et al.*, 2001; Stanley, 2001; Turek, 1994; zur Hausen, 1999; zur Hausen, 2000). A question is: which of these effects are related to malignant conversion of cells and how do these relate to the real purpose of the proteins, which is to aid establishment of the conditions for viral replication?

E6 is an 150 amino acid long nuclear protein. One of its activities is to promote the degradation of p53, which is a crucial cell protein that regulates the G_1/S-phase transition of the cell cycle. In particular, p53 prevents G_1/S transition in circumstances where the cell has sustained DNA damage. Thus, E6 can circumvent this check on cell integrity, forcing the cell into DNA synthesis and allowing the virus to replicate its DNA. It has been suggested that this activity of E6 is required to counterbalance effects by the E2 and E7

Table 12.2 Papillomavirus proteins

Designation	Group	Cellular localization and expression levels	Function	Natural immune response
L1	Late	Nuclear/++++	Major capsid protein (structural)	Antibody in 50–100%, weeks to years after infection
L2	Late	Nuclear/++	Minor capsid protein, assists DNA packaging	Nil
E1	Early	Nuclear/+	Assists episomal replication, DNA helicase	Nil
E2	Early	Nuclear/+	Transcription factor	Cellular responses associated with regressing lesions
E4	Early	Cytoplasmic/+++	Interaction with cell cytoskeleton possibly to promote virion release	Nil
E5	Early	Cytoplasmic/+	Prevents cell differentiation (more important for BPV than HPV)	Nil
E6	Intermediate	Nuclear/+	Prevents cell differentiation, promotes p53 degradation	DTH associated with regressing lesions
E7	Intermediate	Nuclear/++	Prevents cell growth arrest and differentiation, interacts with Rb protein family to block inhibitors of E2F	Antibody associated with invasive cancers

proteins, which enhance p53 activity. Left unchecked the latter would result in cell growth arrest and apoptosis before viral replication occurred. This activity is the probable origin of the contribution E6 makes to the accumulation of mutagenic events and developing aneuploidy in cells undergoing malignant conversion. E6 also regulates transcription from viral and a variety of cell promoters. One such activity that may contribute to infected cell survival is control of production of cytokines IL-6 and IL-8 via E6 inhibition of the NF-κB transcription factor.

The E7 ORF encodes an approximately 100 amino acid nuclear protein, which contains the major transforming activity of HPV. The E7 protein interacts with numerous cell proteins, particularly those related to cell growth regulation. The interaction of E7 with the Rb family (Rb, p107, p130) involves binding to hypo-phosphorylated forms of the proteins, which subsequently disrupts complexes between them and the cell transcription factor E2F. Since E2F activates DNA synthesis, the outcome of E7 activity is the premature transition of cells into S-phase. It has been suggested that the interaction of E7 with the Rb family results in a separation of cell differentiation from the cell cycle thus providing a better environment for viral replication. However, recent evidence suggests that E7 can immortalize cells by means other than Rb interaction.

In the normal viral infectious cycle E6 and E7 act in concert to promote viral replication, which occurs in differentiating, non-dividing cells. By preventing the operation of the signals that block the cell from entering S-phase and inhibiting apoptosis that should follow DNA synthesis without cell division, these viral proteins allow HPV episomal DNA to replicate to high copy number. These episomes are then available for packaging into virions through interaction with the L proteins that are synthesized in the latter stages of differentiation as the cell approaches the top of the epithelial layer.

It is of interest that the E6 and E7 proteins of low risk HPVs perform many of the above functions. However, these viruses display a greatly reduced capacity for cell immortalization and transformation. One reason for this is that the proteins from high-risk types are more active than the corresponding ones encoded by low risk viruses. For example, E7 from high-risk HPV types is more efficient in inactivating and promoting the degradation of Rb. As well, the proteins from high-risk viruses may have activities lacking in low-risk E6 and E7, such as binding to the cell proliferation regulatory proteins exemplified by PDZ, due to absence of a PDZ binding site in low-risk E6 (Munger *et al.*, 2002).

Circumstances arise where the activities of E6 and E7 become unregulated, initiating the events that can lead to malignant conversion of cells. In the normal course of HPV transcription, the E2 protein can act as a repressor of the promoter of the E6 and E7 ORFs (Desaintes *et al.*, 1996; Fuchs *et al.*, 1994). A consistent observation is that in cervical cancer cells and about half of high grade CIN harbouring HPV sequences, transcription of E6 and E7 is unchecked by this mechanism. This is as a consequence of the viral DNA being integrated into the cell genome, which typically results in deletion or disruption of the E2 ORF, thus preventing the repressive effect of the E2 protein. In this circumstance cellular transcription factors interacting with the LCR can activate E6 and E7 transcription. In cases of cancer where HPV DNA is not in an integrated state, E6 and E7 activity may be enhanced by specific deletions in the LCR. These deletions repress the activity of cell transcription factor YY1, which in turn downregulates an E6/E7 silencer in the LCR (Pfister, 1996). Given the importance of E6 and E7 in malignancy, including maintenance of the malignant state, these proteins have been the targets of a number of attempts to develop therapeutic vaccines for cervical precancer and cancer (Stanley, 2003).

The L proteins and in particular L1, the major structural protein of the virus, have been the subject of much investigation over the last decade. This came in the wake of the demonstration that recombinant L1 and L2 or L1 alone could form virus-like particles (VLPs) when expressed in eukaryote expression systems and that, as expected, these VLPs induced neutralizing antibody responses (Christensen *et al.*, 1994; Kirnbauer *et al.*, 1992; Rose *et al.*, 1994; Zhou *et al.*, 1991). The major targets of these antibodies are genotype-specific conformational epitopes (Combita *et al.*, 2002).

Studies of the HPV virion have been aided greatly by the availability of recombinant VLPs for a number of HPV types. Earlier studies relied upon isolation of HPV particles from warts and BPV isolated from bovine fibropapillomas (Baker *et al.*, 1991). The virus particle is an icosahedron made up of 72 pentameric capsomers, each consisting of five copies of the L1 protein, giving a total of 360 copies of L1 per virion. Sixty of the capsomers are hexavalent, contacting six neighbours. The remaining 12 are pentavalent. L1's role in the virus life cycle appears to be restricted to being the major structural protein of the virion including a primary role in viral entry into the cell (Day *et al.*, 2003). The exact number of L2 copies per virion remains controversial with modelling based on BPV suggesting there are 12 copies per virion, each associated with a pentavalent capsomer (Trus *et al.*, 1997). A portion of the L2 protein is on the surface of the viral particle and may have a role in entry into cells (Kawana *et al.*, 2001). As L2 appears to be required for genome encapsidation and binds DNA, it may be in contact with the viral genome in the virion and/or during packaging (Zhou *et al.*, 1994). However, L2 may have a variety of additional roles, interacting with a number of cell proteins and possibly playing a part in intracellular trafficking of viral proteins (Gornemann *et al.*, 2002).

Studies using various animal papillomaviruses have demonstrated that humoral immune responses directed at the structural proteins of the virus are induced by infection and that these apparently provide protection against subsequent virus challenge. Recombinant L1 VLPs of the relevant virus type have been used as immunogens in vaccination studies in dogs [canine oral papillomavirus (COPV)], European rabbits [cottontail rabbit papillomavirus (CRPV)] and cattle (BPV-4). In prophylactic vaccination studies these induced neutralizing antibodies and provide complete or very high levels of protection against challenge with high titre virus (Breitburd *et al.*, 1995; Kirnbauer *et al.*, 1996; Suzich *et al.*, 1995). A role for L2 in induction of protection via humoral immunity is less clear, although data from BPV-4 indicates that L2 induces a neutralizing antibody response and protection against viral challenge (Gaukroger *et al.*, 1996; Roden *et al.*, 1994). However, L2 appears to be a weak immunogen when copresented with L1 during infection or in vaccination using L1/L2 VLPs (Kirnbauer *et al.*, 1996; Roden *et al.*, 1994). Intriguingly, evidence suggests that the portion of HPV L2 which is surface exposed on the virion includes a neutralization epitope which may not be type restricted (Kawana *et al.*, 1999).

IMMUNITY TO HUMAN PAPILLOMAVIRUS INFECTION

Host immune responses eliminate the majority of viral infections. These responses encompass innate (non-antigen specific) responses, including natural killer cells and their associated antiviral cytokines, including interferons. Additionally, virus specific T cells of helper (CD4) or cytotoxic (CD8) phenotype are induced in the course of viral infection, and help to control infection by killing infected cells or secreting proinflammatory or antiviral cytokines.

Immune responses to HPV proteins, with the exception of antibodies directed against the capsid proteins, are hard to detect following HPV infection. This may be partly methodological, as cellular responses are in general hard to detect in the course of viral infection in humans, even when they are sufficient to eliminate infection. However, antibody to viral protein can be used as a surrogate marker for the cellular responses that might be important in eliminating infection. The only consistent feature of the measured immune response to anogenital HPV infection is development of antibody to the E7 protein of HPV16 in patients with invasive cervical cancer.

The lack of immune response to viral non-structural proteins in patients with persistent HPV infection may explain the persistence. Why is so little immune response induced naturally by infection? HPV proteins are expressed only in small amounts and in superficial epithelial cells, and as a consequence are not available to the immune system in large amounts to invoke immunity. Papillomavirus infection is non-lytic, and the local inflammatory response to cells killed by virus infection is one of the major stimuli necessary to induce host immunity. Additionally, the epithelium secretes many cytokines (IL-10, TGF-β) designed to protect epithelial cells against immune damage, since epithelial integrity is a key component of host homeostasis. Thus papillomavirus infection distinguishes itself from many other chronic viral infections. Infection with human immunodeficiency virus, herpes simplex virus, hepatitis B or hepatitis C virus is associated with easily measurable immune responses that in general are insufficient or of an inappropriate quality to eradicate infection. However, ignorance of HPV infection may be the major reason why the host immune system fails to eliminate virus-infected cells.

VACCINES FOR HUMAN PAPILLOMAVIRUS

It is clear from the above that HPV infection and its consequences result in a substantial burden to the health care system in all communities worldwide, and that effective means to prevent and treat HPV-associated disease would potentially have a profound effect on both the health-related and financial impacts of HPV infection. Generally, development of a successful prophylactic vaccine requires induction of virus-neutralizing antibodies that reduce the number of cells infected after challenge with the virus, thus preventing chronic infection. Data from animal experiments pointed to the obvious target antigens for generation of such an immune response being capsid proteins, which provide structure to the virus and are the antigens that are initially presented to the immune system at the time of infection. However, a therapeutic vaccine to eradicate established HPV infection will most probably require generation of a specific T-cell-mediated effector response. As discussed below, evidence suggests that the expression of early proteins in established HPV-associated lesions make these proteins a target for such an approach.

Prophylactic vaccines

Development of a prophylactic vaccine to HPV was initially problematic because of the inability to grow the virus in culture, although evidence was generated that demonstrated the ability of antibodies against L1 capsid protein to neutralize HPV11 in a nude mouse xenograft, identifying it as a key target for a prophylactic vaccine (Christensen et al., 1990). The field was opened up in 1991 after Zhou and colleagues showed that HPV16 L1 capsid protein, expressed in a recombinant vaccinia virus, spontaneously assembled to form virus-like particles (VLPs) that resemble the natural structure of the virion and are devoid of the oncogenic viral genome (Zhou et al., 1991). Subsequent developments have resulted in expression of VLPs from a number of HPV types using a variety of expression systems, including baculovirus, yeast and mammalian cells.

Although the species-specificity of HPV infection meant there was no disease model directly applicable to human disease, preclinical models have helped to establish the immunogenicity and feasibility of preventative vaccination. VLPs formulated on aluminium adjuvants induced a strong virus-neutralizing antibody response in non-human primates (Lowe et al., 1997; Palker et al., 2001). Immunization with purified VLPs generated neutralizing antibodies and protection from experimental challenge with infectious virus in several animal models, including CRPV (Breitburd et al., 1995; Jansen et al., 1995), COPV (Suzich et al., 1995), and BPV (Campo et al., 1993; Kirnbauer et al., 1996). In several of these animal models, vaccination was also able to clear established disease. It should be noted, however, that these models most closely reflect low-risk HPV infection. CRPV causes large, pigmented, exophytic skin warts in rabbits, COPV is associated with warts on the oral mucosa of dogs, and BPV causes papilloma in the digestive tract in cows. Furthermore, challenge is usually carried out by injection of large quantities of virus into the dermis. How relevant might these be to high-risk HPV infection in humans?

Firstly, generation of high levels of neutralizing antibodies and tolerability of HPV VLP vaccination were demonstrated in a number of phase I clinical trials (Brown et al., 2001; Evans et al., 2001b; Harro et al., 2001). Importantly, immunogenicity to individual HPV genotypes was maintained in multivalent VLP preparations. Most crucially, to date, results of a phase II study have demonstrated protection from HPV infection and associated premalignant lesions.

This study, reported by Koutsky *et al.* (2002), was a double-blind trial that treated 2392 women aged 16 to 23 years. Participants received either placebo or yeast-derived HPV16 L1 VLPs vaccine (40 μg VLP protein, formulated with 225 μg of aluminium adjuvant) at day 0, month 2 and month 6 by intramuscular injection. A gynecological examination was conducted to collect samples from the genital tract for HPV16 DNA testing at enrolment, one month after the third injection and every 6 months thereafter. Cytology was routinely conducted, and colposcopy and biopsy were performed when indicated. Blood was collected at the same intervals for HPV16 antibodies. The primary endpoint of the study was persistent HPV16 infection defined as detection of HPV16 in two or more samples collected at least four months apart, cervical biopsy showing high grade CIN, or HPV16 detected in a sample during the last visit prior to being lost to follow up.

At the time of publication, the median follow up was 17.4 months after completion of the vaccination schedule for the 1533 women included in the primary analysis. Those excluded were evenly balanced between groups, and the main reason for exclusion was evidence of HPV16 at enrolment. High levels of neutralizing antibodies after the third vaccination were detected in all women who received HPV16 VLPs, while only low levels were found in the placebo group. Interestingly, the peak titre for the actively treated group was approximately 60 times higher than in those women with HPV16 detected at enrolment.

The remarkable finding was the difference in the rate of persistent HPV16 infection and related pathology. In the placebo group, 41 cases of persistent infection occurred while there were no cases in the vaccine-treated group. This effect provided protection from the risk of persistent infection – there were 10 cases of HPV16-associated CIN in women given placebo and none in those receiving vaccine. The vaccine did not prevent incident infection. 33 women given vaccine had a single positive test for HPV16 DNA compared with 34 women given with placebo. There was a similar incidence of non-HPV16 related CIN in both groups, consistent with prior observations of a lack of cross-reactivity between HPV neutralizing antibodies. As observed in earlier studies, the adverse event profile was similar between placebo and vaccine groups, with the most frequent side-effect being injection site pain.

These results have been extremely encouraging and prompted Merck to conduct phase III clinical trials to assess the efficacy of a quadrivalent HPV vaccine covering HPV types 16, 18, 6 and 11. This study had completed recruitment by the end of 2003. The National Cancer Institute and GlaxoSmithKline have announced commencement of a study of bivalent vaccine of HPV16 and 18 VLPs by the end of 2003 (Billich, 2003).

While it appears that we are fast closing in on having an effective prophylactic vaccine available, there remain a number of challenges and unanswered questions. Extensive debate has occurred about the appropriate endpoints for the phase III studies. The ultimate aim of an HPV vaccine is to prevent cervical cancer, but because of the long latency between infection and the development of malignancy, and the proven benefit of adequate treatment of CIN in preventing cancer, it would be unethical for development of cancer to be the primary endpoint in these studies. The FDA has accepted this point and the guidance is that prevention of high-grade CIN is an appropriate goal.

The duration of protection is still uncertain. The phase II study described above has only a short follow up period and more prolonged observation in this and the phase III studies is required. An additional limitation is that even if the quadrivalent vaccine being developed by Merck is effective, about 30% of HPV-related cervical cancer will still not be prevented. While there is no evidence that other oncogenic HPVs would evolve to become prevalent in the absence of HPV16 and 18, this would still leave a substantial gap in protection from HPV-related malignancy. It remains to be seen whether an effective, more multivalent vaccine can be developed.

An obstacle to the introduction of an HPV vaccine is in determining what age it would be best to vaccinate. In the Koutsky study, approximately one third of women had prior exposure to HPV16. To optimize benefit to the community the vaccine would need to be given prior to the majority of females commencing sexual intercourse, that is, probably by the age of 12 years (Communicable Disease Reports, 2003). Introduction of vaccinations in infants has been a successful public health model, but without knowledge of the duration of protection, it remains uncertain whether this would apply to an HPV vaccine, where the risk of infection occurs many years later. Besides, the schedule for infant vaccination is now very crowded.

If vaccination prevents persistent HPV infection in females, it will obviously not address the other side of the coin, that is, HPV in males. Current studies focus on females because that is where the majority of HPV-related pathology has historically been identified, but eradication of the reservoir of infection in males is also likely to be necessary. Investigations are ongoing that evaluate the epidemiology of HPV in males and where it is carried (probably the scrotum – transmission is not prevented by use of condoms), and consideration is being given to vaccination trials.

If screening is so effective in preventing cervical cancer, what will the likely impact be of a vaccine to HPV on public health? In the developed world, a multivalent vaccine containing the majority of disease-causing HPV types would greatly reduce the need for colposcopy, biopsy and treatment and be quite cost effective (Hughes *et al.*, 2002; Sanders *et al.*, 2003). The caveat to this is that the vaccine would need to be highly effective (as demonstrated in the Koutsky study) and the vaccination programs would need to provide widespread coverage. Even so, complete elimination of Pap-screening programs is unlikely.

Perhaps the greatest public health gain is if a vaccine can be successfully introduced into developing countries, where effective Pap-screening programs have been difficult or impossible to implement. In this situation, a profound impact on cancer incidence is likely to be observed.

Therapeutic vaccines

Prophylactic vaccines, designed to produce neutralizing antibody against a virus, are unlikely to eliminate existing infection, as viral proteins within cells are not accessible to antibody. A beneficial effect of specific antibodies on existing infection is particularly unlikely for HPV infection, as it seems unlikely that HPV spreads within the host to any significant extent after primary infection is established. Rather, the clinical manifestations of infection are the result of transmission of virus from a limited number of infected cells to their progeny. Therefore the aim of a therapeutic vaccine against a chronic viral infection such as HPV should be to achieve an immune response that the host immune system has not been able to mount during the course of natural infection.

When planning any therapeutic vaccine, it is desirable to understand why natural infection has failed to produce a protective immune response, and to consider, in light of the naturally occurring but non-host protective immune response, which viral proteins should be targeted by the vaccine. A wide range of therapeutic modalities have been tested in an attempt to invoke HPV specific immunity capable of eliminating infected cells. Three animal models have been used and in addition several clinical trials have been undertaken in man. The animal models comprise:

- Transplantable tumours expressing one or more papillomavirus proteins, tested in syngeneic recipients, which can be:
    - immunized prior to tumour transfer; or
    - immunized after tumour is established.
- Mice transgenic for papillomavirus proteins, generally targeted to skin:
    - a variant of this is to transfer a skin graft from such an animal to a naïve host.
- Animals which develop disease following exposure to their natural papillomavirus infection, including:
    - beagle dogs, which develop transient oral warts following infection with COPV;
    - cottontail rabbits, which develop skin warts following challenge with CRPV (these warts can become chronic and transform to carcinomas);
    - cows which develop transient skin warts and occasionally facial cancers following infection with bovine PV;
    - rabbits that develop transient tongue warts following infection with rabbit oral papillomavirus (ROPV).

Generally, most immunization regimens which include papillomavirus antigens prevent tumours expressing those antigens growing in mice. While a more restricted set is able to cause regression of established tumour (Tables 12.3–12.5), none have as yet been demonstrated capable of breaking the CD8 tolerance of E7 that is observed in some E7 transgenic mice (Frazer *et al.*, 1998). In addition, most approaches have failed to cause rejection of an E7 expressing graft (Dunn *et al.*, 1997; Frazer *et al.*, 2001), whether immunization occurs prior to or after graft placement. Graft tolerance appears to be local in this model, as the same graft recipients will, following immunization, reject an E7-bearing transplantable tumour.

The animal models (Tables 12.3–12.5) have demonstrated that E1, E2 E6 and E7 are all potential targets for immunotherapy, with some preference for therapy with multiple proteins over monotherapy. However, a comparison of the location of expression of the early proteins of HPV in animal models and human disease (Peh *et al.*, 2002) suggests these proteins will be better presented in basal epithelium in the animal models. This may account for the near complete spontaneous regression rate in the animals, compared with approximately 10% persistence of infection in humans. Ultimately, vaccine development is driven empirically, mandating phase I and II clinical trials of possible effective immunotherapeutics as proof of principle. In this regard, it is worth observing there are no registered therapeutic vaccines, despite extensive laboratory and clinical efforts over several decades in testing such a strategy against cancer and chronic infection.

A number of immunotherapeutic vaccines for persistent HPV infection have been trialed in man (Table 12.6). These approaches have been tested in patients with cervical cancer or with precancer lesions of the anogenital epithelium including vulval intraepithelial neoplasia, cervical intraepithelial neoplasia and anal intraepithelial neoplasia. While there have been concerns raised about the safety of vaccines based on transforming viral proteins, these have generally been allayed by using mutated viral proteins lacking oncogenic potential and/or fusions that lack the functional configuration of the native proteins. T cell responses depend only on the linear sequence of the immunogen and not on its tertiary structure. The clinical studies to date have generally demonstrated some evidence for immunogenicity, inducing humoral and cell-mediated immune responses in at least a percentage of patients. While the results from the studies published to date can be taken positively, with immune responses observed in the majority of immunized subjects, there are currently no generally accepted surrogate laboratory markers of clinical activity. The clinical outcomes in these predominantly uncontrolled, open label trials have been not particularly compelling with outcome measures including partial lesion regression, or failure of progression, rather than cure, or avoidance of recurrence.

The HPV E6 and E7 proteins are obligatorily expressed to maintain the cancer potential of transformed anogenital epithelial cells, but a significant frequency of mutations is observed in the antigen-presenting machinery of the cells of HPV-associated invasive cancer (Cromme *et al.*, 1994; Evans *et al.*, 2001a), rendering these cells potentially resistant to immunotherapy. Thus, while there may be a place for adjuvant immunotherapy in the management of early stage anogenital cancer, HPV immunotherapy is ideally going to be targeted at premalignant disease, in which problems with viral antigen presentation have not been described.

CONCLUSION

VLP-based vaccines, designed to elicit neutralizing antibodies against HPV capsid proteins, may represent efficient prophylactic vaccines. Such vaccines are however, unlikely to control established HPV infections. Thus, therapeutic vaccines targeting HPV E6 and E7 proteins are needed. In this regard, the considerable practical difficulties of comparing multiple candidate vaccines are compounded by the equally practical difficulties of developing clinical trial protocols which test clinically desirable outcomes in a setting which is realistic in the face of the alternative therapies available for the majority of HPV-associated disease of the genital tract. In this regard vulval intraepithelial neoplasia and anal intraepithelial neoplasia are attractive target diseases for testing HPV specific immunotherapy because there are few effective alternate therapies, the risk of progression to neoplasia is recognized and significant, and the rate of spontaneous regression is low. Further, disease state can be relatively easily monitored. Thus, HPV-associated external anogenital lesions may provide the key to development and assessment of effective immunotherapy not only for HPV-associated cervical disease but also for a wider range of chronic viral infections.

Table 12.3 Polynucleotide-based potential HPV therapeutic vaccines employed in animal models

Antigen	Model animal/tumour	Outcome	Reference
CRPV E1, 2, 6, 7	Rabbit/CRPV	Partial protection against progression of established infection to cancer	Han *et al.* (2000)
CRPV E7	Rabbit/CRPV	Partial protection against progression of established infection to cancer	Michel *et al.* (2002)
E7 + LAMP-1	Mouse/TC-1	E7/LAMP-1 fusions gave better regression of established metastatic tumour than E7 alone	Chen *et al.* (1999), Ji *et al.* (1998), Ji *et al.* (1999)
E7–MDV UL49 fusion	Mouse/TC-1	CTL induction and therapeutic effect	Hung *et al.* (2002)
E7 + calreticulin	Mouse/TC-1	CTL and tumour regression, Calreticulin also effective as therapy when delivered as polynucleotide	Cheng *et al.* (2001)
E7 polytope + ubiquitin	Mouse/C3	CTL and tumour regression	Velders *et al.* (2001b)
E7 ± fusion with LAMP	Mouse/TC-1	CTL, partial therapeutic effect with E7 and with E7-LAMP	Smahel *et al.* (2001)
E7 – membrane insertion protein from *P. aeuroginosa*	Mouse/TC-1	CTL tumour regression	Hung *et al.* (2001b)
E7–VP22	Mouse/TC-1	CTL, tumour regression, VP-22 also effective alone	Hung *et al.* (2001a)
E7–flt3Ligand	Mouse/TC-1	CTL, tumour regression	Hung *et al.* (2001c)
E6, E7	HLA A*0201 transgenic mouse/E7 & Ras transformed A*0201 mouse tumour	CTL induction and reduction of tumour growth	Eiben *et al.* (2002)
HSP70 E7 – i.m. v.s i.d. administration	Mouse/TC1	CTL induction and tumour regression better with i.d. than i.m. administration	Trimble *et al.* (2003)

Table 12.4 Virus-based potential HPV therapeutic vaccines tested in animal models

Virus	Encoded protein	Test model	Oucome	Reference
Vaccinia	Listerolysin–E7	Mouse/TC-1	CTL and tumour regression in some animals, VacLLOE7 better than Vac LAMP-1 E7	Lamikanra et al. (2001)
Sindbis	E7 + VP22	Mouse/TC-1	CTL and tumour regression	Cheng et al. (2002)
Alpha	E6–E7 fusion protein	Mouse	CTL induction and tumour regression	Daemen et al. (2002)
Alpha	E7–HSP70	Mouse/TC-1	CTL, tumour regression	Hsu et al. (2001)
Venezualan encephalitis	E7	Mouse/C3	CTL and tumour regression	Velders et al. (2001a)
Venezuelan encephalitis	E6, E7 polytope	HLA A*0201 transgenic mouse/E7 and Ras-transformed A*0201 mouse tumour	CTL induction and reduction of tumour growth	Eiben et al. (2002)
Adeno-associated	E7 CTL epitope-hsp70	Mouse/TC-1	CTL and tumour regression	Liu et al. (2000)

Table 12.5 Other potential HPV therapeutic vaccines tested in animal models

Delivery system	Antigenic proteins	Test model	Outcome	Reference
Salmonella typhimurium	HPV L1 VLPs	Mouse/C3	Tumour regression after mucosal immunisation	Revaz *et al.* (2001)
Listeria	E7–listerolysin fusion	Mouse/TC-1	CTL, 75% tumour regression with LLO, no regression without	Gunn *et al.* (2001)
PV VLP capsomers	L1	Mouse/C3	CTL and regression	Ohlschlager *et al.* (2003)
Peptide + anti-CD137	E7 CTL peptide/Freunds	Mouse/C3, TC-1	CTL and tumour eradication, successful therapy required CD137 expression on the tumour	Wilcox *et al.* (2002)
Peptide + CpG	E7 peptides/CPG	Mouse/C3	Eradication of tumours	Zwaveling *et al.* (2002)
QS21 or MLP	E7	Mouse/TC-1	CTL and tumour regression	Gerard *et al.* (2001a)
SBAS1 adjuvant	E7	Mouse/TC-1	CTL, TH1 response and tumour regression, in E7 tolerant transgenic mice tumour regression without CTL	Gerard *et al.* (2001b)
Dendritic cells	E7 peptides or tumour lysate	Mouse/MK16 transduced with E6/7	CTL, tumour regression	Indrova *et al.* (2001)
HSP fusion	E7	Mouse/TC1	Regression, Th1 response, CTL	Chu *et al.* (2000)
Tat fusion/Quil A	E7	Mouse/C3	CTL and regression better with tat fusion	Giannouli *et al.* (2003)
PROVAX adjuvant	E7	Mouse/E7 transduced melanoma	Slowing of growth, due to CD8 T cells	Hariharan *et al.* (1998)
Suicide gene modified cancer cells	E7	Hamster/E7 transformed cells	Regression of tumour due to bystander effect/immunity?	Vonka *et al.* (1998)
Transfer of T cells	E7	Mouse/C3	Early tumours controlled by NKT cells and other non-antigen specific mechanisms. Well-established tumours respond to E7-specific T cells	Stewart *et al.* (2003)

Table 12.6 Clinical trials of HPV specific immunotherapy

Delivery system	Antigen	Disease group	Immunogenicity	Clinical Outcome	Reference
Fusion protein (TA-CIN, Xenova)	HPV16 L2E6E7 fusion (no adjuvant)	Healthy volunteers	Antibody, T cell proliferation, IFN-γ ELISPOT all detected	Randomised, placebo controlled. No HPV infections	de Jong et al. (2002)
HSP fusion protein (HSPE7, Stressgen)	HPV16E7	Genital warts	Not reported	Open label. Regression of warts, 3/14 CR, 10/14 PR, non-HPV16 specific	Goldstone et al. (2002)
Encapsulated polynucleotide (ZYC101, Zycos)	HPV16 E7 peptide	Anal dysplasia Cervical dysplasia	Majority of subjects ELISPOT positive; induction of E7 specific immunity	Open label. HPV16 positive. Regression of AIN, 3/12 PR. Regression of CIN, 5/15 CR	Klencke et al. (2002), Sheets et al. (2003)
Protein/ISCOMATRIX4 adjuvant (CSL)	E6E7 fusion protein	CIN	Antibody/DTH/CTL	Randomised, placebo controlled HPV type specific reduction in HPV infection. 7/14 CR, 7/14 PR	Frazer et al. (2005)
Vaccinia virus (TA-HPV, Xenova)	E6E7 fusion protein	Cervical cancer	CTL (1/8); antibody (3/8)	Open label. Outcome not documented	Borysiewicz et al. (1996)
Vaccinia virus, (TA-HPV, Xenova)	E6E7 fusion protein	Vulval HPV/ VIN	Antibody, CMI (13/18)	Open label. 50% reduction in VIN 8/18 subjects; loss of viral load in 12/18	Davidson et al. (2003)
Peptide/Oil+water adjuvant	E7 peptide	Cervical cancer	Not stated	Open label. HPV16 by selection, 2/17 SD	van Driel et al. (1999)
Protein/Algammulin adjuvant	E7–GST fusion protein	Cervical cancer	Antibody, DTH	Open label. No alteration in natural history of disease	Frazer et al. (1999)
Peptide + IFA	E7 A0201 peptide	VIN/CIN	CTL 10/16 no DTH	Open label. HPV16 by selection 3/18 CR; 6/18 PR	Muderspach et al. (2000)
VLPs	L1	Genital warts	Antibody and DTH	Open label. Regression of warts. CR 25/33	Zhang et al. (2000)
Dendritic cells	HPV16 and HPV18 E7	Cervical Cancer	Antibody, Proliferation, Elispot (3/11)	Open label. No objective clinical response	Ferrara et al. (2003)

References

Alvarez-Salas, L.M., Arpawong, T.E., and DiPaolo, J.A. 1999. Growth inhibition of cervical tumor cells by antisense oligodeoxynucleotides directed to the human papillomavirus type 16 E6 gene. Antisense Nucleic Acid Drug Dev. 9: 441–450.

Baker, T.S., Newcomb, W.W., Olson, N.H., Cowsert, L.M., Olson, C., and Brown, J.C. 1991. Structures of bovine and human papillomaviruses. Analysis by cryoelectron microscopy and three-dimensional image reconstruction. Biophys. J. 60: 1445–1456.

Beutner, K.R., Wiley, D.J., Douglas, J.M., Tyring, S.K., Fife, K., Trofatter, K., and Stone, K.M. 1999. Genital warts and their treatment. Clin. Infect. Dis. 28 Suppl 1: S37–S56.

Billich, A. 2003. HPV vaccine. MedImmune/GlaxoSmithKline: Curr. Opin. Investig. Drugs 4: 210–213.

Borysiewicz, L.K., Fiander, A., Nimako, M., Man, S., Wilkinson, G.W., Westmoreland, D., Evans, A.S., Adams, M., Stacey, S.N., Boursnell, M.E., Rutherford, E., Hickling, J.K., and Inglis, S.C. 1996. A recombinant vaccinia virus encoding human papillomavirus types 16 and 18, E6 and E7 proteins as immunotherapy for cervical cancer. Lancet 347: 1523–1527.

Bosch, F.X., Lorincz, A., Munoz, N., Meijer, C.J., and Shah, K.V. 2002. The causal relation between human papillomavirus and cervical cancer. J. Clin. Pathol. 55: 244–265.

Breitburd, F., Kirnbauer, R., Hubbert, N.L., Nonnenmacher, B., Trin-Dinh-Desmarquet, C., Orth, G., Schiller, J.T., and Lowy, D.R. 1995. Immunization with viruslike particles from cottontail rabbit papillomavirus (CRPV) can protect against experimental CRPV infection. J. Virol 69: 3959–3963.

Brown, D.R., Bryan, J.T., Schroeder, J.M., Robinson, T.S., Fife, K.H., Wheeler, C.M., Barr, E., Smith, P.R., Chiacchierini, L., DiCello, A., and Jansen, K.U. 2001. Neutralization of human papillomavirus type 11 (HPV-11) by serum from women vaccinated with yeast-derived HPV-11 L1 virus-like particles: correlation with competitive radioimmunoassay titer. J. Infect. Dis. 184: 1183–1186.

Burk, R.D., Kelly, P., Feldman, J., Bromberg, J., Vermund, S.H., DeHovitz, J.A., and Landesman, S.H. 1996. Declining prevalence of cervicovaginal human papillomavirus infection with age is independent of other risk factors. Sex Transm. Dis. 23: 333–341.

Campo, M.S., Grindlay, G.J., O'Neil, B.W., Chandrachud, L.M., McGarvie, G.M., and Jarrett, W.F. 1993. Prophylactic and therapeutic vaccination against a mucosal papillomavirus. J. Gen. Virol .74 (Pt 6): 945–953.

Cannistra, S. A. and Niloff, J.M. 1996. Cancer of the uterine cervix. N. Engl. J. Med. 334: 1030–1038.

Chang, G.J., Berry, J.M., Jay, N., Palefsky, J.M., and Welton, M.L. 2002. Surgical treatment of high-grade anal squamous intraepithelial lesions: a prospective study. Dis. Colon Rectum 45: 453–458.

Chen, C.H., Ji, H., Suh, K.W., Choti, M.A., Pardoll, D.M., and Wu, T.C. 1999. Gene gun-mediated DNA vaccination induces antitumor immunity against human papillomavirus type 16 E7-expressing murine tumor metastases in the liver and lungs. Gene Ther. 6: 1972–1981.

Cheng, G., Icenogle, J.P., Kirnbauer, R., Hubbert, N.L., St Louis, M.E., Han, C., Svare, E.I., Kjaer, S.K., Lowy, D.R., and Schiller, J.T. 1995. Divergent human papillomavirus type 16 variants are serologically cross-reactive. J. Infect. Dis. 172: 1584–1587.

Cheng, W.F., Hung, C.F., Chai, C.Y., Hsu, K.F., He, L., Ling, M., and Wu, T.C. 2001. Tumor-specific immunity and antiangiogenesis generated by a DNA vaccine encoding calreticulin linked to a tumor antigen. J. Clin. Invest. 108: 669–678.

Cheng, W.F., Hung, C.F., Hsu, K.F., Chai, C.Y., He, L., Polo, J.M., Slater, L.A., Ling, M., and Wu, T.C. 2002. Cancer immunotherapy using Sindbis virus replicon particles encoding a VP22–antigen fusion. Hum. Gene Ther. 13: 553–568.

Chin-Hong, P. V. and Palefsky, J.M. 2002. Natural history and clinical management of anal human papillomavirus disease in men and women infected with human immunodeficiency virus. Clin. Infect. Dis. 35: 1127–1134.

Christensen, N.D., Hopfl, R., DiAngelo, S.L., Cladel, N.M., Patrick, S.D., Welsh, P.A., Budgeon, L.R., Reed, C.A., and Kreider, J.W. 1994. Assembled baculovirus-expressed human papillomavirus type 11 L1 capsid protein virus-like particles are recognized by neutralizing monoclonal antibodies and induce high titres of neutralizing antibodies. J. Gen Virol 75 (Pt 9): 2271–2276.

Christensen, N.D., Kreider, J.W., Cladel, N.M., and Galloway, D.A. 1990. Immunological cross-reactivity to laboratory-produced HPV-11 virions of polysera raised against bacterially derived fusion proteins and synthetic peptides of HPV-6b and HPV-16 capsid proteins. Virology 175: 1–9.

Chu, N.R., Wu, H.B., Wu, T., Boux, L.J., Siegel, M.I., and Mizzen, L.A. 2000. Immunotherapy of a human papillomavirus (HPV) type 16 E7-expressing tumour by administration of fusion protein comprising *Mycobacterium bovis* bacille Calmette–Guerin (BCG) hsp65 and HPV16 E7. Clin. Exp. Immunol. 121: 216–225.

Combita, A.L., Touze, A., BoUSA rghin, L., Christensen, N.D., and Coursaget, P. 2002. Identification of two cross-neutralizing linear epitopes within the L1 major capsid protein of human papillomaviruses. J. Virol. 76: 6480–6486.

Communicable Disease Reports 2003. Sexually transmitted infections quarterly report: anogenital warts and HSV infection in England and Wales. Commun Dis. Rep Weekly 13: 1–4.

Cox, J.T. 1999. Management of cervical intraepithelial neoplasia. Lancet 353: 857–859.

Cromme, F.V., Airey, J., Heemels, M.T., Ploegh, H.L., Keating, P.J., Stern, P.L., Meijer, C.J., and Walboomers, J.M. 1994. Loss of transporter protein, encoded by the TAP-1 gene, is highly correlated with loss of HLA expression in cervical carcinomas. J. Exp. Med. 179: 335–340.

Daemen, T., Regts, J., Holtrop, M., and Wilschut, J. 2002. Immunization strategy against cervical cancer involving an alphavirus vector expressing high levels of a stable fusion protein of human papillomavirus 16 E6 and E7. Gene Ther. 9: 85–94.

Davidson, E.J., Boswell, C.M., Sehr, P., Pawlita, M., Tomlinson, A.E., McVey, R.J., Dobson, J., Roberts, J.S., Hickling, J., Kitchener, H.C., and Stern, P.L. 2003. Immunological and clinical responses in women with vulval intraepithelial neoplasia vaccinated with a vaccinia virus encoding human papillomavirus 16/18 oncoproteins. Cancer Res. 63: 6032–6041.

Day, P.M., Lowy, D.R., and Schiller, J.T. 2003. Papillomaviruses infect cells via a clathrin-dependent pathway. Virology 307: 1–11.

de Jong, A., O'Neill, T., Khan, A.Y., Kwappenberg, K.M., Chisholm, S.E., Whittle, N.R., Dobson, J.A., Jack, L.C., Clair Roberts, J.A., Offringa, R., van der Burg, S.H., and Hickling, J.K. 2002. Enhancement of human papillomavirus (HPV) type 16 E6 and E7-specific T-cell immunity in healthy volunteers through vaccination with TA-CIN, an HPV16 L2E7E6 fusion protein vaccine. Vaccine 20: 3456–3464.

Desaintes, C. and Demeret, C. 1996. Control of papillomavirus DNA replication and transcription. Semin. Cancer Biol. 7: 339–347.

Dillner, J., von Krogh, G., Horenblas, S., and Meijer, C.J. 2000. Etiology of squamous cell carcinoma of the penis. Scand. J. Urol. Nephrol. Suppl. 189–193.

DiMaio, D., Guralski, D., and Schiller, J.T. 1986. Translation of open reading frame E5 of bovine papillomavirus is required for its transforming activity. Proc. Natl. Acad. Sci. USA 83: 1797–1801.

Dunn, L.A., Evander, M., Tindle, R.W., Bulloch, A.L., De Kluyver, R.L., Fernando, G.J., Lambert, P.F., and Frazer, I.H. 1997. Presentation of the HPV16E7 protein by skin grafts is insufficient to allow graft rejection in an E7-primed animal. Virology 235: 94–103.

Eiben, G.L., Velders, M.P., Schreiber, H., Cassetti, M.C., Pullen, J.K., Smith, L.R., and Kast, W.M. 2002. Establishment of an HLA-A*0201 human papillomavirus type 16 tumor model to determine the efficacy of vaccination strategies in HLA-A*0201 transgenic mice. Cancer Res. 62: 5792–5799.

Evans, M., Borysiewicz, L.K., Evans, A.S., Rowe, M., Jones, M., Gileadi, U., Cerundolo, V., and Man, S. 2001a. Antigen processing defects in cervical carcinomas limit the presentation of a CTL epitope from human papillomavirus 16 E6. J. Immunol. 167: 5420–5428.

Evans, T.G., Bonnez, W., Rose, R.C., Koenig, S., Demeter, L., Suzich, J.A., O'Brien, D., Campbell, M., White, W.I., Balsley, J., and Reichman, R.C. 2001b. A Phase 1 study of a recombinant viruslike particle vaccine against human papillomavirus type 11 in healthy adult volunteers. J. Infect. Dis. 183: 1485–1493.

Ferrara, A., Nonn, M., Sehr, P., Schreckenberger, C., Pawlita, M., Durst, M., Schneider, A., and Kaufmann, A.M. 2003. Dendritic cell-based tumor vaccine for cervical cancer II: results of a clinical pilot study in 15 individual patients. J. Cancer Res. Clin. Oncol. 129: 521–530.

Frazer, I.H., Fernando, G.J., Fowler, N., Leggatt, G.R., Lambert, P.F., Liem, A., Malcolm, K., and Tindle, R.W. 1998. Split tolerance to a viral antigen expressed in thymic epithelium and keratinocytes. Eur. J. Immunol. 28: 2791–2800.

Frazer, I.H., Tindle, R.W., Fernando, G.J., Malcolm, K., Herd, K., McFadyn, S., Cooper, P.D., and Ward, B. 1999. Safety and immunogenicity of HPV16 E7/Algammulin immunotherapy for cervical cancer. In: Tindle, R.W. (ed.) Vaccines for human papillomavirus infection and anogenital disease. Landes Bioscience 91–104.

Frazer, I.H., De Kluyver, R., Leggatt, G.R., Guo, H.Y., Dunn, L., White, O., Harris, C., Liem, A., and Lambert, P. 2001. Tolerance or immunity to a tumor antigen expressed in somatic cells can be determined by systemic proinflammatory signals at the time of first antigen exposure. J. Immunol. 167: 6180–6187.

Fuchs, P. G. and Pfister, H. 1994. Transcription of papillomavirus genomes.: Intervirology 37: 159–167.

Gaukroger, J.M., Chandrachud, L.M., O'Neil, B.W., Grindlay, G.J., Knowles, G., and Campo, M.S. 1996. Vaccination of cattle with bovine papillomavirus type 4 L2 elicits the production of virus-neutralizing antibodies. J. Gen. Virol. 77 (Pt 7): 1577–1583.

Gerard, C.M., Baudson, N., Kraemer, K., Bruck, C., Garcon, N., Paterson, Y., Pan, Z.K., and Pardoll, D. 2001a. Therapeutic potential of protein and adjuvant vaccinations on tumour growth. Vaccine 19: 2583–2589.

Gerard, C.M., Baudson, N., Kraemer, K., Ledent, C., Pardoll, D., and Bruck, C. 2001b. Recombinant human papillomavirus type 16 E7 protein as a model antigen to study the vaccine potential in control and E7 transgenic mice. Clin. Cancer Res. 7: 838s–847s.

Giannouli, C., Brulet, J.M., Gesche, F., Rappaport, J., Burny, A., Leo, O., and Hallez, S. 2003. Fusion of a tumour-associated antigen to HIV-1 Tat improves protein-based immunotherapy of cancer. Anticancer Res. 23: 3523–3531.

Gillison, M. L. and Shah, K.V. 2003. Chapter 9: Role of mucosal human papillomavirus in nongenital cancers. J. Natl. Cancer Inst. Monogr 57–65.

Giroglou, T., Sapp, M., Lane, C., Fligge, C., Christensen, N.D., Streeck, R.E., and Rose, R.C. 2001. Immunological analyses of human papillomavirus capsids. Vaccine 19: 1783–1793.

Goldie, S.J., Kuntz, K.M., Weinstein, M.C., Freedberg, K.A., Welton, M.L., and Palefsky, J.M. 1999. The clinical effectiveness and cost-effectiveness of screening for anal squamous intraepithelial lesions in homosexual and bisexual HIV-positive men. JAMA 281: 1822–1829.

Goldie, S.J., Kuntz, K.M., Weinstein, M.C., Freedberg, K.A., and Palefsky, J.M. 2000. Cost-effectiveness of screening for anal squamous intraepithelial lesions and anal cancer in human immunodeficiency virus-negative homosexual and bisexual men. Am. J. Med. 108: 634–641.

Goldstone, S.E., Palefsky, J.M., Winnett, M.T., and Neefe, J.R. 2002. Activity of HspE7, a novel immunotherapy, in patients with anogenital warts. Dis. Colon Rectum 45: 502–507.

Gornemann, J., Hofmann, T.G., Will, H., and Muller, M. 2002. Interaction of human papillomavirus type 16 L2 with cellular proteins: identification of novel nuclear body-associated proteins. Virology 303: 69–78.

Gunn, G.R., Zubair, A., Peters, C., Pan, Z.K., Wu, T.C., and Paterson, Y. 2001. Two *Listeria monocytogenes* vaccine vectors that express different Molecular forms of human papilloma virus-16 (HPV-16) E7 induce qualitatively different T cell immunity that correlates with their ability to induce regression of established tumors immortalized by HPV-16. J. Immunol. 167: 6471–6479.

Gunter, J. 2003. Genital and perianal warts: new treatment opportunities for human papillomavirus infection. Am. J. Obstet. Gynecol. 189: S3–11.

Han, R., Cladel, N.M., Reed, C.A., Peng, X., Budgeon, L.R., Pickel, M., and Christensen, N.D. 2000. DNA vaccination prevents and/or delays carcinoma development of papillomavirus-induced skin papillomas on rabbits. J. Virol 74: 9712–9716.

Hariharan, K., Braslawsky, G., Barnett, R.S., Berquist, L.G., Huynh, T., Hanna, N., and Black, A. 1998. Tumor regression in mice following vaccination with human papillomavirus E7 recombinant protein in PROVAX. Int. J. Oncol. 12: 1229–1235.

Harro, C.D., Pang, Y.Y., Roden, R.B., Hildesheim, A., Wang, Z., Reynolds, M.J., Mast, T.C., Robinson, R., Murphy, B.R., Karron, R.A., Dillner, J., Schiller, J.T., and Lowy, D.R. 2001. Safety and immunogenicity trial in adult volunteers of a human papillomavirus 16 L1 virus-like particle vaccine. J. Natl. Cancer Inst. 93: 284–292.

Hart, W.R. 2001. Vulvar intraepithelial neoplasia: historical aspects and current status. Int. J. Gynecol. Pathol. 20: 16–30.

Harwood, C.A., Surentheran, T., McGregor, J.M., Spink, P.J., Leigh, I.M., Breuer, J., and Proby, C.M. 2000. Human papillomavirus infection and non-melanoma skin cancer in immunosuppressed and immunocompetent individuals. J. Med. Virol 61: 289–297.

Ho, G.Y., Bierman, R., Beardsley, L., Chang, C.J., and Burk, R.D. 1998. Natural history of cervicovaginal papillomavirus infection in young women. N. Engl. J. Med. 338: 423–428.

Holly, E.A., Ralston, M.L., Darragh, T.M., Greenblatt, R.M., Jay, N., and Palefsky, J.M. 2001. Prevalence and risk factors for anal squamous intraepithelial lesions in women. J. Natl. Cancer Inst. 93: 843–849.

Holowaty, P., Miller, A.B., Rohan, T., and To, T. 1999. Natural history of dysplasia of the uterine cervix. J. Natl. Cancer Inst. 91: 252–258.

Hsu, K.F., Hung, C.F., Cheng, W.F., He, L., Slater, L.A., Ling, M., and Wu, T.C. 2001. Enhancement of suicidal DNA vaccine potency by linking *Mycobacterium tuberculosis* heat shock protein 70 to an antigen. Gene Ther. 8: 376–383.

Hughes, J.P., Garnett, G.P., and Koutsky, L. 2002. The theoretical population-level impact of a prophylactic human papilloma virus vaccine. Epidemiology 13: 631–639.

Hung, C.F., Cheng, W.F., Hsu, K.F., Chai, C.Y., He, L., Ling, M., and Wu, T.C. 2001b. Cancer immunotherapy using a DNA vaccine encoding the translocation domain of a bacterial toxin linked to a tumor antigen. Cancer Res. 61: 3698–3703.

Hung, C.F., Cheng, W.F., Chai, C.Y., Hsu, K.F., He, L., Ling, M., and Wu, T.C. 2001a. Improving vaccine potency through intercellular spreading and enhanced MHC class I presentation of antigen. J. Immunol. 166: 5733–5740.

Hung, C.F., He, L., Juang, J., Lin, T.J., Ling, M., and Wu, T.C. 2002. Improving DNA vaccine potency by linking Marek's disease virus type 1 VP22 to an antigen. J. Virol. 76: 2676–2682.

Hung, C.F., Hsu, K.F., Cheng, W.F., Chai, C.Y., He, L., Ling, M., and Wu, T.C. 2001c. Enhancement of DNA vaccine potency by linkage of antigen gene to a gene encoding the extracellular domain of Fms-like tyrosine kinase 3-ligand. Cancer Res. 61: 1080–1088.

Indrova, M., Bubenik, J., Simova, J., Vonka, V., Nemeckova, S., Mendoza, L., and Reinis, M. 2001. Therapy of HPV 16-associated carcinoma with dendritic cell-based vaccines: in vitro priming of the effector cell responses by DC pulsed with tumour lysates and synthetic RAHYNIVTF peptide. Int. J. Mol. Med. 7: 97–100.

Jansen, K.U., Rosolowsky, M., Schultz, L.D., Markus, H.Z., Cook, J.C., Donnelly, J.J., Martinez, D., Ellis, R.W., and Shaw, A.R. 1995. Vaccination with yeast-expressed cottontail rabbit papillomavirus (CRPV) virus-like particles protects rabbits from CRPV-induced papilloma formation. Vaccine 13: 1509–1514.

Ji, H., Chang, E.Y., Lin, K.Y., Kurman, R.J., Pardoll, D.M., and Wu, T.C. 1998. Antigen-specific immunotherapy for murine lung metastatic tumors expressing human papillomavirus type 16 E7 oncoprotein. Int. J. Cancer 78: 41–45.

Ji, H., Wang, T.L., Chen, C.H., Pai, S.I., Hung, C.F., Lin, K.Y., Kurman, R.J., Pardoll, D.M., and Wu, T.C. 1999. Targeting human papillomavirus type 16 E7 to the endosomal/lysosomal compartment enhances the antitumor immunity of DNA vaccines against murine human papillomavirus type 16 E7-expressing tumors. Hum. Gene Ther. 10: 2727–2740.

Kawana, K., Yoshikawa, H., Taketani, Y., Yoshiike, K., and Kanda, T. 1999. Common neutralization epitope in minor capsid protein L2 of human papillomavirus types 16 and 6. J. Virol. 73: 6188–6190.

Kawana, Y., Kawana, K., Yoshikawa, H., Taketani, Y., Yoshiike, K., and Kanda, T. 2001. Human papillomavirus type 16 minor capsid protein l2 N-terminal region containing a common neutralization epitope binds to the cell surface and enters the cytoplasm. J. Virol 75: 2331–2336.

Kirnbauer, R., Booy, F., Cheng, N., Lowy, D.R., and Schiller, J.T. 1992. Papillomavirus L1 major capsid protein self-assembles into virus-like particles that are highly immunogenic. Proc. Natl. Acad. Sci. USA 89: 12180–12184.

Kirnbauer, R., Chandrachud, L.M., O'Neil, B.W., Wagner, E.R., Grindlay, G.J., Armstrong, A., McGarvie, G.M., Schiller, J.T., Lowy, D.R., and Campo, M.S. 1996. Virus-like particles of bovine papillomavirus type 4 in prophylactic and therapeutic immunization. Virology 219: 37–44.

Klencke, B., Matijevic, M., Urban, R.G., Lathey, J.L., Hedley, M.L., Berry, M., Thatcher, J., Weinberg, V., Wilson, J., Darragh, T., Jay, N., Da Costa, M., and Palefsky, J.M. 2002. Encapsulated plasmid DNA treatment for human papillomavirus 16-associated anal dysplasia: a Phase I study of ZYC101. Clin. Cancer Res. 8: 1028–1037.

Koutsky, L.A., Holmes, K.K., Critchlow, C.W., Stevens, C.E., Paavonen, J., Beckmann, A.M., DeRouen, T.A., Galloway, D.A., Vernon, D., and Kiviat, N.B. 1992. A cohort study of the risk of cervical intraepithelial neoplasia grade 2 or 3 in relation to papillomavirus infection. N. Engl. J. Med. 327: 1272–1278.

Koutsky, L.A., Ault, K.A., Wheeler, C.M., Brown, D.R., Barr, E., Alvarez, F.B., Chiacchierini, L.M., and Jansen, K.U. 2002. A controlled trial of a human papillomavirus type 16 vaccine. N. Engl. J. Med. 347: 1645–1651.

Kreider, J.W., Howett, M.K., Leure-Dupree, A.E., Zaino, R.J., and Weber, J.A. 1987. Laboratory production in vivo of infectious human papillomavirus type 11. J. Virol. 61: 590–593.

Lamikanra, A., Pan, Z.K., Isaacs, S.N., Wu, T.C., and Paterson, Y. 2001. Regression of established human papillomavirus type 16 (HPV-16) immortalized tumors in vivo by vaccinia viruses expressing different forms of HPV-16 E7 correlates with enhanced CD8(+) T-cell responses that home to the tumor site. J. Virol. 75: 9654–9664.

Liu, D.W., Tsao, Y.P., Kung, J.T., Ding, Y.A., Sytwu, H.K., Xiao, X., and Chen, S.L. 2000. Recombinant adeno-associated virus expressing human papillomavirus type 16 E7 peptide DNA fused with heat shock protein DNA as a potential vaccine for cervical cancer. J. Virol. 74: 2888–2894.

Lowe, R.S., Brown, D.R., Bryan, J.T., Cook, J.C., George, H.A., Hofmann, K.J., Hurni, W.M., Joyce, J.G., Lehman, E.D., Markus, H.Z., Neeper, M.P., Schultz, L.D., Shaw, A.R., and Jansen, K.U. 1997. Human papillomavirus type 11 (HPV-11) neutralizing antibodies in the serum and genital mucosal secretions of African green monkeys immunized with HPV-11 virus-like particles expressed in yeast. J. Infect. Dis. 176: 1141–1145.

McIndoe, W.A., McLean, M.R., Jones, R.W., and Mullins, P.R. 1984. The invasive potential of carcinoma in situ of the cervix. Obstet. Gynecol. 64: 451–458.

McMurray, H.R., Nguyen, D., Westbrook, T.F., and McCance, D.J. 2001. Biology of human papillomaviruses. Int. J. Exp. Pathol. 82: 15–33.

Meyers, C., Frattini, M.G., Hudson, J.B., and Laimins, L.A. 1992. Biosynthesis of human papillomavirus from a continuous cell line upon epithelial differentiation. Science 257: 971–973.

Michel, N., Osen, W., Gissmann, L., Schumacher, T.N., Zentgraf, H., and Muller, M. 2002. Enhanced immunogenicity of HPV 16 E7 fusion proteins in DNA vaccination. Virology 294: 47–59.

Mork, J., Lie, A.K., Glattre, E., Hallmans, G., Jellum, E., Koskela, P., Mol.ler, B., Pukkala, E., Schiller, J.T., Youngman, L., Lehtinen, M., and Dillner, J. 2001. Human papillomavirus infection as a risk factor for squamous-cell carcinoma of the head and neck. N. Engl. J. Med. 344: 1125–1131.

Moscicki, A.B., Shiboski, S., Broering, J., Powell, K., Clayton, L., Jay, N., Darragh, T.M., Brescia, R., Kanowitz, S., Miller, S.B., Stone, J., Hanson, E., and Palefsky, J. 1998. The natural history of human papillomavirus infection as measured by repeated DNA testing in adolescent and young women. J. Pediatr. 132: 277–284.

Muderspach, L., Wilczynski, S., Roman, L., Bade, L., Felix, J., Small, L.A., Kast, W.M., Fascio, G., Marty, V., and Weber, J. 2000. A phase I trial of a human papillomavirus (HPV) peptide vaccine for women with high-grade cervical and vulvar intraepithelial neoplasia who are HPV 16 positive. Clin. Cancer Res. 6: 3406–3416.

Munger, K. and Howley, P.M. 2002. Human papillomavirus immortalization and transformation functions. Virus Res. 89: 213–228.

Munoz, N., Bosch, F.X., de Sanjose, S., Herrero, R., Castellsague, X., Shah, K.V., Snijders, P.J., and Meijer, C.J. 2003. Epidemiologic classification of human papillomavirus types associated with cervical cancer. N. Engl. J. Med. 348: 518–527.

Myers, E.R., McCrory, D.C., Nanda, K., Bastian, L., and Matchar, D.B. 2000. Mathematical model for the natural history of human papillomavirus infection and cervical carcinogenesis. Am J. Epidemiol. 151: 1158–1171.

Nobbenhuis, M.A., Helmerhorst, T.J., van den Brule, A.J., Rozendaal, L., Voorhorst, F.J., Bezemer, P.D., Verheijen, R.H., and Meijer, C.J. 2001. Cytological regression and clearance of high-risk human papillomavirus in women with an abnormal cervical smear. Lancet 358: 1782–1783.

Ohlschlager, P., Osen, W., Dell, K., Faath, S., Garcea, R.L., Jochmus, I., Muller, M., Pawlita, M., Schafer, K., Sehr, P., Staib, C., Sutter, G., and Gissmann, L. 2003. Human papillomavirus type 16 L1 capsomeres induce L1-specific cytotoxic T lymphocytes and tumor regression in C57BL/6 mice. J. Virol. 77: 4635–4645.

Palefsky, J. M. and Holly, E.A. 2003. Chapter 6: Immunosuppression and co-infection with HIV. J. Natl. Cancer Inst. Monogr. 41–46.

Palefsky, J.M., Holly, E.A., Gonzales, J., Berline, J., Ahn, D.K., and Greenspan, J.S. 1991. Detection of human papillomavirus DNA in anal intraepithelial neoplasia and anal cancer. Cancer Res. 51: 1014–1019.

Palefsky, J.M. 2003. Cervical human papillomavirus infection and cervical intraepithelial neoplasia in women positive for human immunodeficiency virus in the era of highly active antiretroviral therapy. Curr. Opin. Oncol. 15: 382–388.

Palefsky, J.M., Holly, E.A., Ralston, M.L., Jay, N., Berry, J.M., and Darragh, T.M. 1998. High incidence of anal high-grade squamous intra-epithelial lesions among HIV-positive and HIV-negative homosexual and bisexual men. AIDS 12: 495–503.

Palker, T.J., Monteiro, J.M., Martin, M.M., Kakareka, C., Smith, J.F., Cook, J.C., Joyce, J.G., and Jansen, K.U. 2001. Antibody, cytokine and cytotoxic T lymphocyte responses in chimpanzees immunized with human papillomavirus virus-like particles. Vaccine 19: 3733–3743.

Pastrana, D.V., Vass, W.C., Lowy, D.R., and Schiller, J.T. 2001. NHPV16 VLP vaccine induces human antibodies that neutralize divergent variants of HPV16. Virology 279: 361–369.

Peh, W.L., Middleton, K., Christensen, N., Nicholls, P., Egawa, K., Sotlar, K., Brandsma, J., Percival, A., Lewis, J., Liu, W.J., and Doorbar, J. 2002. Life cycle heterogeneity in animal models of human papillomavirus-associated disease. J. Virol. 76: 10401–10416.

Pfister, H. 1996. The role of human papillomavirus in anogenital cancer. Obstet. Gynecol. Clin. N. Am. 23: 579–595.

Piketty, C., Darragh, T.M., Da Costa, M., Bruneval, P., Heard, I., Kazatchkine, M.D., and Palefsky, J.M. 2003. High prevalence of anal human papillomavirus infection and anal cancer precursors among HIV-infected persons in the absence of anal intercourse. Ann. Intern. Med. 138: 453–459.

Revaz, V., Benyacoub, J., Kast, W.M., Schiller, J.T., De Grandi, P., and Nardelli-Haefliger, D. 2001. Mucosal vaccination with a recombinant Salmonella typhimurium expressing human papillomavirus type 16 (HPV16) L1 virus-like particles (VLPs) or HPV16 VLPs purified from insect cells inhibits the growth of HPV16-expressing tumor cells in mice. Virology 279: 354–360.

Richardson, H., Kelsall, G., Tellier, P., Voyer, H., Abrahamowicz, M., Ferenczy, A., Coutlee, F., and Franco, E.L. 2003. The natural history of type-specific human papillomavirus infections in female university students. Cancer Epidemiol. Biomarkers Prev. 12: 485–490.

Roden, R.B., Weissinger, E.M., Henderson, D.W., Booy, F., Kirnbauer, R., Mushinski, J.F., Lowy, D.R., and Schiller, J.T. 1994. Neutralization of bovine papillomavirus by antibodies to L1 and L2 capsid proteins. J. Virol. 68: 7570–7574.

Rose, R.C., Reichman, R.C., and Bonnez, W. 1994. Human papillomavirus (HPV) type 11 recombinant virus-like particles induce the formation of neutralizing antibodies and detect HPV-specific antibodies in human sera. J. Gen. Virol .75 (Pt 8): 2075–2079.

Sanders, G. D. and Taira, A.V. 2003. Cost-effectiveness of a potential vaccine for human papillomavirus. Emerg. Infect. Dis. 9: 37–48.

Schiffman, M. and Kjaer, S.K. 2003. Chapter 2: Natural history of anogenital human papillomavirus infection and neoplasia. J. Natl. Cancer Inst. Monogr. 14–19.

Schlecht, N.F., Kulaga, S., Robitaille, J., Ferreira, S., Santos, M., Miyamura, R.A., Duarte-Franco, E., Rohan, T.E., Ferenczy, A., Villa, L.L., and Franco, E.L. 2001. Persistent human papillomavirus infection as a predictor of cervical intraepithelial neoplasia. JAMA 286: 3106–3114.

Schwarz, E., Freese, U.K., Gissmann, L., Mayer, W., Roggenbuck, B., Stremlau, A., and zur, H.H. 1985. Structure and transcription of human papillomavirus sequences in cervical carcinoma cells. Nature 314: 111–114.

Sheets, E.E., Urban, R.G., Crum, C.P., Hedley, M.L., Politch, J.A., Gold, M.A., Muderspach, L.I., Cole, G.A., and Crowley-Nowick, P.A. 2003. Immunotherapy of human cervical high-grade cervical intraepithelial neoplasia with microparticle-delivered human papillomavirus 16 E7 plasmid DNA. Am J. Obstet. Gynecol. 188: 916–926.

Shen, Z.Y., Hu, S.P., Lu, L.C., Tang, C.Z., Kuang, Z.S., Zhong, S.P., and Zeng, Y. 2002. Detection of human papillomavirus in esophageal carcinoma. J. Med. Virol. 68: 412–416.

Sherman, L., Alloul, N., Golan, I., Durst, M., and Baram, A. 1992. Expression and splicing patterns of human papillomavirus type 16 mRNAs in pre-cancerous lesions and carcinomas of the cervix, in human keratinocytes immortalized by HPV 16, and in cell lines established from cervical cancers. Int. J. Cancer 50: 356–364.

Sisk, E. A. and Robertson, E.S. 2002. Clinical implications of human papillomavirus infection: Front Biosci. 7: e77–e84.

Smahel, M., Sima, P., Ludvikova, V., and Vonka, V. 2001. Modified HPV16 E7 Genes as DNA Vaccine against E7-containing oncogenic cells. Virology 281: 231–238.

Stanley, M.A. 2001. Human papillomavirus and cervical carcinogenesis: Best. Pract. Res. Clin. Obstet. Gynaecol. 15: 663–676.

Stanley, M.A. 2003. Progress in prophylactic and therapeutic vaccines for human papillomavirus infection. Expert. Rev. Vaccines. 2: 381–389.

Stewart, T.J., Smyth, M.J., Fernando, G.J., Frazer, I.H., and Leggatt, G.R. 2003. Inhibition of early tumor growth requires J alpha 18-positive (natural killer T) cells. Cancer Res. 63: 3058–3060.

Stubenrauch, F. and Laimins, L.A. 1999. Human papillomavirus life cycle: active and latent phases. Semin. Cancer Biol. 9: 379–386.

Sugase, M. and Matsukura, T. 1997. Distinct manifestations of human papillomaviruses in the vagina. Int. J. Cancer 72: 412–415.

Suzich, J.A., Ghim, S.J., Palmer-Hill, F.J., White, W.I., Tamura, J.K., Bell, J.A., Newsome, J.A., Jenson, A.B., and Schlegel, R. 1995. Systemic immunization with papillomavirus L1 protein completely prevents the development of viral mucosal papillomas. Proc. Natl. Acad. Sci. USA 92: 11553–11557.

Tracking the Hidden Epidemics, Trends in STDs in the United States 2000, 2001. Centers for Disease Control and Prevention, 18–19.

Trimble, C., Lin, C.T., Hung, C.F., Pai, S., Juang, J., He, L., Gillison, M., Pardoll, D., Wu, L., and Wu, T.C. 2003. Comparison of the CD8[+] T cell responses and antitumor effects generated by DNA vaccine administered through gene gun, biojector, and syringe. Vaccine 21: 4036–4042.

Trus, B.L., Roden, R.B., Greenstone, H.L., Vrhel, M., Schiller, J.T., and Booy, F.P. 1997. Novel structural features of bovine papillomavirus capsid revealed by a three-dimensional reconstruction to 9 A resolution. Nature Struct. Biol. 4: 413–420.

Turek, L.P. 1994. The structure, function, and regulation of papillomaviral genes in infection and cervical cancer. Adv. Virus Res. 44: 305–356.

Unckell, F., Streeck, R.E., and Sapp, M. 1997. Generation and neutralization of pseudovirions of human papillomavirus type 33. J. Virol. 71: 2934–2939.

van Driel, W.J., Ressing, M.E., Kenter, G.G., Brandt, R.M., Krul, E.J., van Rossum, A.B., Schuuring, E., Offringa, R., Bauknecht, T., Tamm-Hermelink, A., van Dam, P.A., Fleuren, G.J., Kast, W.M., Melief, C.J., and Trimbos, J.B. 1999. Vaccination with HPV16 peptides of patients with advanced cervical carcinoma: clinical evaluation of a phase I–II trial. Eur. J. Cancer 35: 946–952.

Velders, M.P., McElhiney, S., Cassetti, M.C., Eiben, G.L., Higgins, T., Kovacs, G.R., Elmishad, A.G., Kast, W.M., and Smith, L.R. 2001a. Eradication of established tumors by vaccination with Venezuelan equine encephalitis virus replicon particles delivering human papillomavirus 16 E7 RNA. Cancer Res. 61: 7861–7867.

Velders, M.P., Weijzen, S., Eiben, G.L., Elmishad, A.G., Kloetzel, P.M., Higgins, T., Ciccarelli, R.B., Evans, M., Man, S., Smith, L., and Kast, W.M. 2001b. Defined flanking spacers and enhanced proteolysis is essential for eradication of established tumors by an epitope string DNA vaccine. J. Immunol. 166: 5366–5373.

von Knebel, D.M., Rittmuller, C., zur, H.H., and Durst, M. 1992. Inhibition of tumorigenicity of cervical cancer cells in nude mice by HPV E6-E7 anti-sense RNA. Int. J. Cancer 51: 831–834.

Vonka, V., Sobotkova, E., Hamsikova, E., Smahel, M., Zak, R., Kitasato, H., and Sainerova, H. 1998. Induction of anti-tumour immunity by suicide-gene-modified HPV-16-transformed hamster cells. Int. J. Cancer 77: 470–475.

Walboomers, J.M., Jacobs, M.V., Manos, M.M., Bosch, F.X., Kummer, J.A., Shah, K.V., Snijders, P.J., Peto, J., Meijer, C.J., and Munoz, N. 1999. Human papillomavirus is a necessary cause of invasive cervical cancer worldwide. J. Pathol. 189: 12–19.

Wallin, K.L., Wiklund, F., Angstrom, T., Bergman, F., Stendahl, U., Wadell, G., Hallmans, G., and Dillner, J. 1999. Type-specific persistence of human papillomavirus DNA before the development of invasive cervical cancer. N. Engl. J. Med. 341: 1633–1638.

Wiatrak, B.J. 2003. Overview of recurrent respiratory papillomatosis: Curr. Opin. Otolaryngol. Head Neck Surg. 11: 433–441.

Wilcox, R.A., Flies, D.B., Zhu, G., Johnson, A.J., Tamada, K., Chapoval, A.I., Strome, S.E., Pease, L.R., and Chen, L. 2002. Provision of antigen and CD137 signaling breaks Immunological ignorance, promoting regression of poorly immunogenic tumors. J. Clin. Invest 109: 651–659.

Wiley, D.J., Douglas, J., Beutner, K., Cox, T., Fife, K., Moscicki, A.B., and Fukumoto, L. 2002. External genital warts: diagnosis, treatment, and prevention. Clin. Infect. Dis. 35: S210–S224.

Wright, T.C., Jr., Cox, J.T., Massad, L.S., Carlson, J., Twiggs, L.B., and Wilkinson, E.J. 2003. 2001 consensus guidelines for the management of women with cervical intraepithelial neoplasia. Am J. Obstet. Gynecol. 189: 295–304.

Yeager, M.D., Aste-Amezaga, M., Brown, D.R., Martin, M.M., Shah, M.J., Cook, J.C., Christensen, N.D., Ackerson, C., Lowe, R.S., Smith, J.F., Keller, P., and Jansen, K.U. 2000. Neutralization of human papillomavirus (HPV) pseudovirions: a novel and efficient approach to detect and characterize HPV neutralizing antibodies. Virology 278: 570–577.

Zhang, L.F., Zhou, J., Chen, S., Cai, L.L., Bao, Q.Y., Zheng, F.Y., Lu, J.Q., Padmanabha, J., Hengst, K., Malcolm, K., and Frazer, I.H. 2000. HPV6b virus like particles are potent immunogens without adjuvant in man. Vaccine 18: 1051–1058.

Zhou, J., Sun, X.Y., Stenzel, D.J., and Frazer, I.H. 1991. Expression of vaccinia recombinant HPV 16 L1 and L2 ORF proteins in epithelial cells is sufficient for assembly of HPV virion-like particles. Virology 185: 251–257.

Zhou, J., Stenzel, D.J., Sun, X.Y., and Frazer, I.H. 1993. Synthesis and assembly of infectious bovine papillomavirus particles in vitro. J. Gen. Virol. 74 (Pt 4): 763–768.

Zhou, J., Sun, X.Y., Louis, K., and Frazer, I.H. 1994. Interaction of human papillomavirus (HPV) type 16 capsid proteins with HPV DNA requires an intact L2 N-terminal sequence. J. Virol. 68: 619–625.

zur Hausen, H. 1999. Immortalization of human cells and their malignant conversion by high risk human papillomavirus genotypes. Semin. Cancer Biol. 9: 405–411.

zur Hausen, H. 2000. Papillomaviruses causing cancer: evasion from host-cell control in early events in carcinogenesis. J. Natl. Cancer Inst. 92: 690–698.

Zwaveling, S., Ferreira Mota, S.C., Nouta, J., Johnson, M., Lipford, G.B., Offringa, R., van der Burg, S.H., and Melief, C.J. 2002. Established human papillomavirus type 16-expressing tumors are effectively eradicated following vaccination with long peptides. J. Immunol. 169: 350–358.

Chapter 13

Development of Cancer Vaccines: Current Status

Pamela L. Beatty and Olivera J. Finn

Abstract

The pioneering work leading to the isolation and molecular characterization of tumor antigens has been fundamental to the design of cancer vaccines. It showed that tumor-specific epitopes were presented by tumor cells and cancer vaccine strategies could be developed to prime the immune system to recognize and destroy tumor cells while preserving normal cells. The current challenges to tumor immunologists working on therapeutic and prophylactic vaccines include making the right choices of antigen, delivery systems, adjuvants, and routes of administration, as well as overcoming evasion mechanisms imposed by the tumor. Studies of cancer vaccines in animal models and their testing in small clinical trials have shown promising results, prompting further improvements in their design according to the newest discoveries in immunology. This chapter will highlight various cancer vaccines that are under development as well as review several that are currently in clinical trials.

INTRODUCTION

The main goal of vaccination is to establish long lasting immune memory cells that will enable a faster and more robust immune response to a subsequent challenge, either by an invading pathogen or a cancer cell. Unique to the development of cancer vaccines, as currently applied, is the challenge to generate a robust effector response and a memory response in the presence of the disease and in the context of a suppressed immune system. Immune suppression is a result of the effects exerted by the tumor, the previous therapy, or the advanced age of the patient. The first attempt to treat cancer with immunological methods resembling vaccines occurred more than 100 years ago. The treating physician was William Coley, and his 'vaccines' became known as 'Coley's toxins'. Coley found a correlation between disease remission in sarcoma patients and the development of erysipelas, a severe skin infection that is caused by *Streptococcus pyogenes* (Wiemann *et al.*, 1994; Hobohm, 2001). Coley vaccinated sarcoma patients with a mixture of heat-killed streptococci and *Serratia marrescens*. Although the exact mechanism leading to tumor regression was not known at the time, it was correlated with the presence of fever. With today's knowledge, most of the antitumor effects of Coley's toxins can be attributed to the bacterial products they contained, which produce 'danger signals' (Matzinger, 2002) and are thus potent activators of the immune system.

Danger signals can be given by foreign DNA, RNA, heat shock proteins, and bacterial and viral gene products that are released by infected necrotic or apoptotic cells. Recognition of danger signals is mediated through germ line encoded pattern recognition receptors and

Toll-like receptors (Gordon, 2002; Triantafilou *et al.*, 2002) that are present on or within cells of the innate immune system. Activation of the innate immune system is required for the subsequent activation of antigen specific T cells and B cells that comprise the adaptive immune response (Carroll *et al.*, 1998; Dabbagh *et al.*, 2003). In the absence of danger signals, tumor development can proceed without opposition from the immune system. Many cancer vaccine strategies are incorporating ways to elicit the responses of the innate immune system in order to ensure more robust tumor-specific responses.

Currently, the development of cancer vaccines is moving in two directions and although they share many conceptual and technological challenges (Finn, 2003), they require separate models for testing of their potential and efficacy. One direction is towards the development of therapeutic cancer vaccines that are designed to elicit and/or boost antitumor immunity in patients with minimal residual disease, thereby preventing or prolonging the time to recurrence. Therapeutic cancer vaccines have been tested in animal models and phase I/II human clinical trials. The other direction is towards the development of prophylactic cancer vaccines, which are designed to induce a state of immunity in healthy individuals with a predisposition to cancer (Lollini *et al.*, 2002; Finn, 2003). To date, prophylactic cancer vaccines have only been tested in animal models.

The current challenges for the tumor immunologist in the design of therapeutic and prophylactic vaccines include choices of the best antigens, delivery systems, adjuvants and routes of administration, that would overcome immune evasion mechanisms present in the tumor patient. All of these choices require appropriate models for testing the efficacy of the vaccine.

IMMUNE RESPONSE TO CANCER

Tumor-specific T-cells and antibodies can be found in patients with cancer, suggesting that a mechanism exists that allows the initial recognition of tumor cells. The concept of cancer immunosurveillance was initially proposed by Burnet more than 30 years ago (Burnet, 1970) who suggested for the first time that the immune system had the ability to recognize and eliminate developing tumor cells. In an attempt to give credence to this proposed immune surveillance mechanism and to explain the formation and progression of spontaneous tumor cells, several groups tested the hypothesis that animals with compromised immune systems developed tumors more frequently than immunocompetent animals. Initial experiments that compared chemically induced tumor formation in nude mice versus wild type mice showed no statistically significant difference between the two groups (Stutman, 1974). Subsequent experiments, however, have shown that the basic concept of immunosurveilance is indeed valid and that the many constituents of an intact immune system participate in the recognition and control of primary tumor formation and progression. Tumor development is a multistep process requiring years for a single transformed cell to become a malignant cell mass with distant metastases. During this time, there are many interactions between the tumor and the immune system and the tumor variants that persist do so because they acquire numerous mutations that not only direct their continued growth and survival but also evade the immune destruction. A process termed 'cancer immunoediting' has been proposed that hypothesizes that the immune surveillance system can function to select tumor variants that have found ways to subvert the host immune system (Dunn *et al.*, 2002). This process is analogous to the evasion mechanisms employed by many persistent viral and bacterial infections, where the selective pressure of drug intervention propagates a more virulent outgrowth. The cumulative knowledge gained from this and the early work shows that tumor cells are not passive targets; rather, their interaction with the immune system is a very dynamic process, not unlike that of a pathogen. This supports the idea that vaccines could be designed to enhance the immune system and prevent cancer much the same way that vaccination has been successful for the prevention of many infectious diseases. The crucial message born out of the immunosurveilance concept is that to fight tumor cells it is of fundamental importance to preserve and augment the immune system. It is counterproductive to destroy the immune system to eradicate tumor cells, which unfortunately has been the result of standard cancer therapies, such as chemotherapy and radiation.

Whether an active or a passive process, tumor cells have developed mechanisms to avoid the immune system (Marincola *et al.*, 2000). Some tumors can drastically reduce or lose expression of classical MHC molecules (Garcia-Lora *et al.*, 2001; Maleno *et al.*, 2002) while expressing non-classical MHC molecules, thereby inhibiting both T cell and NK cell activity (Marin *et al.*, 2003). Tumor cells have also been shown to lose expression of tumor antigens (Jager *et al.*, 1997), stressing the requirement in vaccine development to choose a tumor antigen that is critical for the survival of the tumor cell. Loss of TAP transporter proteins has been shown to occur in tumors (Cromme *et al.*, 1994), which interferes with peptide delivery to MHC class I molecules resulting in decreased surface expression of MHC molecules as well as tumor-specific antigens. Apoptosis of activated tumor infiltrating lymphocytes has been shown to occur through the up-regulation of Fas-L on the surface of tumor cells (Strand *et al.*, 1996; Cefai *et al.*, 2001). Tumor cells have also been shown to secrete soluble cytokines that can directly interfere with T-cell function. TGF-β has been shown to suppress T-cell activation and proliferation, as well as increase angiogenesis facilitating tumor growth (Beck *et al.*, 2001; Hasegawa *et al.*, 2001).

Current research in the field of tumor immunology is aimed at elucidating the many mechanisms involved in tumor evasion and when in the process of tumor formation these mechanisms occur. An understanding of the tumor-host interaction will lead to the development of cancer vaccine strategies that can effectively manipulate these mechanisms in favor of the host.

REQUIREMENTS FOR AN EFFECTIVE ANTI-TUMOR IMMUNE RESPONSE

An effective antitumor immune response requires an initial priming step that activates naive T-cells to differentiate into effector T-cells, followed by killing of tumor that is mediated by CD8$^+$ cytotoxic T cells (CTLs). The priming step is critically important for the generation of both effector and memory responses. The initial effector burst size, in addition to determining the strength of the antitumor response, has been correlated with the magnitude of memory that is generated for a subsequent encounter with the same antigen. Tumors can evade the immune system simply by suppressing or avoiding the initial priming phase of the immune response, thus never generating effector T-cells.

Priming immunity to tumor antigens

Tumor cells express a wide variety of proteins that can serve as tumor antigens; some associated with the oncogenic process and others associated with basic cellular functions. For T-cell recognition of tumors, these proteins must be presented to T-cells both as priming antigens and as target antigens for CTL mediated tumor killing. Tumor antigens can be presented to the immune system in one of two ways: antigen-presenting cells (APCs) can phagocytose tumor cells or endocytose proteins derived from tumor cells, and process and present peptide fragments in MHC class I and class II molecules for recognition by CD4[+] helper T cells and CD8[+] cytotoxic T cells (CTLs) respectively. Activated CD4[+] T-cells are rarely involved in direct killing of tumor cells, however, they produce cytokines that are able to direct a cell-mediated immune response. Efficient priming of naïve T-cells requires two signals. Recognition of the tumor peptide–MHC complex through the antigen-specific T-cell receptor (TCR) provides the required first signal for T-cell activation. The second signal is provided by the ligation of CD28 molecule on the surface of the T-cell with costimulatory molecules CD80 (B7.1) and CD86 (B7.2), on the surface of APCs.

The challenge in generating an anti-tumor immune response

The majority of the protein targets from tumor cells are self-antigens. Therefore, in the context of cancer, the majority of peptides presented to the immune system by APCs are derived from self-antigens and serve as signal one to the adaptive immune system. The innate immune system is activated and costimulatory signal two delivered in the presence of danger signals (Matzinger, 2002), which are usually not present during processing and presentation of self-peptides or tumor peptides. Signal one (tumor antigen) in the absence of signal two (costimulation) renders T cells anergic, which could result in tolerance to some tumor antigens. Another factor that influences the initial priming step in tumor-specific immunity is the quality of the available T-cell repertoire. During T-cell maturation in the thymus, T-cells that react to self-peptide/MHC molecules with high affinity are deleted from the T-cell repertoire. Thus, T-cells in the periphery have low affinity TCR for self-antigen. These T-cells are unable to generate or sustain signal one, which results in their inability to mature into effector cells. Although this prevents unwanted autoimmune responses, it leaves a T-cell repertoire that is ill equipped to eliminate tumor cells.

Current research into cancer vaccine development is aimed at manipulating this initial priming process by exploring different antigen delivery systems and adjuvants for APC activation (Cox *et al.*, 1997; Marciani, 2003). Dendritic cells (DCs) have been identified as the most effective antigen-presenting cells for priming the immune system and have been referred to as 'nature's adjuvant' (Banchereau *et al.*, 1998). Under normal, non-disease circumstances, DCs are quite efficient at taking-up and processing antigen in peripheral tissues of the body where they reside as immature DCs. In this immature state, which is characterized by low level expression of costimulatory as well as MHC class I and class II molecules, they are inefficient at presenting antigen. Danger signals promote DC migration to the nearest lymph node, and induce their maturation and expression of costimulatory and MHC molecules, resulting in their ability to deliver signal one and signal two, and prime antigen-specific T-cells (Guermonprez *et al.*, 2002). DCs also possess the ability to present exogenous tumor antigenic peptides in the context of MHC class I or class II molecules. In a process termed cross-priming, the immature DCs capture and process apoptotic or necrotic cells at the site of tumor formation and direct antigens from these cells into the cytoplasm and the MHC class I pathway. This is thought to be the major mechanism of priming naïve CD8[+] T cells, which are the main effector cells in an antitumor immune response.

For this reason, much of the current vaccine research is devoted to finding ways to utilize DCs as vaccine vehicles for the presentation of tumor antigens (Banchereau *et al.*, 1998; Dallal *et al.*, 2000). This includes finding efficient means of targeting tumor antigens to DCs, both *ex vivo* and *in vivo*. Some of the current strategies include: (1) *ex vivo* loading of DCs with peptides or whole tumor cell lysates, (2) transduction of DCs with tumor antigens and/or costimulatory molecules using recombinant viruses or bacteria, and (3) transfection with naked DNA or RNA. Studies performed to date using a variety of DC-based vaccination protocols have shown that the DC biology is quite complex and that DCs not only possess the ability to activate T-cells but can also tolerize T-cells. Currently, extensive research is being applied to better understanding the fundamental biology of different DC subsets and their role in regulating multiple facets of the immune response (Guermonprez *et al.*, 2002).

Importance of the route of immunization

The route of vaccine administration determines the amount of antigen that is delivered and the location of the antigen. Currently, the majority of experiments that compare routes of administration are using DC-based vaccines. Serody *et al.* immunized mice with antigen pulsed DCs delivered either intravenously (i.v.), intradermally (i.d.), or subcutaneously (s.c.). They found that i.d. injection generated the highest frequency of cytotoxic T cells (CTLs), but that the overall antitumor response did not correlate with the specific route of administration (Serody *et al.*, 2000). However, Okada *et al.* found that greater CTL responses were generated from i.d. and s.c. injections versus intraperitoneal (i.p) and i.v. injections (Okada *et al.*, 2001), suggesting that the route of administration can determine the magnitude of a T-cell response. The i.v. route of administration has been shown to generate very efficient antibody responses (Fong *et al.*, 2001a), but not CTLs.

Increased attention is being given to the mucosal route of administration for cancer vaccines. It has been shown that cells primed in a mucosal inductive site may preferentially migrate to mucosal effector sites through a pathway termed the common mucosal system (McGhee, 1999). This may represent an important vaccine strategy for the prevention of adenocarcinomas, as the majority of these tumors originally arise in mucosal sites. This is a relatively new area in cancer vaccine development, but information is beginning to emerge with regard to the migration of lymphocytes and APCs to mucosal sites (von Andrian *et al.*, 2000; Campbell *et al.*, 2002).

THE ROLE OF ADJUVANTS IN CANCER VACCINES

Adjuvants are substances added to vaccines to increase the immunogenicity of antigens that are not very immunogenic on their own, thus enhancing the initial priming step. Adjuvants are also used to preferentially induce Th1 or Th2 responses (McNeela *et al.*, 2001). Activated CD4$^+$ T cells, bound to the same APCs as CD8$^+$ T-cells, can induce increased costimulatory molecules on the surface of the APCs, thus providing the enhanced costimulation needed for CD8$^+$ T cell activation (Ridge *et al.*, 1998). Activated CD4$^+$ T cells initially produce large amounts of IL-2 and differentiate into Th0 cells where they produce both IL-4 and IFN-γ. Depending on the cytokine environment, Th0 cells differentiate along one of two pathways becoming either Th1 or Th2 cells (Murphy *et al.*, 2000). This initial cytokine environment is critically dependent upon the cells of the innate immune system and this is the first step where adjuvants have the ability to shape an immune response. Th1 cells predominantly produce IFN-γ (Szabo *et al.*, 2000), which activates macrophages to produce IL-12. The synergy between IFN-γ and IL-12 enhances the cytotoxic effector functions of CD8$^+$ T cells. Th2 cells predominantly secrete IL-4, IL-5, and IL-10, and enhance humoral immune responses by activating B cells to produce antibody. Although it has become evident that the most efficacious cancer vaccines are those that can elicit multiple components of the immune system, induction of a Th1 dominated immune response has been the important mandate for the majority of cancer vaccines.

Different adjuvants act at different steps of the immunological events that ultimately lead to efficient lymphocyte priming. Adjuvants can exert their activity at the site of injection or in the draining lymph node. They increase the migration of DCs to the site of injection and facilitate antigen up take and transport to the draining lymph node. Adjuvants can also provide a 'depot effect' for prolonged release of antigen. The sustained presence of antigen is important for the duration of the immune response. Lastly, adjuvants can provide danger signals. These induce the release of inflammatory cytokines that direct the course of an immune response and induce DCs to up-regulate their costimulatory molecules enhancing delivery of signal 2.

Adjuvants are generally categorized as particulate or non-particulate, however, some have been found to have properties of both categories (Cox *et al.*, 1997). The mode of action for most non-particulate adjuvants is elicitation of danger signals. Non-particulate adjuvants include bacterial products such as lipopolysaccharide (LPS), cholera toxin (CT), *Escherichia coli* labile toxin (LT), monophosphoryl lipid A (MPL), and saponins (Quil A). Lipopolysaccharide (LPS) from gram-negative bacteria and monophosphoryl lipid A (MPL) from *Salmonella* have been widely used in experimental cancer vaccines and found to be particularly good at activating CTLs. Recently, unmethylated CpG dinucleotides, contained in bacterial DNA, have received much attention for their strong immunostimulatory abilities (Davila *et al.*, 2000).

Particulate adjuvants are microscopic particles that protect encapsulated antigen, serve as 'depots' for antigen release, and facilitate phagocytosis and entry into the MHC class I pathway. These include aluminum salts (alum), water-in-oil-emulsions [incomplete Freund's adjuvant (IFA)], oil-in-water emulsions [squalene, muramyl dipeptide (MDP)], immune stimulating complexes (ISCOMs), and liposomes. Immune-stimulating complexes (ISCOMs) are rigid cage-like structures that form spontaneously when mixing cholesterol, phosphatidylcholine, and saponins. Saponins are detergents that are obtained from the tree bark of *Quillaia saponaria* (Cox *et al.*, 1998). The purified fraction used most often with ISCOMs is termed Quil A. Several antigens can be incorporated into a single ISCOM matrix and the matrix provides protection for the antigen from degradation and a means to concentrate the antigen into a small particle. ISCOMs method of action appears to be their ability to fuse with membranes, which facilitates their uptake by APCs. The detergent properties of Quil A may form pores in the endosomes, thereby delivering the antigen into the cytoplasm. Liposomes are similar to ISCOMs in that they provide a means to protect antigen from degradation and concentrate antigen into a small particle. Liposomes consist of one (unilamellar) or more (multilamellar) phospholipids bilayers, which enclose an aqueous phase (Barratt, 2003). Liposomes have greater cell specificity than ISCOMs in that they target macrophages (Barratt, 2003; Renno *et al.*, 2003). However, peptides have been coupled to their surface to activate B- and T-cells directly (Lundberg *et al.*, 2000). Due to their lipid content, liposomes can readily fuse with plasma membranes and can be designed with a pH sensitive configuration that changes conformation within lysosomes, thereby allowing the encapsulated material to enter the cytoplasm. This is especially important for facilitating antigen processing and presentation in MHC class I pathway.

MOLECULARLY DEFINED TUMOR ANTIGENS AS CANCER VACCINES

Crucial to the field of tumor immunology and cancer vaccination was the development of methods for isolating tumor antigens, leading to the isolation and molecular characterization of the first tumor antigen, MAGE-1 (Van Pel et al., 1982; De Plaen et al., 1988; van der Bruggen et al., 1991). The past two decades of research have been fruitful leading to the identification of a myriad of tumor antigens, which have been used to elucidate many of the basic mechanisms involved in tumor recognition and rejection, and in cancer vaccines composition. Tumor antigens are classified into broad categories based on the nature and origin of the protein. Several review articles describe the categories in detail (Melief et al., 2000; Renkvist et al., 2001; Renno et al., 2003), and an updated list of known tumor antigens and their epitopes is accessible on the Istituto Nazionale Tumori website (www. istitutotumori.mi.it). The list continues to grow as new tumor antigens are discovered. Cyclin B1 is an example of a newly discovered tumor antigen (Kao et al., 2001), which is currently under investigation as a potential target for vaccine therapy. It is over-expressed in many tumors (Yu et al., 2002), and is critical for maintaining tumor cell integrity. A list of the most common tumor antigen categories with selected examples for each category can be found in Table 13.1.

Many of the known tumor antigens are self-proteins that are expressed at low levels in normal tissue but are over-expressed or modified in tumor cells. The self versus non-self distinction highlights the specific challenge facing the development of cancer vaccines, in as much as a self-tumor antigen might require a more potent vaccine to break self-tolerance. There are several key factors that need to be considered when choosing a tumor antigen as a target for the development of a cancer vaccine. First, the selection of a tumor antigen that is expressed by a broad range of tumor types would enable the development of a vaccine that could translate into therapy for a large number of patients. Second, the tumor antigen should have epitopes that can be recognized by $CD4^+$ and $CD8^+$ T cells as well as antibodies. Furthermore, to be efficacious it should be administered in a formulation able to stimulate multiple components of the innate as well as the adaptive immune systems. Third, the tumor antigen should be a protein that is required to maintain the integrity of the tumor cell. This will prevent the tumor cell from selectively eliminating the antigen and subverting the antigen-specific immune response. Lastly, a tumor antigen should be perceived by the immune system as non-self to avoid problems of tolerance and autoimmunity. The fact is, however, that many of the tumor antigens that are expressed in a broad range of tumors and can elicit a tumor-specific response are also self-proteins that are expressed in normal cells. Therefore, one of the important issues in many vaccine designs is finding ways to overcome tolerance, activate the low-affinity T cells to kill tumor cells, and avoid destructive autoimmunity.

DIFFERENT CANCER VACCINE FORMULATIONS

Discovery of numerous tumor antigens has revolutionized the field of tumor immunology by providing potential candidates for antigen-specific cancer vaccines and targets for tumor specific immunity. Cancer vaccines have been designed utilizing many forms of antigen depending on the tumor type as well as the type of the desired immune response.

Table 13.1 Tumor antigens

Cancer/testis antigens (these antigens result from reactivation of genes that are normally silent in adult tissue)

MAGE family

BAGE family

GAGE family

NY-ESO-1

Differentiation antigens (these antigens are tissue specific and shared between tumors and normal tissue from which the tumor arose)

MART-1/Melan-A

Gp100

PSA

Tyrosinase

Overexpressed antigens (these antigens are expressed in normal tissue and overexpressed in tumors)

CEA

HER2/neu

MUC1

RU1

Tumor-specific antigens (these antigens are unique to tumors and generally arise from point mutations or abnormal expression of normal genes)

β-Catenin

CDK4

ELF2M

Cyclin B1

p53

Fusion proteins (these antigens are a result of translocation of chromosomes)

bcr-abl

Pml/RARa

Viral tumor antigens (viruses can induce the transformation of many cell types which then express the viral proteins)

EBV Epstein–Barr virus

HBV hepatitis B virus

HPV human papillomavirus

Peptide and adjuvant vaccines

Synthetic peptides as antigens in vaccines are attractive alternatives to many other forms of antigen because they are easily manufactured, chemically stable, and can provide greater control in specific targeting of an antitumor immune response. The first generation of peptide vaccines consisted of synthetic peptides administered via subcutaneous or epidermal injections (Salgaller *et al.*, 1995). This strategy uses the inherent endocytic ability of immature DCs that reside in the skin, to process and present tumor antigens to T-cells. In early trials, some clinical responses were observed, but induction of antigen-specific T-cells rarely occurred. Subsequent studies demonstrated that peptides in solution were rapidly degraded and eliminated before they reached DCs and coadministration with an adjuvant could facilitate their delivery to DCs, resulting in antigen-specific T-cell responses. A second generation of peptide vaccines incorporated various adjuvants such as oil–water emulsions [incomplete Freund's adjuvant (IFA)], alum precipitates, microspheres, liposomes, and ISCOMs. Initial experiments with MAGE-3 peptide resulted in some objective clinical responses (Marchand *et al.*, 1995). In another trial with the same peptide combined with IFA, T-cell responses could be detected (Weber *et al.*, 1999). A number of small pilot trials have been conducted using other peptides such as MART-1/MelanA, gp100, and tyrosinase (Salgaller *et al.*, 1996), and these early results showed minimal toxicity and the induction of CTL immune responses associated with this vaccination strategy. Cytokines have also been included in second generation peptide vaccines to enhance T-cells activity. These include IL-2, IL-12 and GM-CSF. Rosenberg *et al.* reported that vaccination of melanoma patients with synthetic peptide and IFA produced tumor regression in patients only if IL-2 was coadministered (Rosenberg *et al.*, 1998). Many vaccines based on peptide/adjuvant combinations have been evaluated in phase I/II clinical trials (Table 13.2). Induction of a more robust immunity remains one of the main challenges facing peptide vaccines.

The overall poor immunogenicity of peptides has led to other strategies to increase the potency of vaccines based on these epitopes. First, substitutions have been made of

Table 13.2 Examples of peptide and adjuvant vaccines

Type of cancer	Vaccine	Route	Reference
Melanoma	HSPPC-gp100	i.d./s.c.	Belli *et al.* (2002)
Melanoma	Shed tumor antigens + adjuvant	i.d.	Reynolds *et al.* (2003)
Melanoma	Gp100(210M) + tyrosinase (370D) + Montanide ± GM-CSF	s.c.	Weber *et al.* (2003)
Melanoma	Gp100(210M) + tyrosinase (370D) + montanide or QS-21 or GM-CSF	i.d. or s.c.	Schaed *et al.* (2002)
Melanoma	MART-1 (27L) + gp100 (210M) + tyrosinase (370D) + montanide + progenipoietin	s.c.	Pullarkat *et al.* (2003)
Breast	HER-2/neu peptides + flt3 ± GM-CSF	s.c.	Disis *et al.* (2002)
Breast and ovarian	HER-2/neu + GM-CSF	i.d.	Murray *et al.* (2002)
Prostate	HER-2/neu peptide + Flt3	s.c.	McNeel *et al.* (2003)
Prostate	Liposomal PSA + GM-CSF	s.c.	Meidenbauer *et al.* (2000)
Adenocarcinoma	MUC1 peptide + BCG	i.d.	Goydos *et al.* (1996)
Pancreatic	Ras peptide + GM-CSF	i.d.	Gjertsen *et al.* (2001)
Pancreatic	MUC1 + SB-AS2	i.m	Ramanathan *et al.* (2004)
Colon	Autologous tumor + BCG	i.d.	Harris *et al.* (2000)
Colorectal	HSPPC-gp96	i.d.	Mazzaferro *et al.* (2003)
CEA expressing	CEA protein ± GM-CSF	s.c.	Samanci *et al.* (1998)
CML	Bcr-abl peptide + QS-21	s.c.	Cathcart *et al.* (2003)
NY-ESO-1 expressing	NY-ESO-1 peptides ± GM-CSF	i.d.	Jager *et al.* (2000)
Various	HSPPC-gp96	s.c.	Janetzki *et al.* (2000)

HSPPC-gp96 = heat shock protein-gp96 peptide, Montanide = incomplete Freund's adjuvant, GM-CSF = granulocyte monocyte colony stimulating factor, Progenipoietin = agonist of granulocyte colony stimulating factor and Flt3 ligand, BCG = bacillus Calmette–Guerin, CEA = carcinoembryonic antigen, i.d. = intradermal, s.c. = subcutaneous.

residues at the MHC anchor positions to improve binding affinity of the tumor peptide for a given MHC molecule. It has been shown that the immunogenicity of a peptide is correlated with its affinity for an MHC molecule (van der Burg *et al.*, 1996). Second, substitutions can be made of peptide residues that directly contact the TCR. Tolerance to a self tumor antigen may be reversed by using peptide analogues with single amino acid substitutions, generating an epitope that is more immunogenic and still able to mediate T-cell responses. Rivoltini *et al.* found that using a variant of MART-1/MelanA peptide, containing a Leu instead of Ala in position 1, induced MART-1/MelanA-specific T-cells with enhanced immunological function (Rivoltini *et al.*, 1999). Peripheral blood lymphocytes from HLA-A2 melanoma patients were stimulated *in vitro* with either the native peptide or the peptide analogue. The analogue-primed T-cells lysed MART-1/MelanA targets with higher efficiency than cells primed with the native peptide. Analogue-primed T-cells were also capable of earlier and higher release of IFN-γ than T-cells generated from the native peptide. Although it is not possible to predict the effects of a single amino acid substitutions on T-cell affinity, computer programs are available that can predict epitopes with high affinity binding to MHC class I molecules. This strategy for modifying natural tumor epitopes has been tested in several clinical trials with promising results (Tables 13.2 and 13.3).

Tumor-derived heat shock proteins are gaining attention as potential cancer vaccines and are currently being evaluated in clinical trials (Mazzaferro *et al.*, 2003). Heat shock proteins (HSP) are a family of glycoproteins that form noncovalent complexes with peptides and can function as chaperones for antigenic tumor peptides (Srivastava *et al.*, 2001). These complexes can be purified from tumor tissue and injected as a vaccine. The HSP complex binds to and is internalized via the CD91 HSP-receptors on DCs, and the chaperoned peptides are processed within DCs and presented by MHC molecules to T cells. It has been shown that the tumor-derived HSP complex is tumor specific (Manjili *et al.*, 2002; Mazzaferro *et al.*, 2003) and that HSP can provide danger signals to DCs, inducing their migration, maturation, and secretion of inflammatory cytokines (Srivastava *et al.*, 2001; Manjili *et al.*, 2002).

DC-BASED VACCINES

In order to eliminate the problems associated with delivering peptides to DCs *in vivo,* such as peptide degradation and absence of DC migration at the injection site, many laboratories found ways to grow DCs *ex vivo*. They have become a useful tool for the study of various vaccination strategies (Nestle *et al.*, 2001). An important advantage to using DCs as a mode of vaccination is their ability to bypass inherent deficiencies in antigen presentation in the host. Tumor antigens can be loaded *ex vivo* into the MHC molecules of DCs by directly pulsing DCs with synthetic peptides or using whole tumor cell lysates, the prior being used for a defined T-cell epitope (Schuler-Thurner *et al.*, 2002) and the latter used for undefined epitopes (Zitvogel *et al.*, 1996; Asavaroengchai *et al.*, 2002). In murine models, *ex vivo* loaded DCs with peptides corresponding to T-cell epitopes were shown to elicit protective immunity as well as tumor regression (Zitvogel *et al.*, 1996; Mayordomo *et al.*, 1997; Soares *et al.*, 2001; Heimberger *et al.*, 2002). Based on the results obtained from animal studies, many clinical trials have been initiated, some of them providing promising preliminary results (Table 13.3).

In addition to defined tumor antigens, whole tumor cell lysates have become an attractive antigen source for cancer vaccines. This is based on the premise that using one

Table 13.3 Examples of dendritic cell vaccines

Type of cancer	Vaccine	Route	References
Melanoma	Peptide pulsed or tumor lysate pulsed DC + KLH	i.n.	Nestle *et al.* (1998)
Melanoma	DC + MelanA/MART-1 + tyrosinase + MAGE-3 + gp100 + Flu-MP + KLH	s.c.	Banchereau *et al.* (2001)
Melanoma	DC + tumor lysate + KLH	i.d.	Chang *et al.* (2002)
Melanoma	DC + tumor lysate	i.d.	Chakraborty *et al.* (1998)
Melanoma	DC + MAGE-3	s.c.	Schuler-Thurner *et al.* (2002)
Melanoma	DC + gp100 + tyrosinase + tetanus	i.v./s.c.	Slingluff *et al.* (2003)
Melanoma	DC + gp100 (210M) + tyrosinase (370D)	i.v.	Lau *et al.* (2001)
Breast or ovarian	DC + HER-2/neu or MUC1	s.c.	Brossart *et al.* (2000)
Prostate	DC + PSMA peptides	i.v.	Tjoa *et al.* (1999)
Prostate	DC + PAP/GM-CSF	i.v.	Small *et al.* (2000)
Bladder	DC + MAGE-3	s.c.	Nishiyama *et al.* (2001)
Gastric	DC + HER-2/neu peptide	i.d.	Kono *et al.* (2002)
CEA expressing	DC + Cap1 (6D) + KLH	i.v.	Fong *et al.* (2001)
CEA expressing	DC + Cap1	i.v. or i.d.	Morse *et al.* (1999)

DC = dendritic cell, KLH = keyhole limpet hemocyanin, PSMA = prostate-specific membrane antigen, PAP = prostatic acid phosphatase, CEA = carcinoembryonic antigen, i.n. = intranodal, i.v. = intravenous, i.d. = intradermal, s.c. = subcutaneous, i.m. = intramuscular.

unique protein or peptide for immunization may limit the T-cell repertoire for an antitumor response and that tumor cell lysates provide multiple tumor antigens. This has been tested in animal models and in clinical trials in order to enhance antigen-specific T-cells that can mediate protective immunity (Chakraborty *et al.*, 1998; Nestle *et al.*, 1998; Ni *et al.*, 2001). However, when using whole tumor cell lysates, DCs are expected to present in an immunogenic fashion many normal antigens in addition to tumor-specific antigens, which has the potential to elicit unwanted immune responses and destructive autoimmunity, as has been shown to occur in animal models (Ludewig *et al.*, 2000).

Fusion of tumor cells with DCs has also been shown to induce potent tumor immunity in animal models (Lespagnard *et al.*, 1998; Wang *et al.*, 1998; Tanaka *et al.*, 2001; Xia *et al.*, 2003). Much like using whole tumor cell lysates, this method provides another strategy to induce polyclonal T-cell responses against known and unidentified tumor antigens. This method has utilized syngeneic DC fused with syngeneic or allogeneic tumor cells, but also allogeneic DCs with syngeneic tumor cells. The rational for using an allogeneic fusion partner is based on the ability of a high frequency of naïve T-cells to proliferate in response to alloantigens, which could provide a stimulating environment for the generation of tumor specific responses. Tanaka *et al.* showed that in a mouse model the fusion with allogeneic DCs elicited higher proliferation of T cells than did the syngeneic DCs (Tanaka *et al.*, 2001). Krause *et al.* vaccinated melanoma patients with autologous tumor cells fused to allogeneic DCs and found only minimal signs of antitumor activity (Krause *et al.*, 2002) suggesting that the success of this vaccine strategy may vary with the type of cancer.

DNA VACCINES

DNA vaccination is receiving much attention on both the infectious disease and the cancer vaccine fronts (Gurunathan *et al.*, 2000). DNA vaccines consist of the gene(s) of interest cloned into a bacterial plasmid that is engineered for optimal expression in mammalian cells. It has been shown that this method of introducing gene(s) into cells results in protein expression as well as the induction of antibody and cellular immunity (Ulmer *et al.*, 1993). One of the methods used to enhance the potency of DNA vaccination includes targeting antigens to the MHC class II or class I compartments. This can be done by constructing chimeric genes that link the gene of interest with signal sequences that can direct normally cytoplasmic proteins to the endosome/lysosome compartments for enhanced MHC class II presentation (Ji *et al.*, 1999), or designing chimeric genes that can enhance intercellular spreading of an antigen and enhance MHC class I presentation (Hung *et al.*, 2001). Dendritic cells are the predominant cells involved in the immune response to DNA vaccination. They can be directly transfected by injection of DNA to present peptides in MHC class I molecules, or they can endocytose the secreted protein produced by other transfected cells and present peptides within MHC class II molecules (Gurunathan *et al.*, 2000). DNA vaccines have also been shown to have a strong propensity to induce Th1 immune responses due to the CpG motifs in the bacterial plasmid (Gurunathan *et al.*, 2000).

Tumor cells have been used as vehicles to deliver their antigens, either unmodified or transduced to express other genes of interest, such as cytokines or costimulatory molecules. Cavallo *et al.* did a comparative study in a murine model, evaluating the ability of genetically modified tumor cells to release cytokines and elicit an immune response against the parental tumor (Cavallo *et al.*, 1997). This study found varied responses from IL-4, IL-10, and IL-12 modified tumor cells. Several clinical trials have looked at the immunostimulatory potential of tumor cells genetically modified to produce GM-CSF and the costimulatory molecule B7.1 (Soiffer *et al.*, 1998; Jaffee *et al.*, 2001; Antonia *et al.*, 2002; Salgia *et al.*, 2003) and have demonstrated promising results.

IN VIVO TESTING OF CANCER VACCINES

Animal models

Transplantable tumors have been used for evaluating many antitumor vaccines based on various tumor antigens. However, the more appropriate model would be a spontaneous tumor that more closely resembles neoplastic progression in humans, and much of the current effort in vaccine development is directed toward the development of relevant animal models. HER-2/neu is a member of the epidermal growth factor receptor family and encodes a transmembrane growth factor receptor with tyrosine kinase activity (Karunagaran *et al.*, 1996). The HER-2/neu protein is expressed in tumor and normal cells, however, the gene is amplified in 30% of primary human breast and ovarian cancer cases (Ko *et al.*, 2003). Thus, vaccination strategies against HER-2/neu need to be evaluated in models where natural mechanisms of T-cell deletion or peripheral tolerance are expected to occur. There are two of HER-2/neu transgenic mouse models that have been developed. One model expresses the proto-oncogene rat *neu* cDNA under the control of the mouse mammary promoter (Guy *et al.*, 1992) resulting in mice that develop spontaneous mammary carcinomas. The second model expresses the activated *neu* oncogene where a point mutation renders the gene product constitutively active and these animals develop rapid spontaneous mammary tumors (Muller *et al.*, 1988). These different models based on the same tumor antigen allow for vaccine strategies to be tested in a preventative setting where tumor growth is a slower process, or a therapeutic setting where tumor growth is more aggressive. A number of vaccines have been tested in these mice with varied results (Reilly *et al.*, 2000; Rovero *et al.*, 2000; Pupa *et al.*, 2001). Rovero *et al.* immunized BALB-neuT mice transgenic for rat Her-2/neu, with a plasmid encoding the extracellular and transmembrane domain of rat Her-2/neu oncogene. They found that only when immunizations were started at early time points in tumor formation could protection be conferred. Furthermore, when animals were immunized and then challenged with transplantable tumors expressing rat Her-2/neu oncogene, these mice were unable to reject tumors. This suggests that the mechanisms required for rejection of transplantable tumors differ from those required to inhibit slow progression of carcinogenesis (Rovero *et al.*, 2000).

Carcinoembryonic antigen (CEA) is an oncofetal glycoprotein that is expressed in many cancer types, including colorectal, gastric and pancreatic carcinomas (Thompson *et al.*, 1991). Circulating CEA can be detected in the majority of patients with CEA-positive tumors and is used as a marker to monitor patient responses to therapy. Human CEA transgenic mice have been generated that express the transgene under its own promoter (Eades-Perner *et al.*, 1994; Thompson *et al.*, 1997; Clarke *et al.*, 1998). This model has been used to evaluate CEA vaccines and it has been shown that CEA transgenic mice show a certain degree of tolerance compared with wild-type mice. A colorectal cancer mouse model has been established by crossing CEA transgenic mice with Apc1638N mice, which have a mutation inserted into the Apc gene, resulting in formation of an inactive truncated protein. The resulting double transgenic mice develop CEA-expressing tumors of the gastrointestinal tract and represent a model for evaluating CEA-specific immunity and therapy (Horig *et al.*, 2001).

Prostate cancer cells express a tumor antigen, prostate-specific antigen (PSA), which is used clinically as a marker for prostate cancer. PSA has a highly restricted tissue distribution, being primarily expressed in normal and neoplastic epithelial cells of the prostate gland (Barratt, 2003). A transgenic mouse expressing human PSA can be used to study the degree of PSA tolerance (Wei *et al.*, 1997), or can be crossed with a transgenic mouse that develops cancer in the prostate (Greenberg *et al.*, 1995) to evaluate the efficacy of PSA directed vaccines. Another mouse model, TRAMP (transgenic adenocarcinoma mouse prostate), has been developed to study prostate cancer. These mice express SV40 T antigen under the probasin promoter that is regulated by androgens and is restricted to prostate epithelial cells, and has been shown to cause prostate tumor progression that resembles this process in humans (Gingrich *et al.*, 1996).

MUC1 is a tumor antigen that is expressed on normal and transformed ductal epithelial cells. MUC1 transgenic mice express the entire human MUC1 gene driven by its own promoter. MUC1 tumor antigen is found on adenocarcinomas derived from various tissues, including breast, pancreas, lung, colon, ovaries, and prostate. MUC1 transgenic mice can be crossed with several transgenic tumor models that express the SV-40 large T antigen under various tissue specific promoters and develop tissue specific tumors expressing MUC1. One model, MET mice, has been used to study MUC1-expressing pancreatic tumors (Mukherjee *et al.*, 2000), and a second model, which crossed MUC1 transgenic mice with PyV mT transgenic mice, develop MUC1 expressing mammary tumors (Mukherjee *et al.*, 2003).

There are numerous transgenic mouse models that develop spontaneous tumors in the breast, pancreas, stomach, prostate, lung, and colon. Other transgenic mouse models have been developed that express human tumor antigens that are observed in many human tumors. Mice that develop spontaneous cancers that express specific tumor antigens are ideal models to study the efficacy of newly developed cancer vaccine strategies and provide the field of cancer vaccines with physiologically relevant information about the mechanisms that are used by tumors to evade the immune system and how they might be overcome.

CLINICAL TRIALS

Early studies of therapeutic cancer vaccines in animal models and small clinical trials have shown marginal but promising results, prompting the design of larger phaseI/II clinical trials. This section will summarize some of the recent findings obtained from various clinical trials (Tables 13.2–13.4).

Peptide vaccine trials

Two recent trials showed promising results from vaccination using heat shock proteins (Belli *et al.*, 2002; Mazzaferro *et al.*, 2003). Belli *et al.* vaccinated 42 melanoma patients with heat shock protein gp-96-peptide complex (HSPPC-96; Oncophage). Of the 42 patients, 21 had no disease progression and received the second cycle of vaccination. ELISPOT assay was used in 23 out of 42 patients, to detect antigen-specific T-cell responses. Significant increases in melanoma-specific T-cells were found in 11 out of the 23 tested patients, with clinical responders displaying a high frequency of increased T-cell activity. This study demonstrated that vaccination with autologous HSPPC-96 was devoid of significant toxicity and induced clinical and tumor-specific T-cell responses in a majority of the patients (Belli *et al.*, 2002).

HSPPC-96 vaccination has also been tested in colorectal cancer patients with modest but encouraging results (Mazzaferro *et al.*, 2003). Patients were treated with two cycles of i.d. vaccination with HSPPC-96 derived from tumor cell suspensions of liver metastases from colon carcinoma and an increase in T-cell responses was observed.

Her-2/neu peptide E75 has been evaluated in trials in advanced breast, ovarian, and prostate cancer patients with disappointing results (Murray *et al.*, 2002; McNeel *et al.*, 2003). Murray *et al.* demonstrated the induction of CTL, but their frequency was extremely low (Murray *et al.*, 2002). McNeel *et al.* used the same peptide coadministered with flt3 ligand as a systemic adjuvant to augment the number of DCs attracted to the site of injection (McNeel *et al.*, 2003). However, they also showed an absence of a robust peripheral immune response. In contrast, Brossart *et al.* used DCs pulsed with the same peptide and showed induction of antigen-specific T-cell responses (Brossart *et al.*, 2000) suggesting that a DC vaccination may be a better strategy for this peptide.

NY-ESO-1 peptide vaccination has been shown to have promising results in melanoma patients. Jager *et al.* demonstrated that antigen-specific T-cells can be induced and disease stabilization and objective tumor regression observed in some patients (Jager *et al.*, 2000).

DC vaccine trials

Several clinical trials using DCs as vaccine vehicles, have been initiated for melanoma patients and have provided promising results. Banchereau *et al.* used DCs pulsed with a cocktail of four melanoma peptides derived from MelanA/MART-1, tyrosinase, MAGE-3, and gp100 and reported enhanced immunity in 16 of 18 patients (Banchereau *et al.*, 2001).

Table 13.4 Examples of DNA vaccines

Type of cancer	Vaccine	Route	Reference
Melanoma	rV–B7.1	i.l.	Kaufman *et al.* (2000)
Melanoma	rV–Tricom	i.l.	Kaufman *et al.* (2001)
Melanoma	Tumor cells transfected with GM-CSF	i.d. or s.c.	Soiffer *et al.* (1998)
Melanoma	rfowlpox + gp100	i.v. or i.m.	Rosenberg *et al.* (2003)
Prostate	rV-PSA ±GM-CSF	i.d. or s.c.	Eder *et al.* (2000)
Prostate	DC transfected with PSA	i.v.	Heiser *et al.* (2002)
Pancreatic	Tumor cells expressing GM-CSF	i.d.	Jaffee *et al.* (2001)
Ns.c.LC	Tumor cells adenoviral GM-CSF	i.d.	Salgia *et al.* (2003)
Cervical	rV-HPVE7 + rV-HPVE6	Scarification	Kaufmann *et al.* (2002)
Colorectal	ALVAC–p53	i.v.	van der Burg *et al.* (2002)
CEA expressing	ALVAC–CEA	i.m.	Marshall *et al.* (1999)
CEA expressing	ALVAC–CEA/B7.1	i.d. or i.m.	Horig *et al.* (2000); von Mehren *et al.* (2000)
CEA expressing	rV–CEA + avipox-CEA ± GM-CSF	i.d./s.c.	Marshall *et al.* (2000)
CEA expressing	rV–CEA	i.d.	Conry *et al.* (1999); Conry *et al.* (2000)

rV = recombinant vaccinia virus, Tricom = B7.1, ICAM-1, LFA-1, GM-CSF = granulocyte–monocyte colony-stimulating factor, PSA = prostate-specific antigen, HPV = human papillomavirus, ALVAC = canarypox virus, CEA = carcinoembryonic antigen, Ns.c.LC = non-small cell lung carcinoma, i.v. = intravenous, i.d. = intradermal, s.c. = subcutaneous, i.m. = intramuscular, i.l. = intralesion.

Nestle *et al.* used DCs pulsed with either melanoma cell lysates or peptide cocktails and found immune responses measured by delayed-type sensitivity (DTH) skin reactions in 11 out of 16 patients, and tumor regression characterized by two complete responses, three partial responses, and 1 minor response (Nestle *et al.*, 1998). Shuler-Thurner *et al.* vaccinated melanoma patients with the MAGE-3 peptide and found peptide-specific T-cell responses in 12 out of 16 patients (Schuler-Thurner *et al.*, 2002).

Peptide-DC vaccines have been extended to other malignancies as well. In a small trial, bladder cancer patients were vaccinated with DCs pulsed with MAGE-3 peptide and significant reduction in the size of lymph node metastases and/or liver metastasis was found in three out of four patients (Nishiyama *et al.*, 2001). DCs pulsed with CEA peptide CAP-1 have been used in vaccination of patients with CEA-expressing malignancies (Morse *et al.*, 1999), and recently, a modified CEA peptide with aspartate substituting for asparagine at position 610D has shown promise as a vaccine strategy (Fong *et al.*, 2001b). Patients were vaccinated with the Flt3 expanded DCs pulsed with the CEA variant and 8 out of 12 patients showed an increase in CTL responses (Fong *et al.*, 2001b). Modified peptide sequences for gp100 and tyrosinase have also provided promising results. Melanoma patients vaccinated with both gp100 and tyrosinase variants resulted in one patient with complete remission, two patients with stable disease, and two patients with mixed responses (Lau *et al.*, 2001).

Brossart *et al.* (2000). vaccinated breast and ovarian cancer patients with DCs pulsed with HER-2/neu or MUC-1 peptides and in 5 out of 10 patients peptide-specific CTLs could be detected in the peripheral blood. Kono *et al.* (2002) also demonstrated Her-2/neu-peptide specific recognition in six out of nine patients vaccinated with Her-2/neu peptide pulsed DCs. This was in contrast to other clinical trials using HER-2/neu as a peptide vaccine without DCs (Murray *et al.*, 2002; McNeel *et al.*, 2003), where only minimal CTL induction occurred.

DCs pulsed with whole tumor cell lysates have also been evaluated in clinical trials. This vaccine strategy has not given as promising results as the DC pulsed with peptide vaccines. Chakraborty *et al.* and Chang *et al.* have shown that T-cell responses can be induced with this type of vaccine strategy (Chakraborty *et al.*, 1998; Chang *et al.*, 2002), but additional manipulations are needed to optimize the utility of this vaccine.

DNA vaccine trials

Several clinical trials have been designed to evaluate the utility of recombinant viral vectors as a strategy to deliver tumor antigen genes to the immune system of cancer patients. Eder *et al.* vaccinated prostate cancer patients with a recombinant vaccinia virus encoding prostate-specific antigen (rV-PSA). This study demonstrated promising results with enhanced PSA-specific T-cell responses after one vaccine administration and stabilization of serum PSA levels. However, there was eventual rise in PSA levels in most patients suggesting that the immune responses elicited by this vaccine was short lived (Eder *et al.*, 2000). The results of this trial have led to the initiation of a phase II clinical trial using a prime and boost regime with rV–PSA used for priming and recombinant fowlpox encoding PSA (rfowlpox–PSA) used for boosting.

Marshall *et al.* vaccinated patients with CEA-expressing cancers using a canarypox vector (ALVAC) encoding carcinoembryonic antigen (CEA), which can infect human cells but does not replicate. The results of this study were disappointing with no objective antitumor responses and induction of CEA-specific CTLs in some patients only (Marshall *et al.*, 1999). The same group initiated another clinical trial to compare priming with rV–CEA and boosting with ALVAC–CEA or the other way around (Marshall *et al.*, 2000). This trial demonstrated more promising results showing that rV–CEA was more effective at priming the immune system then ALVAC–CEA and that future trials should use rV–CEA followed by ALVAC–CEA.

Rosenberg *et al.* used recombinant fowlpox virus (rfowlpox) encoding three different forms of gp100 in three different clinical trials in melanoma patients (Rosenberg *et al.*, 2003). Fowlpox virus is a member of the avipox family and represents an attractive vector because it can encode large gene fragments and can infect, but does not replicate in mammalian cells. The first rfowlpox encoded full-length gp100 molecule. The second rfowlpox encoded full-length gp100 with two amino acid modifications to enhance MHC binding. The third rfowlpox encoded a shorter peptide gp100 with a single amino acid modification. Only one in seven patients had immune responses after vaccination with the native molecule. In contrast, 10 of 14 patients had immune responses after vaccination with the modified full-length gp100. The greatest responses were observed in the modified peptide group, in which 12 of 16 patients had immune responses. These data clearly demonstrated the potential benefit of using modified peptides in vaccines.

CONCLUSION

Recent advances in tumor immunology have provided a lengthy and comprehensive list of tumor antigen candidates for cancer vaccines that cover many different tumor types, and the understanding of the immune mechanisms that recognize these antigens and destroy tumor cells. The future direction of cancer vaccine development is to understand the best approaches to control the dynamics that exist between the tumor and the host immune system, and determine the most efficacious means to immunize in order to bias this interaction in favor of the immune system.

References

Antonia, S.J., Seigne, J., Diaz, J., Muro-Cacho, C., Extermann, M., Farmelo, M.J., Friberg, M., Alsarraj, M., Mahany, J.J., Pow-Sang, J., Cantor, A., and Janssen, W. 2002. Phase I trial of a B7–1 (CD80) gene modified autologous tumor cell vaccine in combination with systemic interleukin 2 in patients with metastatic renal cell carcinoma. J. Urol. 167: 1995–2000.

Asavaroengchai, W., Kotera, Y., and Mule, J.J. 2002. Tumor lysate-pulsed dendritic cells can elicit an effective antitumor immune response during early lymphoid recovery. Proc. Natl. Acad. Sci. USA 99: 931–936.

Banchereau, J., Palucka, A.K., Dhodapkar, M., Burkeholder, S., Taquet, N., Rolland, A., Taquet, S., Coquery, S., Wittkowski, K.M., Bhardwaj, N., Pineiro, L., Steinman, R., and Fay, J. 2001. Immune and clinical responses in patients with metastatic melanoma to CD34(+) progenitor-derived dendritic cell vaccine. Cancer Res. 61: 6451–6458.

Banchereau, J., and Steinman, R.M. 1998. Dendritic cells and the control of immunity. Nature 392: 245–252.

Barratt, G. 2003. Colloidal drug carriers: achievements and perspectives. Cell. Mol. Life Sci. 60: 21–37.

Beck, C., Schreiber, H., and Rowley, D. 2001. Role of TGF-beta in immune-evasion of cancer. Microscopy. Res. Technique 52: 387–395.

Belli, F., Testori, A., Rivoltini, L., Maio, M., Andreola, G., Sertoli, M.R., Gallino, G., Piris, A., Cattelan, A., Lazzari, I., Carrabba, M., Sci.ta, G., Santantonio, C., Pilla, L., Tragni, G., Lombardo, C., Arienti, F., Marchiano, A., Queirolo, P., Bertolini, F., Cova, A., Lamaj, E., Ascani, L., Camerini, R., Corsi, M., Cascinelli, N., Lewis, J.J., Srivastava, P., and Parmiani, G. 2002. Vaccination of metastatic melanoma patients with autologous tumor-derived heat shock protein gp96-peptide complexes: clinical and Immunologic findings. J. Clin. Oncol. 20: 4169–4180.

Brossart, P., Wirths, S., Stuhler, G., Reichardt, V.L., Kanz, L., and Brugger, W. 2000. Induction of cytotoxic T-lymphocyte responses in vivo after vaccinations with peptide-pulsed dendritic cells. Blood 96: 3102–3108.

Burnet, F.M. 1970. The concept of Immunological surveillance. Prog. Exp. Tumor Res. 13: 1–27.

Campbell, D.J., and Butcher, E.C. 2002. Rapid acquisition of tissue-specific homing phenotypes by CD4(+) T cells activated in cutaneous or mucosal lymphoid tissues. J. Exp. Med. 195: 135–141.

Carroll, M.C. and Prodeus, A.P. 1998. Linkages of innate and adaptive immunity. Curr. Opin. Immunol. 10: 36–40.

Cathcart, K., Pinilla-Ibarz, J., Korontsvit, T., Schwartz, J., Zakhaleva, V., Papadopoulus, E.B., and Scheinberg, D.A. 2003. A multivalent bcr-abl fusion peptide vaccination trial in patients with chronic myeloid leukemia. Blood 3: 1037–1042.

Cavallo, F., Signorelli, P., Giovarelli, M., Musiani, P., Modesti, A., Brunda, M.J., Colombo, M.P., and Forni, G. 1997. Antitumor efficacy of adenocarcinoma cells engineered to produce interleukin 12 (IL-12) or other cytokines compared with exogenous IL-12. J. Natl. Cancer Inst. 89: 1049–1058.

Cefai, D., Favre, L., Wattendorf, E., Marti, A., Jaggi, R., and Gimmi, C.D. 2001. Role of Fas ligand expression in promoting escape from immune rejection in a spontaneous tumor model. Int. J. Cancer 91: 529–537.

Chakraborty, N.G., Sporn, J.R., Tortora, A.F., Kurtzman, S.H., Yamase, H., Ergin, M.T., and Mukherji, B. 1998. Immunization with a tumor-cell-lysate-loaded autologous-antigen-presenting-cell-based vaccine in melanoma. Cancer Immunol. Immunother. 47: 58–64.

Chang, A.E., Redman, B.G., Whitfield, J.R., Nickoloff, B.J., Braun, T.M., Lee, P.P., Geiger, J.D., and Mule, J.J. 2002. A phase I trial of tumor lysate-pulsed dendritic cells in the treatment of advanced cancer. Clin. Cancer Res. 8: 1021–1032.

Clarke, P., Mann, J., Simpson, J.F., Rickard-Dickson, K., and Primus, F.J. 1998. Mice transgenic for human carcinoembryonic antigen as a model for immunotherapy. Cancer Res. 58: 1469–1477.

Conry, R.M., Allen, K.O., Lee, S., Moore, S.E., Shaw, D.R., and LoBuglio, A.F. 2000. Human autoantibodies to carcinoembryonic antigen (CEA) induced by a vaccinia-CEA vaccine. Clin. Cancer Res. 6: 34–41.

Conry, R.M., Khazaeli, M.B., Saleh, M.N., Allen, K.O., Barlow, D.L., Moore, S.E., Craig, D., Arani, R.B., Schlom, J., and LoBuglio, A.F. 1999. Phase I trial of a recombinant vaccinia virus encoding carcinoembryonic antigen in metastatic adenocarcinoma: comparison of intradermal versus subcutaneous administration. Clin. Cancer Res. 5: 2330–2337.

Cox, J.C., and Coulter, A.R. 1997. Adjuvants – a classification and review of their modes of action. Vaccine 15: 248–256.

Cox, J.C., Sjolander, A., and Barr, I.G. 1998. ISCOMs and other saponin based adjuvants. Adv. Drug Deliv. Rev. 32: 247–271.

Cromme, F.V., Airey, J., Heemels, M.T., Ploegh, H.L., Keating, P.J., Stern, P.L., Meijer, C.J., and Walboomers, J.M. 1994. Loss of transporter protein, encoded by the TAP-1 gene, is highly correlated with loss of HLA expression in cervical carcinomas. J. Exp. Med. 179: 335–340.

Dabbagh, K., and Lewis, D.B. 2003. Toll-like receptors and T-helper-1/T-helper-2 responses. Curr. Opin. Infect. Dis. 16: 199–204.

Dallal, R.M., and Lotze, M.T. 2000. The dendritic cell and human cancer vaccines. Curr. Opin. Immunol. 12: 583–588.

Davila, E., and Celis, E. 2000. Repeated administration of cytosine-phosphorothiolated guanine-containing oligonucleotides together with peptide/protein immunization results in enhanced CTL responses with anti-tumor activity. J. Immunol. 165: 539–547.

De Plaen, E., Lurquin, C., Van Pel, A., Mariame, B., Szikora, J.P., Wolfel, T., Sibille, C., Chomez, P., and Boon, T. 1988. Immunogenic (tum-) variants of mouse tumor P815: cloning of the gene of tum- antigen P91A and identification of the tum- mutation. Proc. Natl. Acad. Sci. USA 85: 2274–2278.

Disis, M.L., Rinn, K., Knutson, K.L., Davis, D., Caron, D., dela Rosa, C., and Schiffman, K. 2002. Flt3 ligand as a vaccine adjuvant in association with HER-2/neu peptide-based vaccines in patients with HER-2/neu-overexpressing cancers. Blood 99: 2845–2850.

Dunn, G.P., Bruce, A.T., Ikeda, H., Old, L.J., and Schreiber, R.D. 2002. Cancer immunoediting: from immunosurveillance to tumor escape. Nature Immunol. 3: 991–998.

Eades-Perner, A.M., van der Putten, H., Hirth, A., Thompson, J., Neumaier, M., von Kleist, S., and Zimmermann, W. 1994. Mice transgenic for the human carcinoembryonic antigen gene maintain its spatiotemporal expression pattern. Cancer Res. 54: 4169–4176.

Eder, J.P., Kantoff, P.W., Roper, K., Xu, G.X., Bubley, G.J., Boyden, J., Gritz, L., Mazzara, G., Oh, W.K., Arlen, P., Tsang, K.Y., Panicali, D., Schlom, J., and Kufe, D.W. 2000. A phase I trial of a recombinant vaccinia virus expressing prostate-specific antigen in advanced prostate cancer. Clin. Cancer Res. 6: 1632–1638.

Finn, O.J. 2003. Cancer vaccines: between the idea and the reality. Nature Rev. Immunol. 3: 630–641.

Fong, L., Brockstedt, D., Benike, C., Wu, L., and Engleman, E.G. 2001a. Dendritic cells injected via different routes induce immunity in cancer patients. J. Immunol. 166: 4254–4259.

Fong, L., Hou, Y., Rivas, A., Benike, C., Yuen, A., Fisher, G.A., Davis, M.M., and Engleman, E.G. 2001b. Altered peptide ligand vaccination with Flt3 ligand expanded dendritic cells for tumor immunotherapy. Proc. Natl. Acad. Sci. USA 98: 8809–8814.

Garcia-Lora, A., Algarra, I., Gaforio, J.J., Ruiz-Cabello, F., and Garrido, F. 2001. Immunoselection by T lymphocytes generates repeated MHC class I-deficient metastatic tumor variants. Int. J. Cancer 91: 109–119.

Gingrich, J.R., Barrios, R.J., Morton, R.A., Boyce, B.F., DeMayo, F.J., Finegold, M.J., Angelopoulou, R., Rosen, J.M., and Greenberg, N.M. 1996. Metastatic prostate cancer in a transgenic mouse. Cancer Res. 56: 4096–4102.

Gjertson, M.K., Buanes, T., Rosseland, A.R., Bakka, A., Gladhaug, I., Soreide, O., Eriksen, J.A., Moller, M., Baksaas, I., Lothe, R.A., Saeterdal, I., and Gaudernack, G. 2001. Intradermal ras peptide vaccination with granulocyte–macrophage colony-stimulating factor as adjuvant: Clinical and immunological responses in patients with pancreatic adenocarcinoma. Int. J. Cancer 92: 441–450.

Gordon, S. 2002. Pattern recognition receptors: doubling up for the innate immune response. Cell 111: 927–930.

Goydos, J.S., Elder, E., Whiteside, T.L., Finn, O.J., and Lotze, M.T. 1996. A phase I trial of a synthetic mucin peptide vaccine. Induction of specific immune reactivity in patients with adenocarcinoma. J. Surg. Res. 63: 298–304.

Greenberg, N.M., DeMayo, F., Finegold, M.J., Medina, D., Tilley, W.D., Aspinall, J.O., Cunha, G.R., Donjacour, A.A., Matusik, R.J., and Rosen, J.M. 1995. Prostate cancer in a transgenic mouse. Proc. Natl. Acad. Sci. USA 92: 3439–3443.

Guermonprez, P., Valladeau, J., Zitvogel, L., Thery, C., and Amigorena, S. 2002. Antigen presentation and T cell stimulation by dendritic cells. Annu. Rev. Immunol. 20: 621–667.

Gurunathan, S., Klinman, D.M., and Seder, R.A. 2000. DNA vaccines: Immunology, application, and optimization. Annu. Rev. Immunol. 18: 927–974.

Guy, C.T., Webster, M.A., Schaller, M., Parsons, T.J., Cardiff, R.D., and Muller, W.J. 1992. Expression of the neu protooncogene in the mammary epithelium of transgenic mice induces metastatic disease. Proc. Natl. Acad. Sci. USA 89: 10578–10582.

Harris, J.E., Ryan, L., Hoover, H.C., Jr., Stuart, R.K., Oken, M.M., Benson, A.B., 3rd, Mansour, E., Haller, D.G., Manola, J., and Hanna, M.G., Jr. 2000. Adjuvant active specific immunotherapy for stage II and III colon cancer with an autologous tumor cell vaccine: Eastern Cooperative Oncology Group Study E5283. J. Clin. Oncol. 18: 148–157.

Hasegawa, Y., Takanashi, S., Kanehira, Y., Tsushima, T., Imai, T., and Okumura, K. 2001. Transforming growth factor-beta1 level correlates with angiogenesis, tumor progression, and prognosis in patients with nonsmall cell lung carcinoma. Cancer 91: 964–971.

Heimberger, A.B., Archer, G.E., Crotty, L.E., McLendon, R.E., Friedman, A.H., Friedman, H.S., Bigner, D.D., and Sampson, J.H. 2002. Dendritic cells pulsed with a tumor-specific peptide induce long-lasting immunity and are effective against murine intracerebral melanoma. Neurosurgery 50: 158–164: discussion 164–156.

Heiser, A., Coleman, D., Dannull, J., Yancey, D., Maurice, M.A., Lallas, C.D., Dahm, P., Niedzwiecki, D., Gilboa, E., and Vieweg, J. 2002. Autologous dendritic cells transfected with prostate-specific antigen RNA stimulate CTL responses against metastatic prostate tumors. J. Clin. Invest. 109: 409–417.

Hobohm, U. 2001. Fever and cancer in perspective. Cancer Immunol. Immunother. 50: 391–396.

Horig, H., Wainstein, A., Long, L., Kahn, D., Soni, S., Marcus, A., Edelmann, W., Kucherlapati, R., and Kaufman, H.L. 2001. A new mouse model for evaluating the immunotherapy of human colorectal cancer. Cancer Res. 61: 8520–8526.

Horig, H., Wainstein, A., Long, L., Kahn, D., Soni, S., Marcus, A., Edelmann, W., Kucherlapati, R., and Kaufman, H.L. 2001. A new mouse model for evaluating the immunotherapy of human colorectal cancer. Cancer Res. 61: 8520–8526.

Hung, C.F., Cheng, W.F., Chai, C.Y., Hsu, K.F., He, L., Ling, M., and Wu, T.C. 2001. Improving vaccine potency through intercellular spreading and enhanced MHC class I presentation of antigen. J. Immunol. 166: 5733–5740.

Jaffee, E.M., Hruban, R.H., Biedrzycki, B., Laheru, D., Schepers, K., Sauter, P.R., Goemann, M., Coleman, J., Grochow, L., Donehower, R.C., Lillemoe, K.D., O'Reilly, S., Abrams, R.A., Pardoll, D.M., Cameron, J.L., and Yeo, C.J. 2001. Novel allogeneic granulocyte-macrophage colony-stimulating factor-secreting tumor vaccine for pancreatic cancer: a phase I trial of safety and immune activation. J. Clin. Oncol. 19: 145–156.

Jager, E., Gnjatic, S., Nagata, Y., Stockert, E., Jager, D., Karbach, J., Neumann, A., Rieckenberg, J., Chen, Y.T., Ritter, G., Hoffman, E., Arand, M., Old, L.J., and Knuth, A. 2000. Induction of primary NY-ESO-1 immunity: CD8+ T lymphocyte and antibody responses in peptide-vaccinated patients with NY-ESO-1+ cancers. Proc. Natl. Acad. Sci. USA 97: 12198–12203.

Jager, E., Ringhoffer, M., Altmannsberger, M., Arand, M., Karbach, J., Jager, D., Oesch, F., and Knuth, A. 1997. Immunoselection in vivo: independent loss of MHC class I and melanocyte differentiation antigen expression in metastatic melanoma. Int. J. Cancer. 71: 142–147.

Janetzki, S., Palla, D., Rosenhauer, V., Lochs, H., Lewis, J.J., Srivastava, P.K. 2000. Immunization of cancer patients with autologous cancer-derived heat shock protein gp96 preparations: a pilot study. Int. J. Cancer 88: 232–238.

Ji, H., Wang, T.L., Chen, C.H., Pai, S.I., Hung, C.F., Lin, K.Y., Kurman, R.J., Pardoll, D.M., and Wu, T.C. 1999. Targeting human papillomavirus type 16 E7 to the endosomal/lysosomal compartment enhances the antitumor immunity of DNA vaccines against murine human papillomavirus type 16 E7-expressing tumors. Hum. Gene Ther. 10: 2727–2740.

Kao, H., Marto, J.A., Hoffmann, T.K., Shabanowitz, J., Finkelstein, S.D., Whiteside, T.L., Hunt, D.F., and Finn, O.J. 2001. Identification of cyclin B1 as a shared human epithelial tumor-associated antigen recognized by T cells. J. Exp. Med. 194: 1313–1323.

Karunagaran, D., Tzahar, E., Beerli, R.R., Chen, X., Graus-Porta, D., Ratzkin, B.J., Seger, R., Hynes, N.E., and Yarden, Y. 1996. ErbB-2 is a common auxiliary subunit of NDF and EGF receptors: implications for breast cancer. EMBO J. 15: 254–264.

Kaufman, H.L., DeRaffele, G., Divito, J., Horig, H., Lee, D., Panicali, D., and Voulo, M. 2001. A phase I trial of intralesional rV-Tricom vaccine in the treatment of malignant melanoma. Hum. Gene Ther. 12: 1459–1480.

Kaufmann, A.M., Stern, P.L., Rankin, E.M., Sommer, H., Nuessler, V., Schneider, A., Adams, M., Onon, T.S., Bauknecht, T., Wagner, U., Kroon, K., Hickling, J., Boswell, C.M., Stacey, S.N., Kitchener, H.C., Gillard, J., Wanders, J., Roberts, J.S., and Zwierzina, H. 2002. Safety and immunogenicity of TA-HPV, a recombinant vaccinia virus expressing modified human papillomavirus (HPV)-16 and HPV-18 E6 and E7 genes, in women with progressive cervical cancer. Clin. Cancer Res. 8: 3676–3685.

Ko, B.K., Kawano, K., Murray, J.L., Disis, M.L., Efferson, C.L., Kuerer, H.M., Peoples, G.E., and Ioannides, C.G. 2003. Clinical studies of vaccines targeting breast cancer. Clin. Cancer Res. 9: 3222–3234.

Kono, K., Takahashi, A., Sugai, H., Fujii, H., Choudhury, A.R., Kiessling, R., and Matsumoto, Y. 2002. Dendritic cells pulsed with HER-2/neu-derived peptides can induce specific T-cell responses in patients with gastric cancer. Clin. Cancer Res. 8: 3394–3400.

Krause, S.W., Neumann, C., Soruri, A., Mayer, S., Peters, J.H., and Andreesen, R. 2002. The treatment of patients with disseminated malignant melanoma by vaccination with autologous cell hybrids of tumor cells and dendritic cells. J. Immunother. 25: 421–428.

Lau, R., Wang, F., Jeffery, G., Marty, V., Kuniyoshi, J., Bade, E., Ryback, M.E., and Weber, J. 2001. Phase I trial of intravenous peptide-pulsed dendritic cells in patients with metastatic melanoma. J. Immunother. 24: 66–78.

Lespagnard, L., Mettens, P., Verheyden, A.M., Tasiaux, N., Thielemans, K., van Meirvenne, S., Geldhof, A., De Baetselier, P., Urbain, J., Leo, O., and Moser, M. 1998. Dendritic cells fused with mastocytoma cells elicit therapeutic antitumor immunity. Int. J. Cancer. 76: 250–258.

Lollini, P.L., and Forni, G. 2002. Antitumor vaccines: is it possible to prevent a tumor? Cancer Immunol. Immunother. 51: 409–416.

Ludewig, B., Ochsenbein, A.F., Odermatt, B., Paulin, D., Hengartner, H., and Zinkernagel, R.M. 2000. Immunotherapy with dendritic cells directed against tumor antigens shared with normal host cells results in severe autoimmune disease. J. Exp. Med. 191: 795–804.

Lundberg, B.B., Griffiths, G., and Hansen, H.J. 2000. Specific binding of sterically stabilized anti-B-cell Immunol.iposomes and cytotoxicity of entrapped doxorubicin. Int. J. Pharm. 205: 101–108.

McGhee, J., Lamm, ME., and Strober, W. 1999. Mucosal Immune Responses. In: Ogra P., et al., ed. Mucosal Immunology. Academic Press, pp. 485–506.

McNeel, D.G., Knutson, K.L., Schiffman, K., Davis, D.R., Caron, D., and Disis, M.L. 2003. Pilot study of an HLA-A2 peptide vaccine using flt3 ligand as a systemic vaccine adjuvant. J. Clin. Immunol. 23: 62–72.

McNeela, E.A., and Mills, K.H. 2001. Manipulating the immune system: humoral versus cell-mediated immunity. Adv. Drug Deliv. Rev. 51: 43–54.

Maleno, I., Lopez-Nevot, M.A., Cabrera, T., Salinero, J., and Garrido, F. 2002. Multiple mechanisms generate HLA class I altered phenotypes in laryngeal carcinomas: high frequency of HLA haplotype loss associated with loss of heterozygosity in chromosome region 6p21. Cancer Immunol. Immunother. 51: 389–396.

Manjili, M.H., Henderson, R., Wang, X.Y., Chen, X., Li, Y., Repasky, E., Kazim, L., and Subjeck, J.R. 2002. Development of a recombinant HSP110-HER-2/neu vaccine using the chaperoning properties of HSP110. Cancer Res. 62: 1737–1742.

Marchand, M., Weynants, P., Rankin, E., Arienti, F., Belli, F., Parmiani, G., Cascinelli, N., Bourlond, A., Vanwijck, R., Humblet, Y., et al. 1995. Tumor regression responses in melanoma patients treated with a peptide encoded by gene MAGE-3. Int. J. Cancer. 63: 883–885.

Marciani, D.J. 2003. Vaccine adjuvants: role and mechanisms of action in vaccine immunogenicity. Drug Discov. Today 8: 934–943.

Marin, R., Ruiz-Cabello, F., Pedrinaci, S., Mendez, R., Jimenez, P., Geraghty, D.E., and Garrido, F. 2003. Analysis of HLA-E expression in human tumors. Immunogenetics 54: 767–775.

Marincola, F.M., Jaffee, E.M., Hicklin, D.J., and Ferrone, S. 2000. Escape of human solid tumors from T-cell recognition: Molecular mechanisms and functional significance. Adv. Immunol. 74: 181–273.

Marshall, J.L., Hawkins, M.J., Tsang, K.Y., Richmond, E., Pedicano, J.E., Zhu, M.Z., and Schlom, J. 1999. Phase I study in cancer patients of a replication-defective avipox recombinant vaccine that expresses human carcinoembryonic antigen. J. Clin. Oncol. 17: 332–337.

Marshall, J.L., Hoyer, R.J., Toomey, M.A., Faraguna, K., Chang, P., Richmond, E., Pedicano, J.E., Gehan, E., Peck, R.A., Arlen, P., Tsang, K.Y., and Schlom, J. 2000. Phase I study in advanced cancer patients of a diversified prime-and-boost vaccination protocol using recombinant vaccinia virus and recombinant nonreplicating avipox virus to elicit anti-carcinoembryonic antigen immune responses. J. Clin. Oncol. 18: 3964–3973.

Matzinger, P. 2002. The danger model: a renewed sense of self. Science 296: 301–305.

Mayordomo, J.I., Zorina, T., Storkus, W.J., Zitvogel, L., Garcia-Prats, M.D., DeLeo, A.B., and Lotze, M.T. 1997. Bone marrow-derived dendritic cells serve as potent adjuvants for peptide-based antitumor vaccines. Stem Cells 15: 94–103.

Mazzaferro, V., Coppa, J., Carrabba, M.G., Rivoltini, L., Schiavo, M., Regalia, E., Mariani, L., Camerini, T., Marchiano, A., Andreola, S., Camerini, R., Corsi, M., Lewis, J.J., Srivastava, P.K., and Parmiani, G. 2003. Vaccination with autologous tumor-derived heat-shock protein gp96 after liver resection for metastatic colorectal cancer. Clin. Cancer Res. 9: 3235–3245.

Meidenbauer, N., Harris, D.T., Spitler, L.E., Whiteside, T.L. 2002. Generation of PSA-reactive effector cells after vaccination with a PSA-based vaccine in patients with prostate cancer. Prostate 43: 88–100.

Melief, C.J., Toes, R.E., Medema, J.P., van der Burg, S.H., Ossendorp, F., and Offringa, R. 2000. Strategies for immunotherapy of cancer. Adv. Immunol. 75: 235–282.

Morse, M.A., Deng, Y., Coleman, D., Hull, S., Kitrell-Fisher, E., Nair, S., Schlom, J., Ryback, M.E., and Lyerly, H.K. 1999. A Phase I study of active immunotherapy with carcinoembryonic antigen peptide (CAP-1)-pulsed, autologous human cultured dendritic cells in patients with metastatic malignancies expressing carcinoembryonic antigen. Clin. Cancer Res. 5: 1331–1338.

Mukherjee, P., Ginardi, A.R., Madsen, C.S., Sterner, C.J., Adriance, M.C., Tevethia, M.J., and Gendler, S.J. 2000. Mice with spontaneous pancreatic cancer naturally develop MUC-1-specific CTLs that eradicate tumors when adoptively transferred. J. Immunol. 165: 3451–3460.

Mukherjee, P., Madsen, C.S., Ginardi, A.R., Tinder, T.L., Jacobs, F., Parker, J., Agrawal, B., Longenecker, B.M., and Gendler, S.J. 2003. Mucin 1-specific immunotherapy in a mouse model of spontaneous breast cancer. J. Immunother. 26: 47–62.

Muller, W.J., Sinn, E., Pattengale, P.K., Wallace, R., and Leder, P. 1988. Single-step induction of mammary adenocarcinoma in transgenic mice bearing the activated c-neu oncogene. Cell 54: 105–115.

Murphy, K.M., Ouyang, W., Farrar, J.D., Yang, J., Ranganath, S., Asnagli, H., Afkarian, M., and Murphy, T.L. 2000. Signaling and transcription in T helper development. Annu. Rev. Immunol. 18: 451–494.

Murray, J.L., Gillogly, M.E., Przepiorka, D., Brewer, H., Ibrahim, N.K., Booser, D.J., Hortobagyi, G.N., Kudelka, A.P., Grabstein, K.H., Cheever, M.A., and Ioannides, C.G. 2002. Toxicity, immunogenicity, and induction of E75-specific tumor-lytic CTLs by HER-2 peptide E75 (369–377) combined with granulocyte macrophage colony-stimulating factor in HLA-A2+ patients with metastatic breast and ovarian cancer. Clin. Cancer Res. 8: 3407–3418.

Nestle, F.O., Alijagic, S., Gilliet, M., Sun, Y., Grabbe, S., Dummer, R., Burg, G., and Schadendorf, D. 1998. Vaccination of melanoma patients with peptide- or tumor lysate-pulsed dendritic cells. Nature Med. 4: 328–332.

Nestle, F.O., Banchereau, J., and Hart, D. 2001. Dendritic cells: On the move from bench to bedside. Nature Med. 7: 761–765.

Ni, H.T., Spellman, S.R., Jean, W.C., Hall, W.A., and Low, W.C. 2001. Immunization with dendritic cells pulsed with tumor extract increases survival of mice bearing intracranial gliomas. J. Neurooncol. 51: 1–9.

Nishiyama, T., Tachibana, M., Horiguchi, Y., Nakamura, K., Ikeda, Y., Takesako, K., and Murai, M. 2001. Immunotherapy of bladder cancer using autologous dendritic cells pulsed with human lymphocyte antigen-A24-specific MAGE-3 peptide. Clin. Cancer Res. 7: 23–31.

Okada, N., Tsujino, M., Hagiwara, Y., Tada, A., Tamura, Y., Mori, K., Saito, T., Nakagawa, S., Mayumi, T., Fujita, T., and Yamamoto, A. 2001. Administration route-dependent vaccine efficiency of murine dendritic cells pulsed with antigens. Br. J. Cancer. 84: 1564–1570.

Pullarkat, V., Lee, P.P., Scotland, R., Rubio, V., Groshen, S., Gee, C., Lau, R., Snively, J., Sian, S., Woulfe, S.L., Wolfe, R.A., and Weber, J.S. 2003. A Phase I trial of SD-9427 (progenipoietin) with a multipeptide vaccine for resected metastatic melanoma. Clin. Cancer Res. 9: 1301–1312.

Pupa, S.M., Invernizzi, A.M., Forti, S., Di Carlo, E., Musiani, P., Nanni, P., Lollini, P.L., Meazza, R., Ferrini, S., and Menard, S. 2001. Prevention of spontaneous neu-expressing mammary tumor development in mice transgenic for rat proto-neu by DNA vaccination. Gene Ther. 8: 75–79.

Ramanathan, R.K., Lee, K.M., McKolanis, J., Hiltbold, E., Schraut, W., Moser, A.J., Warnick, E., Whiteside, T., Osborne, J., Kim, H., Day, R., Troetschel, M., and Finn, O.J. 2004. Phase I study of a MUC1 vaccine composed of different doses of MUC1 peptide with SB-AS2 adjuvant in resected and locally advanced pancreatic cancer. Cancer. Immunol. Immunother. (in press)

Reilly, R.T., Gottlieb, M.B., Ercolini, A.M., Machiels, J.P., Kane, C.E., Okoye, F.I., Muller, W.J., Dixon, K.H., and Jaffee, E.M. 2000. HER-2/neu is a tumor rejection target in tolerized HER-2/neu transgenic mice. Cancer Res. 60: 3569–3576.

Renkvist, N., Castelli, C., Robbins, P.F., and Parmiani, G. 2001. A listing of human tumor antigens recognized by T cells. Cancer Immunol. Immunother. 50: 3–15.

Renno, T., Lebecque, S., Renard, N., Saeland, S., and Vicari, A. 2003. What's new in the field of cancer vaccines? Cell. Mol. Life Sci. 60: 1296–1310.

Reynolds, S.R., Zeleniuch-Jacquotte, A., Shapiro, R.L., Roses, D.F., Harris, M.N., Johnston, D., and Bystryn, J.C. 2003. Vaccine-induced CD8+ T cell responses to MAGE-3 correlate with clinical outcome in patients with melanoma. Clin. Cancer Res. 9: 657–662.

Ridge, J.P., Di Rosa, F., and Matzinger, P. 1998. A conditioned dendritic cell can be a temporal bridge between a CD4+ T-helper and a T-killer cell. Nature 393: 474–478.

Rivoltini, L., Squarcina, P., Loftus, D.J., Castelli, C., Tarsini, P., Mazzocchi, A., Rini, F., Viggiano, V., Belli, F., and Parmiani, G. 1999. A superagonist variant of peptide MART1/Melan A27–35 elicits anti-melanoma CD8+ T cells with enhanced functional characteristics: implication for more effective immunotherapy. Cancer Res. 59: 301–306.

251

Rosenberg, S.A., Yang, J.C., Schwartzentruber, D.J., Hwu, P., Marincola, F.M., Topalian, S.L., Restifo, N.P., Dudley, M.E., Schwarz, S.L., Spiess, P.J., Wunderlich, J.R., Parkhurst, M.R., Kawakami, Y., Seipp, C.A., Einhorn, J.H., and White, D.E. 1998. Immunologic and therapeutic evaluation of a synthetic peptide vaccine for the treatment of patients with metastatic melanoma. Nature Med. 4: 321–327.

Rosenberg, S.A., Yang, J.C., Schwartzentruber, D.J., Hwu, P., Topalian, S.L., Sherry, R.M., Restifo, N.P., Wunderlich, J.R., Seipp, C.A., Rogers-Freezer, L., Morton, K.E., Mavroukakis, S.A., Gritz, L., Panicali, D.L., and White, D.E. 2003. Recombinant fowlpox viruses encoding the anchor-modified gp100 melanoma antigen can generate antitumor immune responses in patients with metastatic melanoma. Clin. Cancer Res. 9: 2973–2980.

Rovero, S., Amici, A., Carlo, E.D., Bei, R., Nanni, P., Quaglino, E., Porcedda, P., Boggio, K., Smorlesi, A., Lollini, P.L., Landuzzi, L., Colombo, M.P., Giovarelli, M., Musiani, P., and Forni, G. 2000. DNA vaccination against rat her-2/Neu p185 more effectively inhibits carcinogenesis than transplantable carcinomas in transgenic BALB/c mice. J. Immunol. 165: 5133–5142.

Salgaller, M.L., Afshar, A., Marincola, F.M., Rivoltini, L., Kawakami, Y., and Rosenberg, S.A. 1995. Recognition of multiple epitopes in the human melanoma antigen gp100 by peripheral blood lymphocytes stimulated in vitro with synthetic peptides. Cancer Res. 55: 4972–4979.

Salgaller, M.L., Marincola, F.M., Cormier, J.N., and Rosenberg, S.A. 1996. Immunization against epitopes in the human melanoma antigen gp100 following patient immunization with synthetic peptides. Cancer Res. 56: 4749–4757.

Salgia, R., Lynch, T., Skarin, A., Lucca, J., Lynch, C., Jung, K., Hodi, F.S., Jaklitsch, M., Mentzer, S., Swanson, S., Lukanich, J., Bueno, R., Wain, J., Mathisen, D., Wright, C., Fidias, P., Donahue, D., Clift, S., Hardy, S., Neuberg, D., Mulligan, R., Webb, I., Sugarbaker, D., Mihm, M., and Dranoff, G. 2003. Vaccination with irradiated autologous tumor cells engineered to secrete granulocyte-macrophage colony-stimulating factor augments antitumor immunity in some patients with metastatic non-small-cell lung carcinoma. J. Clin. Oncol. 21: 624–630.

Samanci, A., Yi, Q., Fagerberg, J., Strigard, K., Smith, G., Ruden, U., Wahren, B., and Mellstedt, H. 1998. Pharmacological administration of granulocyte/macrophage-colony-stimulating factor is of significant importance for the induction of a strong humoral and cellular response in patients immunized with recombinant carcinoembryonic antigen. Cancer Immunol. Immunother. 47: 131–142.

Schaed, S.G., Klimek, V.M., Panageas, K.S., Musselli, C.M., Butterworth, L., Hwu, W.J., Livingston, P.O., Williams, L., Lewis, J.J., Houghton, A.N., and Chapman, P.B. 2002. T-cell responses against tyrosinase 368-376(370D) peptide in HLA*A0201+ melanoma patients: randomized trial comparing incomplete Freund's adjuvant, granulocyte macrophage colony-stimulating factor, and QS-21 as immunological adjuvants. Clin. Cancer Res. 8: 967–972.

Schuler-Thurner, B., Schultz, E.S., Berger, T.G., Weinlich, G., Ebner, S., Woerl, P., Bender, A., Feuerstein, B., Fritsch, P.O., Romani, N., and Schuler, G. 2002. Rapid induction of tumor-specific type 1 T helper cells in metastatic melanoma patients by vaccination with mature, cryopreserved, peptide-loaded monocyte-derived dendritic cells. J. Exp. Med. 195: 1279–1288.

Serody, J.S., Collins, E.J., Tisch, R.M., Kuhns, J.J., and Frelinger, J.A. 2000. T cell activity after dendritic cell vaccination is dependent on both the type of antigen and the mode of delivery. J. Immunol. 164: 4961–4967.

Slingluff, C.L., Jr., Petroni, G.R., Yamshchikov, G.V., Barnd, D.L., Eastham, S., Galavotti, H., Patterson, J.W., Deacon, D.H., Hibbitts, S., Teates, D., Neese, P.Y., Grosh, W.W., Chianese-Bullock, K.A., Woodson, E.M., Wiernasz, C.J., Merrill, P., Gibson, J., Ross, M., and Engelhard, V.H., 2003. Clinical and immunologic results of a randomized phase II trial of vaccination using four melanoma peptides either administered in granulocyte-macrophage colony-stimulating factor in adjuvant or pulsed on dendritic cells. J. Clin. Oncol. 21: 4016–4026.

Small, E.J., Fratesi, P., Reese, D.M., Strang, G., Laus, R., Peshwa, M.V., and Valone, F.H., 2000. Immunotherapy of hormone-refractory prostate cancer with antigen-loaded dendritic cells. J. Clin. Oncol. 18: 3894–3903.

Soares, M.M., Mehta, V., and Finn, O.J. 2001. Three different vaccines based on the 140-amino acid MUC1 peptide with seven tandemly repeated tumor-specific epitopes elicit distinct immune effector mechanisms in wild-type versus MUC1-transgenic mice with different potential for tumor rejection. J. Immunol. 166: 6555–6563.

Soiffer, R., Lynch, T., Mihm, M., Jung, K., Rhuda, C., SchMol.linger, J.C., Hodi, F.S., Liebster, L., Lam, P., Mentzer, S., Singer, S., Tanabe, K.K., Cosimi, A.B., Duda, R., Sober, A., Bhan, A., Daley, J., Neuberg, D., Parry, G., Rokovich, J., Richards, L., Drayer, J., Berns, A., Clift, S., Dranoff, G., et al. 1998. Vaccination with irradiated autologous melanoma cells engineered to secrete human granulocyte-macrophage colony-stimulating factor generates potent antitumor immunity in patients with metastatic melanoma. Proc. Natl. Acad. Sci. USA 95: 13141–13146.

Srivastava, P.K., and Amato, R.J. 2001. Heat shock proteins: the 'Swiss Army Knife' vaccines against cancers and infectious agents. Vaccine 19: 2590–2597.

Strand, S., Hofmann, W.J., Hug, H., Muller, M., Otto, G., Strand, D., Mariani, S.M., Stremmel, W., Krammer, P.H., and Galle, P.R. 1996. Lymphocyte apoptosis induced by CD95 (APO-1/Fas) ligand-expressing tumor cells – a mechanism of immune evasion? Nature Med. 2: 1361–1366.

Stutman, O. 1974. Tumor development after 3-methylcholanthrene in Immunologically deficient athymic-nude mice. Science 183: 534–536.

Szabo, S.J., Kim, S.T., Costa, G.L., Zhang, X., Fathman, C.G., and Glimcher, L.H. 2000. A novel transcription factor, T-bet, directs Th1 lineage commitment. Cell 100: 655–669.

Tanaka, Y., Koido, S., Chen, D., Gendler, S.J., Kufe, D., and Gong, J. 2001. Vaccination with allogeneic dendritic cells fused to carcinoma cells induces antitumor immunity in MUC1 transgenic mice. Clin. Immunol. 101: 192–200.

Thompson, J.A., Eades-Perner, A.M., Ditter, M., Muller, W.J., and Zimmermann, W. 1997. Expression of transgenic carcinoembryonic antigen (CEA) in tumor-prone mice: an animal model for CEA-directed tumor immunotherapy. Int. J. Cancer. 72: 197–202.

Thompson, J.A., Grunert, F., and Zimmermann, W. 1991. Carcinoembryonic antigen gene family: Molecular biology and clinical perspectives. J. Clin. Lab. Anal. 5: 344–366.

Tjoa, B.A., Simmons, S.J., Elgamal, A., Rogers, M., Ragde, H., Kenny, G.M., Troychak, M.J., Boynton, A.L., and Murphy, G.P. 1999. Follow-up evalation of a phase II prostate cancer vaccine trial. Prostate 40: 125–129.

Triantafilou, M., Brandenburg, K., Gutsmann, T., Seydel, U., and Triantafilou, K. 2002. Innate recognition of bacteria: engagement of multiple receptors. Crit. Rev. Immunol. 22: 251–268.

Ulmer, J.B., Donnelly, J.J., Parker, S.E., Rhodes, G.H., Felgner, P.L., Dwarki, V.J., Gromkowski, S.H., Deck, R.R., DeWitt, C.M., Friedman, A., et al. 1993. Heterologous protection against influenza by injection of DNA encoding a viral protein. Science 259: 1745–1749.

van der Bruggen, P., Traversari, C., Chomez, P., Lurquin, C., De Plaen, E., Van den Eynde, B., Knuth, A., and Boon, T. 1991. A gene encoding an antigen recognized by cytolytic T lymphocytes on a human melanoma. Science 254: 1643–1647.

van der Burg, S.H., Visseren, M.J., Brandt, R.M., Kast, W.M., and Melief, C.J. 1996. Immunogenicity of peptides bound to MHC class I molecules depends on the MHC–peptide complex stability. J. Immunol. 156: 3308–3314.

van der Burg, S.H., Menon, A.G., Redeker, A., Bonnet, M.C., Drijfhout, J.W., Tollenaar, R.A., van de Velde, C.J., Moingeon, P., Kuppen, P.J., Offringa, R., and Melief, C.J. 2002. Induction of p53-specific immune responses in colorectal cancer patients receiving a recombinant ALVAC-p53 candidate vaccine. Clin. Cancer Res. 8: 1019–1027.

Van Pel, A., and Boon, T. 1982. Protection against a nonimmunogenic mouse leukemia by an immunogenic variant obtained by mutagenesis. Proc. Natl. Acad. Sci. USA 79: 4718–4722.

von Andrian, U.H., and Mackay, C.R. 2000. T-cell function and migration. Two sides of the same coin. N. Engl. J. Med. 343: 1020–1034.

von Mehren, M., Arlen, P., Tsang, K.Y., Rogatko, A., Meropol, N., Cooper, H.S., Davey, M., McLaughlin, S., Schlom, J., and Weiner, L.M. 2000. Pilot study of a dual gene recombinant avipox vaccine containing both carcinoembryonic antigen and B7.1 transgenes in patients with recurrent CEA-expressing adenocarcinomas. Clin. Cancer Res. 6: 2219–2228.

Wang, J., Saffold, S., Cao, X., Krauss, J., and Chen, W. 1998. Eliciting T cell immunity against poorly immunogenic tumors by immunization with dendritic cell-tumor fusion vaccines. J. Immunol. 161: 5516–5524.

Weber, J., Sondak, V.K., Scotland, R., Phillip, R., Wang, F., Rubio, V., Stuge, T.B., Groshen, S.G., Gee, C., Jeffery, G.G., Sian, S., and Lee, P.P. 2003. Granulocyte-macrophage-colony-stimulating factor added to a multipeptide vaccine for resected Stage II melanoma. Cancer 97: 186–200.

Weber, J.S., Hua, F.L., Spears, L., Marty, V., Kuniyoshi, C., and Celis, E. 1999. A phase I trial of an HLA-A1 restricted MAGE-3 epitope peptide with incomplete Freund's adjuvant in patients with resected high-risk melanoma. J. Immunother. 22: 431–440.

Wei, C., Willis, R.A., Tilton, B.R., Looney, R.J., Lord, E.M., Barth, R.K., and Frelinger, J.G. 1997. Tissue-specific expression of the human prostate-specific antigen gene in transgenic mice: implications for tolerance and immunotherapy. Proc. Natl. Acad. Sci. USA 94: 6369–6374.

Wiemann, B., and Starnes, C.O. 1994. Coley's toxins, tumor necrosis factor and cancer research: a historical perspective. Pharmacol. Ther. 64: 529–564.

Xia, J., Tanaka, Y., Koido, S., Liu, C., Mukherjee, P., Gendler, S.J., and Gong, J. 2003. Prevention of spontaneous breast carcinoma by prophylactic vaccination with dendritic/tumor fusion cells. J. Immunol. 170: 1980–1986.

Yu, M., Zhan, Q., and Finn, O.J. 2002. Immune recognition of cyclin B1 as a tumor antigen is a result of its overexpression in human tumors that is caused by non-functional p53. Mol. Immunol. 38: 981–987.

Zitvogel, L., Mayordomo, J.I., Tjandrawan, T., DeLeo, A.B., Clarke, M.R., Lotze, M.T., and Storkus, W.J. 1996. Therapy of murine tumors with tumor peptide-pulsed dendritic cells: dependence on T cells, B7 costimulation, and T helper cell 1-associated cytokines. J. Exp. Med. 183: 87–97.

Chapter 14

Antigen-specific Immunotherapy for Allergies

Claude André

Abstract

Specific immunotherapy has been performed since the beginning of the twentieth century with the objective of preventing the development of allergic reactions following contact of a sensitized organism with common allergens from the environment. This approach is effective for the treatment of rhinoconjunctivitis and allergic asthma, but is associated with rare adverse events that can sometimes be severe after injection. Immunotherapy is being developed along several lines in order to improve efficacy and safety. This includes sublingual administration of allergens in tablet form, preparation of major allergens by genetic recombination and immunomodulation based on the understanding of mechanisms responsible for allergy.

INTRODUCTION

As a result of genetic and environmental factors, an increasingly large share of the world population develops an inappropriate immune response when exposed to common antigens, such as pollens, mites, animal epithelia, moulds and food. The initial contact triggers production of antibodies belonging to the immunoglobulin E class, a response normally observed in parasite infestations, particularly with helminths. Subsequent exposure to allergens (i.e. antigens recognized by and generating immunoglobulin E) can be responsible for various diseases, including atopic dermatitis, rhinitis, allergic asthma, and allergic conjunctivitis. Only two aetiological treatments for allergy are available: avoidance, which is not always feasible and which remains imperfect, and specific immunotherapy, previously referred to as hyposensitization or desensitization.

Despite a few earlier reports, Noon (1911) is generally considered to be the father of allergy vaccination. In the current age of preventive as well as curative vaccines, the title of Noon's article 'Prophylactic inoculation against hayfever' appears to be ahead of its time. By pure chance, the same year, Wells and Osborne reported that guinea-pigs previously fed with corn could no longer be sensitized by injections of zein (a corn protein). This constitutes the first experimental demonstration of the possibility to induce immune tolerance via a transmucosal pathway. However, this local vaccination was performed on immunologically naive animals. It was only much later that Lafont (Lafont *et al.*, 1982) showed that oral administration of an allergen could also suppress a specific immune response, including IgE production. The paucity of preclinical data available can in part account for the slow development of transmucosal allergen vaccination. It can also explain the lack of definition of the optimal therapeutic dose, which is still a subject of debate.

For a long time, the imperfect knowledge of the pathophysiology of allergic disease – IgE was only discovered in 1966 – led to a number of treatments inappropriate both in terms of their indications (e.g. uveitis, mycosis, atopic dermatitis) and of the antigens used (e.g. total hymenoptera bodies, bacteria, *Candida albicans*) to name a few. Good medical practices validated by expert consensus now confines the application of allergen vaccination to rhinoconjunctivitis and allergic asthma, with the exclusion of severe asthma. Hymenoptera venom anaphylaxis is also obviously a major indication. This review will successively analyse the efficacy of allergen vaccination, the nature of allergens used for desensitization and their standardization, the safety profile of allergy immunotherapy, the known or supposed mechanisms of action and finally the future prospects for this treatment modality.

EFFICACY OF SPECIFIC IMMUNOTHERAPY

In asthma

Asthma is a disease for which the efficacy of injection immunotherapy has been the most frequently denied, probably due to the administration of mixtures containing excessive numbers of allergens (Adkinson *et al.*, 1997), which obviously resulted in a significant dilution of each individual component. Many molecules, particularly in mould extracts, also exert a proteolytic enzyme activity which denatures other antigens, and as such should not be mixed with other allergens for desensitization purposes.

Confirmation of the efficacy of parenteral immunotherapy in asthma was formally provided by a recent meta-analysis (Abramson, 1999). The authors conducted a systematic Cochrane meta-analysis, including data from 54 trials published between 1954 and 1997, and concluded that subjects randomized to immunotherapy (i) exhibited significantly fewer asthma symptoms, (ii) required significantly less asthma medication, and (iii) demonstrated reduced allergen-specific and non-specific bronchial hyperreactivity compared with those randomized to placebo.

Allergen-specific immunotherapy has been administered orally, bronchially, nasally and sublingually. The oral route was not adopted in the absence of data supporting its efficacy, and the bronchial route was excluded because it is based on anecdotal evidence and could potentially be dangerous. Nasal administration and sublingual-swallow treatment have been recently recognized by national and international bodies as effective treatments for adults and children with allergic asthma (Bousquet *et al.*, 1998). However, it must be emphasized that the nasal route was used almost exclusively by Italian clinicians, and is currently less popular. Sublingual immunotherapy, when not associated with swallowing the allergen extract, called sublingual-spit, has not been specifically validated in view of the limited number of studies conducted as of today.

In rhinoconjunctivitis

Allergic rhinitis and allergic conjunctivitis, which are often associated, do not represent serious clinical manifestations, but their impact on the patient's quality of life can be greater than that of moderately severe asthma. Injection immunotherapy for allergic rhinoconjunctivitis has been evaluated in a large number of studies. A review of these studies (Malling, 1998) also demonstrated the efficacy of active immunotherapy versus placebo both on the reduction of clinical symptoms and on the residual medication consumption. Fewer studies have been devoted to sublingual immunotherapy (SLIT), but enough data was generated in human studies to allow a Cochrane meta-analysis (Wilson *et al.*, 2003). The 22 studies analysed led to the same conclusions: SLIT exhibited a statistically significant efficacy versus placebo, both for reduction of symptoms and reduction of symptomatic medication consumption.

Other benefits of specific immunotherapy

Apart from its curative role on reduction of symptoms during the treatment period, immunotherapy also provides three other therapeutic advantages: a carry-over effect after discontinuation of treatment, the prevention of the development of polysensitization in monosensitized patients, and also prevention of progression from rhinitis to asthma.

The carry-over effect of injection immunotherapy has been known for a number of years (Mosbech and Osterballe, 1988). These authors showed, in 1988, that the efficacy of timothy grass immunotherapy administered over a period of two and a half years in 40 patients suffering from rhinitis was maintained 6 years after stopping treatment. These results have been confirmed for house-dust mite rhinitis and asthma (Des Roches *et al.*, 1996). Forty patients receiving this type of immunotherapy for 12 to 96 months were assessed 3 years after stopping treatment. The recurrence rate for asthma or rhinitis was inversely proportional to the duration of immunotherapy. The differences observed in such recurrence rates were significant as soon as immunotherapy was administered for more than 3 years. Other studies have confirmed the carry-over effect of injection immunotherapy, using either tree pollens (Jacobsen *et al.*, 1997) administered for 3 years with a follow-up of 6 years, or grass pollens (Durham *et al.*, 1999). The long-term benefit of specific immunotherapy against HDM or grass-pollen allergies was also documented in asthmatic children (Cools *et al.*, 2000). Insufficient data are available in this regard concerning the use of sublingual immunotherapy, but preliminary data are promising (Di Rienzo *et al.*, 2003). As immunotherapy is contraindicated or less effective in polysensitized subjects, the fact that injection immunotherapy can prevent the development of polysensitization also constitutes a major advantage. Three studies reported results documenting such an effect (Des Roches *et al.*, 1997; Purello-D'Ambrosio *et al.*, 2001; Pajno *et al.*, 2001). These studies were conducted in adults and children with asthma or rhinitis due to pollens or mites. However, a fourth (Asero, 2003) and a fifth study (Tella *et al.*, 2003), evaluating injection and sublingual immunotherapy, respectively albeit at a very low therapeutic dose (Di Rienzo *et al.*, 2003), did not confirm these results. Finally, injection immunotherapy in patients with rhinitis prevents transformation of rhinitis into asthma, provided a sufficient therapeutic dose is administered (Johnstone, 1957). This preliminary study performed on a small series of patients was confirmed on a much larger population, in which progression to asthma was reduced by 50% (Jacobsen *et al.*, 1997; Möller *et al.*, 2002).

ALLERGENS AND STANDARDIZATION

As immunotherapy is indicated in patients producing IgE antibodies and therefore susceptible to present intense clinical reactions following the administration of allergens, allergy vaccines must be administered at gradually increasing concentrations and volumes (titration phase). During maintenance therapy, when the patient receives a monthly injection for several years, the extract must have the same biological activity, even when a new batch of vaccine is used. However, in the past this was not always the case, as the first extracts were simply characterized on the basis of their protein nitrogen content.

Although aqueous solutions of allergen extracts have always been used in North America, allergen extracts adsorbed onto mineral salts, aluminium hydroxide or calcium phosphate, are predominantly used in Europe. In the past, the justification for these additives was based on a hypothetical adjuvant effect. Allergoids are very popular in some countries. Allergoids, for which a large proportion of B epitopes are eliminated by the poorly reproducible chemical process occurring during manufacture, appear to induce fewer adverse events. This is hardly surprising, but the efficacy of this type of product, generally studied on small populations of patients, also appears to be lower. There is a widely held belief that adsorbed allergen extracts are much safer than aqueous extracts, but this does not take into account the fact that, for the same manufacturer and the same allergen, the concentration of aqueous extracts can be up to tenfold higher than the maximum concentration of adsorbed extracts. There is also no evidence to suggest that the anaphylactic reactivity of an adsorbed allergen is delayed compared with that of a nonadsorbed allergen. Studies conducted in a related field, that of infection vaccines, show that the physiological extracellular concentration of human albumin very rapidly displaces antigen adsorbed on aluminum hydroxide. We can therefore conclude that adsorbed allergen extracts do not possess a significant pharmacokinetically delayed effect. However, this erroneous information has led some authors to reject the use of adsorbed extracts based on the fact that effective adsorption would require a long observation period after injection to monitor the patient for signs of adverse events. The 20 to 30 minutes of medical surveillance required by good clinical practice may therefore not be sufficient. We now know that this is not the case.

Biological standardization of allergens by skin tests resulted in extracts, which initially appeared to induce more adverse events than previous allergen extracts. However, these extracts are simply more potent and the initial drawbacks of these extracts have been resolved by clinical experience. The various methods used for the standardization of allergen extracts, ensuring a constant potency differ in Europe and the USA. In the USA, the patient's cutaneous reactivity is assessed by an intradermal reaction and by measuring the area of flare induced. In Europe, skin prick-tests are performed and the power of the extract is determined following evaluation of the size of the wheal. However, different units of measurement are used by allergen extract manufacturers. Even if the various unit systems can be compared by assaying the content in major allergens of each extract, these extracts produced by distinct manufacturers are not interchangeable.

Safety of allergy immunotherapy

As the efficacy of injection immunotherapy (Haugaard, 1992) and sublingual immuno-therapy (André et al., 2003) is determined by the cumulative dose administered during maintenance treatment, there is a risk of adverse events, especially as it is recommended to administer the maximum dose tolerated. Since some adverse events can be fatal, either due to an asthma attack or anaphylactic shock, safety obviously remains a constant preoccupation of clinicians. In Great Britain, in 1986, analysis of the conditions of onset of 26 deaths led to the introduction of a set of rules, which contributed to almost complete disappearance of immunotherapy in this country (Committee on Safety of Medicines, 1986). However, the risk factors for adverse events following immunotherapy are now well known: dosage errors, concomitant administration of contraindicated treatments such as beta-blockers, and especially the treatment of severe and unstable asthma. The mortality rate associated with the current modalities of injection immunotherapy is estimated to be 1 per 2 million injections. However, not all adverse events can be explained by treatment errors. The other more frequent adverse events consist of skin reactions at the injection site or a syndromic reaction consisting of reactivation of the disease. Another possible complication of allergen immunotherapy is macrophagic myofasciitis, a recently described clinical entity, possibly induced by the aluminum adjuvant, which, to date, has only been incriminated in the context of vaccines against infectious diseases. This muscle disease is secondary to intramuscular injections, while injection specific immunotherapy only uses the subcutaneous route. Another risk related to aluminum hydroxide gel consists of exceptional 'allergic' reactions to aluminum. A more frequent complication is the development of granulomas, that may sometimes take a long time to resolve, and which correspond to common foreign body reactions caused by intradermal injection (Vogelbruch *et al.*, 2000). Sublingual immunotherapy is particularly safe, as the only adverse events observed consist of pruritus or oral oedema or transient abdominal pain. Syndromic reactions are rare and no cases of anaphylactic shock or death have been reported to date, based on review of clinical both studies (André *et al.*, 2000), post-marketing surveillance studies (Di Rienzo *et al.*, 1999) and the Cochrane meta-analysis (Wilson *et al.*, 2003).

MECHANISMS OF ACTION OF IMMUNOTHERAPY

Studies investigating the mechanisms of action of immunotherapy are just as numerous as the proposed explanations for the pathophysiology of allergy. The proposed mechanisms of action vary according to the latest scientific theory. There does not appear to be any difference between the phenomena observed in the context of injection immunotherapy and those observed in the context of sublingual immunotherapy. A reduction of immediate or semi-delayed cutaneous reactivity and an elevation of reactivity thresholds on bronchial, conjunctival or nasal provocation tests are generally, but not always observed. These findings account for the improvement observed on other target organs.

Elevation of the IgA antibody titre, and especially the IgG_4 titre, in the form of blocking antibodies, is one of the mechanisms that has been proposed for a long time to account for desensitization for successful desentization. Elevation of IgG_4 actually reflects intense and prolonged contact with the allergen, regardless of the route of administration. However, the possible role of these blocking antibodies remains uncertain, as, after discontinuation of wasp venom immunotherapy, IgG_4 antibodies rapidly disappear, whereas the subject remains protected against subsequent wasp stings.

The same decreased reactivity is observed at the cellular level for degranulation of circulating basophils, but also eosinophils. Immunotherapy therefore decreases the release of eosinophil cationic protein, known to be toxic to bronchial epithelial cells.

These findings are perfectly concordant with the latest hypothesis concerning the pathogenesis of allergy: an imbalance between Th1 lymphocytes and Th2 lymphocytes. Very simply, Th1 lymphocytes produce interleukin 2 (IL-2) and interferon γ, a cytokine which inhibits IgE production. Th2 lymphocytes produce several cytokines, including IL-4 and IL-5. IL-4 promotes IgE production, while IL-5 promotes eosinophils recruitment and activation. Allergic patients present a Th1 deficiency and increased Th2 activity compared with healthy subjects.

The explanation for the efficacy of immunotherapy is possibly a restoration of a normal Th1/Th2 balance with a reduction of Th2 activity and an increase of Th1 activity or even

Th0 activity. Unfortunately, depending on the study, modifications of both types or only a single type of lymphocyte are observed, suggesting that this hypothesis is not sufficient to explain the mechanism of action of immunotherapy. It is clearly oversimplistic to attribute allergic disease to a simple Th2 hyperreactivity. Asthma attacks occur after contact with an allergen, a Th2 phenomenon, but also in the context of bacterial infections related to the action of lipopolysaccharides, a Th1 phenomenon. The latest explanations for homeostasis of the normal state or the mechanism of action of immunotherapy are much more realistic (Jutel *et al.*, 2003). The normal physiological state is maintained by regulatory T cells, detected by the presence of $CD4^+$ $CD25^+$ markers. These cells exert a suppressor effect on both proinflammatory Th1 mechanisms and proallergic Th2 mechanisms. The mediators produced by these regulatory cells include IL-10, necessary for the production of IgG_4 and TGF-β, necessary for the production of IgA. These cytokines are produced in the context of effective immunotherapy (Jutel *et al.*, 2003). This last hypothesis also appears to integrate all the various phenomena observed. More specifically in relation to sublingual immunotherapy, the initial step consists of phagocytosis of allergens by Langerhans cells present in abundance in the sublingual mucosa. Following allergen capture, the dendritic cell migrates to lymph nodes draining the region, where it induces immune tolerance.

CONCLUSIONS: THE FUTURE OF IMMUNOTHERAPY
In competition with other treatment modalities, with which it nevertheless remains complementary, the efficacy of immunotherapy must be maintained or improved, while reducing the risks of adverse events. Various approaches are under investigation to achieve these objectives.

Sublingual tablets
A double placebo-controlled study comparing injection immunotherapy and sublingual immunotherapy (Khinchi *et al.*, 2004) demonstrated comparable efficacy of the two methods compared with placebo with an advantage in terms of the benefit/risk ratio for sublingual immunotherapy. Due to its simplicity, safety, and its acceptance by the child, the sublingual route should therefore replace injections, but the doses used need to be more clearly defined and a galenic presentation that would be more user-friendly than drops needs to be developed, for example tablets (André *et al.*, 2003).

Hypoallergenic antigens
Hypoallergenic antigens are already used in the form of allergoids. The allergen extract is denatured, for example by glutaraldehyde, and bound to tyrosine. Modifications of allergenicity are therefore not specific for particular epitopes and industrial reproducibility is difficult to achieve. Denaturation precludes the precise characterization of the finished product. In practice, these products are not superior to classical extracts, but it remains an interesting approach. Peptides, such as the peptide corresponding to a T cell epitope from Fel d1, the cat major allergen, represented another alternative, but their development has been stopped.

Recombinant allergens
Technological progress now allows the production of only those molecules of immunological interest present in an extract. The production of these molecules in the pure state would allow the injection or sublingual administration of much more precise doses. The efficacy

and safety should also be improved, but no results of clinical trials are yet available. If necessary, a complementary development would include directed mutagenesis of the epitopes responsible for residual adverse events, thereby creating hypoallergenic forms of the molecules.

Adjuvants

The use of adjuvants to treat the allergen may appear paradoxical, but these molecules, usually mineral salts, are used to facilitate a protective immunological response, but are no longer required for booster injections. In allergic patients requiring immunotherapy, the immune response is already present and it would be illogical to try to amplify this response. Most of the published studies in this field are derived from the USA, where immunotherapy generally uses simple aqueous allergen extracts. The same applies to all studies devoted to sublingual immunotherapy.

The adjuvants currently in use consist of calcium phosphate and especially aluminum hydroxide, but these additives have never been shown to be superior to aqueous extracts.

The data reported for aluminum hydroxide also raise the problem of transposition of animal data to man. Aluminum hydroxide has been shown to be a very effective adjuvant of IgE responses in experimental murine models. No enhancement of allergy symptoms has been observed with the use of aluminum hydroxide in human. A similar finding was observed for human reactivity to pertussis vaccine, while *Bordetella pertussis* is the other effective adjuvant for IgE production in rodents.

Bacterial lipopolysaccharide derivatives, particularly MPL or monophosphoryl lipid A (Drachenberg *et al.*, 2001), have not been shown to increase the immunogenicity of classical extracts. This type of approach is designed to restore the Th1/Th2 balance. Another approach with a similar objective consists in using allergens conjugated to bacterial CpG (Dieudonné *et al.*, 2001), but no clinical results are yet available.

Other original approaches include the use of liposome-encapsulated allergens (Galvain *et al.*, 1999). Unfortunately, no improvement justifying further development was observed with this type of approach, which was also associated with delayed cutaneous hypersensitivity to lipids.

In light of recent hypotheses, immunomodulators distinct from adjuvants should be used to target regulatory cells in order to induce an allergen-specific activity. As for any type of manipulation of the lymphocyte system, the major prerequisite is the short-term and long-term specificity and safety of this immunomodulation.

References

Abramson, M., Puy, R., and Weiner, J. 1999. Immunotherapy in asthma: an updated systematic review. Allergy 54: 1022–1041.

Adkinson, N.F., Eggleston, P.A., and Eney, D. 1997. A controlled trial of immunotherapy for asthma in allergic children. N. Engl. J. Med. 336: 324–331.

Asero, R. 2003. Injection immunotherapy with different airborne allergens did not prevent de novo sensitization to ragweed and birch pollen north of Milan. Int. Arch. Allergy Immunol 133: 49–54.

André, C., Vatrinet, C., Galvain, S., Carat, F., and Sicard, H. 2000. Safety of sublingual-swallow immunotherapy in children and adults. Int. Arch. Allergy Immunol. 121: 229–234.

André, C., Perrin-Fayolle, M., Grosclaude, M., Couturier, P., Basset, D., Cornillon, J., Piperno, D., Girodet, B., Sanchez, R., Vallon, C., Bellier, P., and Nasr, M. 2003. A double-blind placebo-controlled evaluation of sublingual immunotherapy with a standardized ragweed extract in patients with seasonal rhinitis. Int. Arch. Allergy Immunol 131: 111–118.

Bousquet, J. Lockey, R.F., and Malling, H.J. 1998. Allergen immunotherapy- therapeutic vaccines for allergic diseases. Allergy 53 suppl 44: 4–42.

Cools, M., Van Bever, H.P., and Weyler, J.J. 2000. Long-term effects of specific immunotherapy, administered during childhood, in asthmatic patients allergic to either house-dust mite or to both house-dust mite and grass pollen. Allergy 55: 69–73.

Committee on Safety of Medicines update. 1986. Desensitizing vaccines. Br. Med. J. 293: 948.

Des Roches, A., Paradis, L., Knani, J., Heijouani, A., Dhivert, H., Chanez, P., and Bousquet, J. 1996. Immunotherapy with a standardized Dermatophagoides pteronyssinus extract. V. Duration of the efficacy of immunotherapy after its cessation. Allergy 51: 430–433.

Des Roches, A., Paradis, L., Menardo, J.L., Bouges, S., Daurès, J.P., and Bousquet, J. 1997. Immunotherapy with a standardized *Dermatophagoides pteronyssinus* extract. VI. Specific immunotherapy prevents the onset of new sensitizations in children. J. Allergy Clin. Immunol. 99: 450–453.

Di Rienzo, V., Pagani, A., Parmiani, S., Passalacqua, G., and Canonica, G.W. 1999. Post-marketing surveillance study on the safety of sublingual immunotherapy in pediatric patients. Allergy 54: 1110–1113.

Di Rienzo, V., Marcucci, F., and Puccinelli, P. 2003. Long-lasting effect of sublingual immunotherapy in children with asthma due to house dust mite: a 10-year prospective study. Clin. Exp. Allergy 33: 206–210.

Dieudonné, F., Vital Durand., Eiden, J., Tuck, S., Van Nest, G., Raz, E., Hamilton, R., Creticos, P.S., and André, C. 2001. ISS linked to Amb a 1 allergen (AIC) stimulates IgG response to Amb a 1 by ragweed-allergic humans. J. Allergy Clin. Immunol.107: 933.

Drachenberg, K.J., Wheeler, A.W. Stuebner, P., and Horak, F. 2001. A well tolerated grass pollen-specific allergy vaccine containing a novel adjuvant, monophosphoryl lipid A, reduces allergic symptoms after four preseasonal injections. Allergy 56: 498–505.

Durham, S.R. Walker, S.M., and Varga, E.M. 1999. Long-term clinical efficacy of grass-pollen immunotherapy. N. Engl. J. Med. 341: 468–475.

Galvain, S., André, C., Vatrinet, C., and Villet, B. 1999. Safety and efficacy studies of liposomes in specific immunotherapy Curr. Ther. Res. 60: 278–294.

Haugaard, L., Dahl, R., and Jacobsen, L. 1992. A controlled dose–response of immunotherapy with standardized, partially purified extract of house dust mite. Clinical efficacy and side-effects. J. Allergy Clin. Immunol. 91: 709–722.

Jacobsen, L., Nuchel Petersen, B., and Wihl, J.A. 1997. Immunotherapy with partially purified and standardized tree pollen extract. IV. Results from long-term (6 year) follow-up. Allergy 52: 914–920.

Jacobsen, L. 1997. Preventive allergy treatment as part of allergy disease management. J. Invest. Allergy. Clin. Immunol. 7: 367–368.

Johnstone, D.E. 1957. Study of the role of antigen dosage in the treatment of pollenosis and pollen asthma. AMA J. Dis. Child. 94: 1–5.

Jutel, M., Akdis, M., Budak, F., Aebisher-Casaulta, C., Wrzyszcz, M., Blaser, K., and Akdis, C.A. 2003. IL-10 and TGFB cooperate in the regulatory T cell response to mucosal allergens in normal immunity and specific immunotherapy. Eur. J. Immunol. 33: 1205–1214.

Khinchi, M.S., Poulsen, L.K., Carat, F., André, C., Hansen, A.B., and Malling, H-J. 2004. Clinical efficacy of sublingual and subcutaneous birch pollen allergen-specific immunotherapy: a randomized, placebo-controlled, double-blind, double dummy study. Allergy 59: 45–53.

Lafont, S., André, C., André, F., Gillon, J., and Eargier, M.C. 1982. Abrogation by subsequent feeding of antibody response, including IgE, in parenterally immunized mice. J. Exp. Med. 155: 1573–1578.

Malling, H.J. 1998. Immunotherapy as an effective tool in allergy treatment. Allergy 53: 461–472.

Moller, C., Dreborg, S., and Ferdousi, H.A. 2002. Pollen immunotherapy reduce the development of asthma in children with seasonal rhino conjunctivitis (the PAT-Study). J. Allergy Clin. Immunol. 109: 251–256.

Mosbech, H., and Osterballe, O. 1988. Does the effect of immunotherapy last after termination of treatment? Allergy 43: 523–529.

Noon, L., 1911. Prophylactic inoculation against hay fever. Lancet 1: 1572–1573.

Pajno, G.B., Barberio, G, and DeLuca, F. 2001. Prevention of new sensitizations in asthmatic children monosensitized to house dust mite by specific immunotherapy. A six-year follow-up study. Clin. Exp. Allergy 31: 1392–1397.

Purello-D'Ambrosio, F., Gangemi, S., and Merendino, R.A. 2001. Prevention of new sensitizations in monosensitized subjects submitted to specific immunotherapy or not. A retrospective study. Clin. Exp. Allergy 31: 1295–1302.

Tella, R., Bartra, J., SanMiguel, M., Olona, M., Bosque, H, Graig, P., and Garcia-Ortea, P. 2003. Allergy Immunopathol. 31: 221–225.

Vogelbruch, M., Nuss, B., Körner, M, Kapp, A., Kiehl, P., and Bohm, W. 2000. Aluminium-induced granulomas after inaccurate intradermal hyposensitization injections of aluminium-adsorbed depot preparations. Allergy 55: 883–887.

Wells, H.G., and Osborne, T.B., 1911. The biological reactions to the vegetable proteins. I. Anaphylaxis. J. Infect. Dis. 8: 66–74.

Wilson, D.R., Torres Lima, M., and Durham, S.E. 2003. Sublingual immunotherapy for allergic rhinitis. The Cochrane Library, issue 2, Oxford: Update Software Ltd.

Index

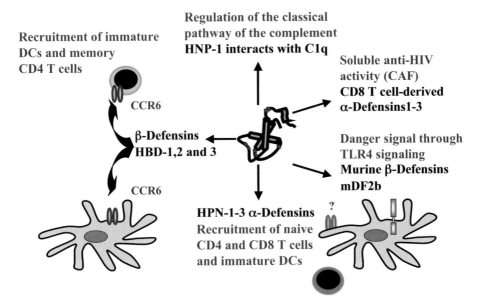

Figure 3.1 Immunoregulatory functions displayed by mouse and human Defensins. Defensins are not only lytic antimicriobial peptides, but they can also modulate some effector phase s of innate immunity such as the conventional pathway of complement or the recruitment of immunocompetent cells such as DCs and T cells. They may act as danger signals through Toll-like receptor-4 and some of them may also possess some anti-HIV activities.

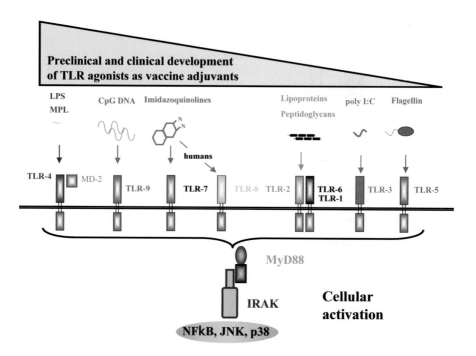

Figure 3.2 Toll-like receptors (TLR) and their ligands. TLR specifically recognize pathogen-derived ligands (PAMPS) or host derived compounds that are induced by inflammation or other stress stimuli. The triggering of single or combinations of TLRs create a repertoire for pathogen recognition. Several natural or synthetic ligands for TLRs are being evaluated and developed as vaccine adjuvants. This includes (from the most to the least developmentally advanced for vaccine application): monophosphoryl lipid A analogues (TLR4), CpG sequences (TLR9), Imidazoquinolines (TLR7), lipopetides (TLR1/2/6), polyI:C like compounds (TLR3) and flagellin (TLR5). All TLRs share a common core MyD88/NFκB activation pathway but additional and more specific signaling components have been identified for most of them.

No PAMPS: no danger: no TLR mediated activation

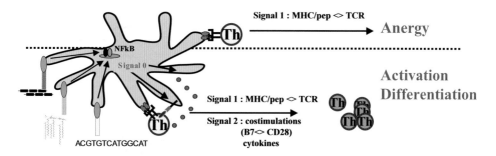

PAMPS = danger signal → activation through TLRs
(specific combinations → accurately tuned effectors)

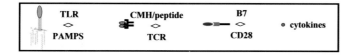

Figure 3.3 TLR ligands-conditioned APCs can then deliver potent costimulatory signals to cognate antigen specific T cells. Antigen presentation to T cells by APCs that have not previously been accurately conditioned usually leads to anergy. Ligands of TLRs deliver potent activation signals to APCs (signal 0) that induce the up regulation of costimulatory molecules and the production of cytokines. APCs are then licensed to present antigen derived peptides (signal 1) in an accurate costimulation context (signal 2) that will lead to the induction of a fully functional immune response. Delivery of various pathogen-derived signals through specific TLRs and combinations thereof (molecular pattern) constitutes a first level of identification of the nature of the invading microbe. This might allow for a more adapted conditioning of APCs in order to optimize the activation of the cognate T cells.

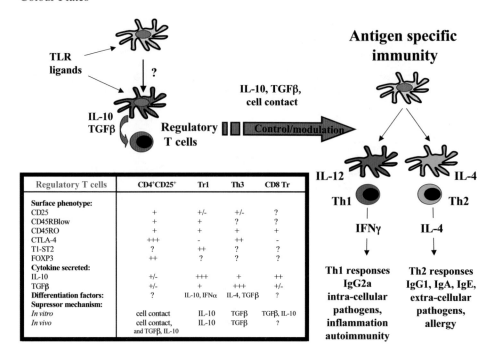

Regulatory T cells	CD4⁺CD25⁺	Tr1	Th3	CD8 Tr
Surface phenotype:				
CD25	+	+/-	+/-	?
CD45RBlow	+	+	?	?
CD45RO	+	+	+	+
CTLA-4	+++	-	++	-
T1-ST2	?	++	?	?
FOXP3	++	?	?	?
Cytokine secreted:				
IL-10	+/-	+++	+	++
TGFβ	+/-	+	+++	+/-
Differentiation factors:	?	IL-10, IFNα	IL-4, TGFβ	?
Supressor mechanism:				
In vitro	cell contact	IL-10	TGFβ	TGFβ, IL-10
In vivo	cell contact, and TGFβ, IL-10	IL-10	TGFβ	?

Figure 3.4 Vaccine adjuvants to manipulate Regulatory T cells? Considering their role in the regulation of the balance between tolerance and immunity against self as well as foreign antigens, it is tempting to speculate that it will be useful to target subsets of regulatory T cells with vaccine adjuvants. This may allow better control over vaccine-induced immunity against infectious pathogens (intensity, diversity and Th1 versus Th2 polarization) but also the prevention of harmful immunopathological situations associated with exacerbated or inappropriate responses. Specific TLR ligands or any other adjuvants that can trigger the production of IL-10, TGFβ or engage ICOSL should be tested for their ability to control the function of regulatory T cells in the context of an antigen-specific immune response.

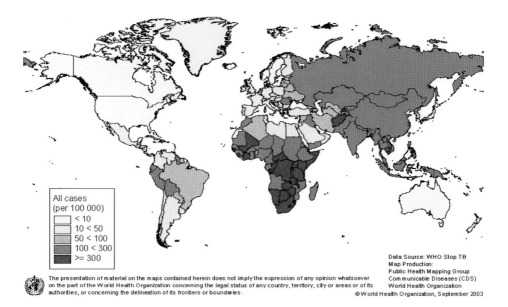

Figure 10.1 Global estimates of TB disease (WHO, 2001).